Prosthetic Rehabilitation of Head and Neck Cancer Patients

Prosthetic Rehabilitation of Head and Neck Cancer Patients

Edited by

PANKAJ PRAKASH KHARADE

Faculty Member, Department of Prosthodontics, Dr. Z A Government Dental College
Aligarh Muslim University, Aligarh, Uttar Pradesh, India
Maulana Azad Institute of Dental Sciences, New Delhi, Delhi, India
Tata Memorial Hospital, Mumbai, Maharashtra, India
Japan Prosthodontic Society, Okayama University, Okayama, Japan
National Academy of Medical Sciences, New Delhi, Delhi, India

ELSEVIER

Publisher: Sarah Barth
Acquisitions Editor: Jessica McCool
Editorial Project Manager: Barbara Makinster
Production Project Manager: Selvaraj Raviraj
Cover Designer: Vicky Pearson Esser

3251 Riverport Lane
St. Louis, Missouri 63043

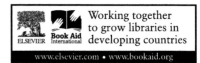

Working together to grow libraries in developing countries

www.elsevier.com • www.bookaid.org

Contributors

Himanshi Aggarwal, MDS
Department of Restorative Sciences
Division of Prosthodontics
University of Alabama at Birmingham
AL, United States

Sangeeta Agarwal, MDS
Department of Dentistry
B J Government Medical College & Hospital
Pune, Mumbai, India

Gorakh Ahire
Tata Memorial Hospital
Mumbai, India

Akiyama, PhD
Faculty Member
Department of Oral Rehabilitation and
    Regenerative Medicine
Okayama School of Medicine
Dentistry and Pharmaceutical Sciences
Okayama University
Okayama, Japan

Andleeb, PhD
Department of Social Work
Aligarh Muslim University
Aligarh, Uttar Pradesh, India

Deeksha Arya, MDS
Department of Prosthodontics
Faculty of Dental Sciences
King George's Medical University UP
Lucknow, Uttar Pradesh, India

Gurmit Kaur Bachher, PhD
Former Head
Department of Speech Therapy
Tata Memorial Hospital
Mumbai, Maharashtra, India

Ardhendu Banerjee, MDS
Department of Prosthodontics
Dr. R Ahmed Dental College
Kolkata, West Bengal, India

Saurav Banerjee, MDS
Associate Professor
Department of Prosthodontics
Dr. R Ahmed Dental College
Kolkata, West Bengal, India

Tridib Banerjee
Associate Professor
Department of Prosthodontics
Dr. R Ahmed Dental College
Kolkata, West Bengal, India

Karthik Bhat, MDS
Department of Dental & Prosthetic Surgery
Tata Memorial Hospital
Mumbai, India

Pravin Bhirangi, D. MECH
Department of Dental & Prosthetic Oncology
Tata Memorial Hospital
Mumbai, India

Department of Prosthodontics
Government Dental College
Mumbai, India

Sunita Bisht, MS
Department of Otorhinolaryngology
Military Hospital Allahabad
Allahabad, Uttar Pradesh, India

Nirmalya Chaterjee
Associate Professor
Department of Prosthodontics
Dr. R Ahmed Dental College
Kolkata, West Bengal, India

Arati Chougule
Technician
Department of Dental and Prosthetic Surgery &
    Oncology
Tata Memorial Hospital
Mumbai, Maharashtra, India

**Cynthia Bernardo D'Lima, BSc,
DIP. Tissue Banking**
Tata Memorial Hospital
Tissue Bank
Mumbai, India

A.K. Dcruz, MS, DNB, FRCS (Hon)
Director Oncology
Apollo Hospitals
President
Union International Cancer Control (UICC) Geneva
Germany

Former Director & Chief Head Neck Services
Tata Memorial Hospital
Mumbai, Maharashtra, India

Tapan Kumar Giri, MDS
Dr. R Ahmed Dental College and Hospital
Kolkata, West Bengal, India

Ahire Gorakh, D. MECH
Department of Dental & Prosthetic Oncology
Tata Memorial Hospital
Mumbai, India

Tapas Gupta
Department of Prosthodontics
Dr. R Ahmed Dental, College
Kolkata, West Bengal, India

Jangala Hari, MDS
Secretary
Indian Prosthodontic Society

**Mohammed Zahedul Islam Nizami, PhD,
GDCSC, BDS**
Restorative Dental Sciences
Faculty of Dentistry
The University of Hong Kong
Hong Kong, China

Saidul Islam, MDS
Senior Maxillofacial Surgeon
Life Line Hospital
Kolkata, West Bengal, India

Anumeha Jha, MDS
Department of Prosthodontics
Government Dental College
Raipur, India

Saumya Kapoor, MDS
School of Dentistry
University of Michigan
Michigan, United States

Rakesh Katna, MS, FHBNI
Department of Surgical Oncology
Lilavati Hospital & Research Centre
Mumbai, India

Jaslok Hospital
Mumbai India

Tata Memorial Hospital
Mumbai, India

Mohsin Khan, MD
Department of Radiation Oncology
JN Medical College
Aligarh Muslim University
Aligarh, Uttar Pradesh, India

Arlingstone Khogshei
Consultant Prosthodontist
Shilong, Meghalaya, India

Malay Kundu, MDS
Consultant Prosthodontist
Kolkata, West Bengal, India

Pankaj Prakash Kharade, MDS, FJPS
Department of Prosthodontics
Dr. Z A Dental College
AMU
India

**Mohammed Fahud Khurram, MBBS, MS, MCH,
DNB Plastic Surgery**
JN Medical College, Aligarh Muslim University,
Aligarh, Uttar Pradesh, India

Surender Kumar
Associate Professor
Department of Prosthodontics
RIMS
Ranchi, Jharkhand, India

Rupali Mondal, MDS
Associate Professor
R G Kar Medical College
Kolkata, West Bengal, India

Kumiko Nawachi, PhD
Faculty Member
Department of Oral Rehabilitation and
    Regenerative Medicine
Okayama School of Medicine
Dentistry and Pharmaceutical Sciences
Okayama University
Okayama, Japan

Sesha Reddy, MDS
Professor
Department of Prosthodontics
Government Dental College & Hospital
Kadapa, Andhra Pradesh, India

Harendra Shahi
Professor
Mithila Minority Dental College & Hospital
Kolkata, West Bengal, India

Jyoti Sharma, MD
Department of Pathology
Military Hospital Amritsar
Amritsar, Punjab, India

Mohit Sharma, MD
Former Senior Registrar
Medical Oncology
Tata Memorial Centre
Mumbai, Maharashtra, India

Medical Oncologist
Fortis Escorts Hospital
Faridabad, Haryana, India

Swati Sharma, MDS
Department of Conservative Dentistry & Endodontics
Institute of Dental Education and Studies
Gwalior, India

Vithal Shendge, MD, MRCSED
Department of Orthopaedic Surgery and Trauma
University of Toledo Medical Centre
Toledo, OH, United States

Shahid A. Siddiqui, MD
Department of Radiation Oncology
JN Medical College, Aligarh Muslim University
Aligarh, Uttar Pradesh, India

Yasir Dilshad Siddiqui, BDS, MSC, PhD
Department of Preventive Dentistry
College of Dentistry
Jouf University
Sakaka, Saudi Arabia

Saumyendra V. Singh, MDS
Department of Prosthodontics
Faculty of Dental Sciences
King George's Medical University UP
Lucknow, Uttar Pradesh, India

Sandeep Tayal, MDS
Former Consultant Prosthodontist
Indian Army Dental Corps
India

Rajendra Kumar Tewari, MDS
Conservative Dentistry & Endodontics
Dr. Z A Dental College
AMU
India

Prabha Yadav, MCh
Former Professor & Head
Department of Plastic Surgery
Tata Memorial Hospital
Mumbai, Maharashtra, India

Foreword

I am delighted to write the foreword for this recent book on prosthetic rehabilitation of head and neck malignancy patients. Prosthetic rehabilitation has evolved into a highly predictable clinical procedure with improved treatment outcome to enhance the quality of life for patients suffering with head and neck malignancy. Prosthodontist in coordination with oncosurgeon, plastic surgeon, medical oncologist, speech therapist, and social workers can deliver better treatment to restore nutrition as well as important functions like mastication, deglutition, and speech. This textbook presents evidence-based information related to the management of head–neck cancer patients in combination with numerous clinical photographs of routine as well as complicated case by means of suitable illustrations.

Dr. Pankaj Prakash Kharade is one of the elite clinicians in the field of maxillofacial prosthesis. He has completed his research fellowship under my supervision and I have found him very capable. He is a combination of dedicated clinician and enthusiastic academician. I am fairly confident that he will go a long way with his enthusiasm and academic credentials.

A devoted team of academicians, clinicians, and researchers from several premier institutes of different countries has worked hard for the completion of this book. They have explained various clinical procedures related to rehabilitation of head and neck cancer in a precise and simplified manner. The importance of interdisciplinary approach to restore the quality of life for cancer patient has been endorsed by this team. I congratulate Dr. Pankaj and his entire team of coauthors for their marvelous effort. I am sure that this book will help the students who are pursuing their career in the field of medicine. All authors have shared their knowledge and experience for this book which will benefit many patients in future.

I congratulate and wish good luck to Dr. Pankaj and the entire team of coauthors.

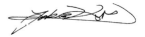

Prof. Takuo KUBOKI, DDS, PhD
Chair and Professor, Department of Oral Rehabilitation
and Regenerative Medicine, Okayama University Faculty
of Medicine, Dentistry and Pharmaceutical Sciences
Dental Section Director,
Okayama University Hospital, Japan
Vice Executive Director, Okayama University, Japan
President, Japan Prosthodontic Society (JPS)

Foreword

I am enchanted to write the foreword for this book about prosthetic rehabilitation of head and neck cancer patients. Evidence-based management of head–neck cancer patients has been discussed in this book. Prosthetic rehabilitation has a positive impact on the patient's quality of life. Multidisciplinary treatment will not only restore nutrition but also important functions such as mastication, deglutition, and speech.

Dr. Pankaj Prakash Kharade has received extensive training in the field of maxillofacial prosthesis. Dr. Pankaj is a blend of good clinician and passionate academician. This book is an outcome of the combined efforts of experts from various institutions from different countries associated with him. I am confident that this book will be helpful for clinicians dealing with rehabilitation of head and neck cancer.

Innumerable clinical procedures regarding rehabilitation of head and neck cancer have been explained in this book with the help of several clinical photographs. I congratulate Dr. Pankaj and the team of coauthors for their wonderful efforts.

I wish good luck to Dr. Pankaj and the entire team of coauthors for their upcoming endeavour.

Prof. Kenji Maekawa
Chair, Department of Removable
Prosthodontics and Occlusion
Osaka Dental University, Japan

Preface

This book represents a comprehensive overview of various forms prosthetic treatments in combination with other medical as well as social managements for successful rehabilitation of head and neck cancer patients. Recent advances in the field of maxillofacial prosthetics have an instrumental role in the improvement of quality of life for head and neck cancer patients. Development in the field of surgical management of tumors necessitates coordination with prosthodontist to perk up the prognosis of the treatment. This book explains about various prosthodontic, surgical, and associated procedures for particular clinical situation related to head and neck cancer patients. Rehabilitation of patients suffering with defects in the region of head and neck is extremely strenuous which demands keen inputs by experts from diverse health disciplines. Interdisciplinary approach can help such patients to lead the routine life in almost normal mode. In the presence of surgical limitations, prosthetic rehabilitation can ensure restoration of speech and other oral functions if there is a scope of improvement from physiological and neurological point of view. Precision toward the clinical procedures in an exemplary manner can restore the psychological status of the patients by improving the overall quality of life. This book will help the clinicians to clarify about the line of treatment after surgical management of tumors in the head and neck region as a wide range of maxillofacial defects and their management has been included in this endeavor. It will facilitate endorsement as well as incorporation of shifting trends in the field of maxillofacial prosthodontics at institutional as well as private practice level.

I am delighted to acknowledge the team of authors who have contributed their experience in the form of chapters for this book which will assist to raise the awareness regarding the management of defects in the head and neck region. I am thankful to them for their dedication and vigor in making this literature multidisciplinary with their expertise. I have witnessed the difficulties faced by head—neck cancer patients after surgery while working at various premier institutes which has inspired me to write this book. I am thankful to my mentors Prof. Ardhendu Banerjee, Prof. Mahesh Verma, and my wife Dr. Swati Sharma for the support as well as motivation.

Contents

CHAPTER 1

Introduction to Maxillofacial Rehabilitation

PANKAJ PRAKASH KHARADE, MDS

Malignancy of the head and neck can be shattering in its influence on vital structures of body as well as various functions related to affected parts, causing severely compromised quality of life. Prosthetic rehabilitation of patients due to surgical resection of tumor as well as congenital defects is extremely demanding task as maxillofacial deformities affect physical, psychological, and social status tremendously.[1] Psychological distress is manifested usually secondary to surgical resection of vital anatomical structures. Such kind of rehabilitation necessitates very kin interaction amid the interdisciplinary squad working or dedicated toward precise management of these deformities. Even though oral healthcare professionals are predominantly involved in rehabilitation of masticatory as well as deglutition function, it is very much essential to have precise coordination of prosthodontist with oncosurgeon, radiotherapist, social worker, speech therapist, and other health science experts. Maxillofacial defects can be congenital, which occur due to malformation as well as developmental disturbances or acquired type caused by surgical management of pathologies, tumors, or trauma as shown in Chart 1.1.[2] The disabilities range from minor cosmetic disfigurements to a major functional disability united with cosmetic disfigurement. The deliverer of treatment must be cognizant of variations in therapy that considerably improve the process of rehabilitation. In addition to being experts in their respective field of responsibility, all members of the interdisciplinary team must be well acquainted with the expertise of the other members of the team so that the process of rehabilitation will be smooth.

Even though plastic surgery is preferred reconstruction of certain maxillofacial defects, several defects necessitate prosthetic rehabilitation for better treatment outcome.[3,4] In the absence of provision for prosthetic rehabilitation, masticatory function may drastically get affected (Fig. 1.1). The basic objectives of prosthetic rehabilitation are to restore deglutition, mastication, cosmetic appearance, speech, and psychological health.[5,6] Several congenital and acquired defects can be restored with prosthetic rehabilitation.[3] In 1953, Ackerman has defined maxillofacial prostheses as the specialty of dentistry that restores and replaces parts of the face artificially after trauma or surgical resection. This definition does not incorporate the use of prostheses for restoration congenital craniofacial deformities to improve facial esthetics.[7,8] In the absence of interdisciplinary team approach, functional as well as cosmetic aspects may remain compromised affecting psychosocial behavior of the patient (Fig. 1.2).

Recent advances in the field of maxillofacial prosthetic rehabilitation such as CAD-CAM technology are helping out for better treatment outcome apart from replacement of lost vital structures of the craniomaxillofacial region (Fig. 1.3). Nowadays, maxillofacial rehabilitation has several other applications such as restoration of form, support in surgical procedures, and reduction in morbidity following surgical procedures as well as reestablishment of lost function due to surgical resection. Also these prosthesis may be prescribed simply for cosmetic as well as psychosocial motives or to maintain the position and safeguard adjacent facial structures during radiotherapy for head and neck region in cancer survivors.[9] With several progresses in the field of plastic surgery, esthetic corrections of such defects are possible. On the other hand, if surgery is contraindicated for certain patients or the defect is very extensive where complete closure of the defect is not possible, maxillofacial prosthetics appear to be a sustainable option. Maxillofacial prosthodontics plays an important role in several cases where the patient is reluctant to undergo another surgical procedure.[10–12]

Maxillofacial prosthodontics today offer a range of prospects right from simple surgical stents and splints,

Prosthetic Rehabilitation of Head and Neck Cancer Patients. https://doi.org/10.1016/B978-0-323-82394-4.00008-2

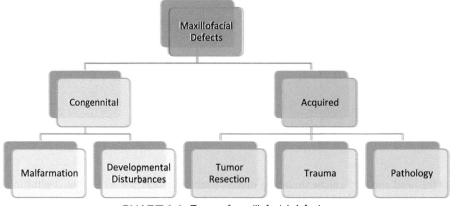

CHART 1.1   Types of maxillofacial defects.

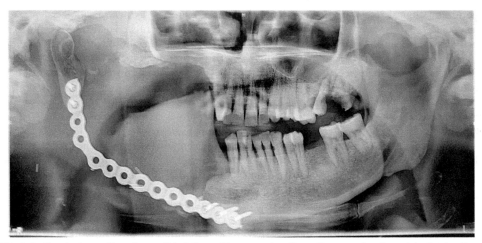

FIG. 1.1   Surgical resection of mandible followed by reconstruction with reconstruction plate. Lack of bone grafting during reconstruction of mandible affects the prosthetic rehabilitation.

laryngectomy devices, tracheostomy aids, maxillectomy obturators, cranial plates, auricular prosthesis, ocular prosthesis, nasal prosthesis, breast as well as vaginal prosthesis to the present-day commercially oriented body doubles. These avenues in the form of less commonly used miscellaneous maxillofacial prosthesis in addition to the newfangled panoramas available to prosthodontists today have led to redefining of maxillofacial prosthodontics in a multidisciplinary treatment approach. Maxillofacial prosthetics and advances in materials used to fabricate these prosthesis have currently laid the path for a surplus of opportunities to prosthodontists to serve the humankind and also to develop interdisciplinary treatment options with the help of our colleagues in the specialty of medicine, surgery in addition to allied specialties. The foremost objective of maxillofacial prosthodontic treatment is

not limited to rehabilitation of the postresection defect but also to restore self-esteem and improve the quality of life of every patient.[13] The main advantage of prosthetic rehabilitation is that it can be fabricated for defect located in any region of the face, jaws as well as the cranial deformity irrespective of the size of the defect. Apart from that, the prosthesis allows for regular examination and observing of the defect site, which is very helpful in early detection of any recurrences.[14,15]

Objectives: Maxillofacial prosthetics has the following significant objectives:

(a) Restoration of esthetics or cosmetic appearance of patient.
(b) Restoration of function.
(c) Protection of tissue.
(d) Therapeutics or healing effect.
(e) Psychological therapy.

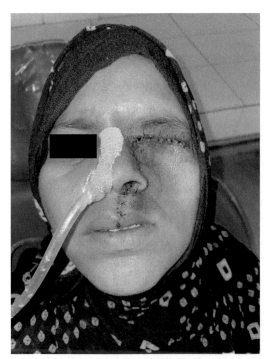

FIG. 1.2 Orbital defect primarily closed leading to poor treatment outcome towards prosthesis.

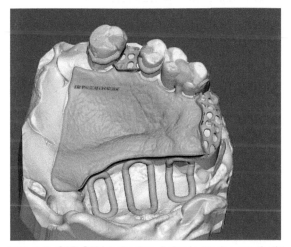

FIG. 1.3 CAD CAM technology helps in precise prosthetic rehabilitation of the surgical defect.

When these objectives are successfully fulfilled in a patient during the rehabilitation, successful treatment outcome can be achieved.[16,17]

History: Several materials have been used in the past in various countries to fabricate artificial eye, ear, and nose.[18] Ambrose Pare has mentioned about fabrication of prosthetic nose in a detailed manner.[19] In 1880, Kingsley described regarding fabrication of prosthetic appliances for restoration of congenital as well as acquired defects of palate, nose as well as orbit.[20]

Obturators can be prescribed for congenital as well as acquired defects. For congenital defects, simple plate type prosthesis will aid in feeding. Along with simple plate, palatal lift prosthesis or an overlay denture can also be fabricated for congenital defects.[21-23] Apart from that, obturators are also fabricated to rehabilitate the defect created due to surgery.[24]

Tetamore in 1894 has discussed about a case series of nasal defects rehabilitated with prosthesis where he had used very light plastic material to produce final prosthesis with life-like appearance, which was retained by bow spectacles. Claude Martin had described diverse prosthetic replacements including porcelain nose prosthesis, which had an intraoral retention mechanism in 1889. Extensive oral tumors necessitates resection of nasal or orbital structures in several situations where prosthodontist has to plan for combination of intraoral as well as extraoral retention. Bourdet has recommended use of silk ligatures attached to natural teeth to support metal sheet for the obturation of defect in 1757. Till date, several materials have been used to fabricate the prosthesis for rehabilitation of various head—neck defects.

Summary: Maxillofacial prostheses reinstate several types of maxillofacial deformities as well as vital functions lost due to those deformities. Even though it is a very challenging process, constant practice will help to achieve expertise toward rehabilitation of complex maxillofacial defects. Precise rehabilitation improves the patient's quality of life up to greater extent. Recent advances in the field of maxillofacial prosthesis have led to enhanced expectations for the future. An increasing number of head—neck cancer patients need meticulous management of maxillofacial defects with suitable prosthesis to restore speech, mastication, and deglutition. Multidisciplinary planning and management is mandatory for rehabilitation of complex maxillofacial defects to achieve superior treatment outcome. While planning the treatment, psychological aspect needs to be handled appropriately as such patients are often associated with deprived psychosocial status.

REFERENCES

1. Goiato MC, Dos Santos DM, Bannwart LC, et al. Psychosocial impact on anophthalmic patients wearing ocular prosthesis. *Int J Oral Maxillofac Surg*. 2013;42(1):113—119.
2. Coas VR, Neves ACC, Rode SDM. Evaluation of the etiology of ocular globe atrophy or loss. *Braz Dent J*. 2005; 16(3):243—246.

3. Dos Santos DM, de Caxias FP, Bitencourt SB, Turcio KH, Pesqueira AA, Goiato MC. Oral rehabilitation of patients after maxillectomy: a systematic review. *Br J Oral Maxillofac Surg.* 2018;56(4):256–266.

4. Costa H, Zenha H, Sequeira H, et al. Microsurgical reconstruction of the maxilla: algorithm and concepts. *J Plast Reconstr Aesthetic Surg.* 2015;68(5):e89–e104.

5. Taylor TD. Psychological management of the maxillofacial prosthetic patients. In: *Clinical Maxillofacial Prosthetics.* Quintessence publishing Co Inc; 2000.

6. Umino S, Masuda G, Ono S, et al. Speech intelligibility following maxillectomy with and without a prosthesis: an analysis of 54 cases. *J Oral Rehabil.* 1998;25:153–158.

7. Ackerman AJ. Maxillofacial prosthesis. Oral surgery, oral medicine. *Oral Pathology.* 1953;6(1):176–200. https://doi.org/10.1016/0030-4220(53)90152-2.

8. Barreto D, Rangel R, Morales J, Gutierrez P. Epiplating in auricular defects as a facial reconstruction method: case series. *J Oral Maxillofac Surg.* 2019;77(1):183.

9. Gopi A. The emerging role of maxillofacial prosthodontics beyond the realms of the maxillofacial region. *J Ind Prosthodont Soc.* November 2018;18(Suppl 2):S88. https://doi.org/10.4103/0972-4052.246549.

10. Thorne Charles H. *Grabb and Smith's Plastic Surgery.* 7th ed. Philadelphia: Lippincott Williams & Wilkins, a Wolters Kluwer Business; 2014.

11. Rodriguez Eduardo D, Losee Joseph E. *Plastic Surgery: Craniofacial Head and Neck Surgery, Pediatric Plastic Surgery.* 3rd ed Vol. 3. China: Saunders an imprint of Elsevier Inc.; 2013.

12. Dolan Robert W. *Facial Plastic, Reconstructive and Trauma Surgery.* 1st ed. 270 Madison Ave., New York: Marcel Dekker Inc.; 2003.

13. Chalian VA. *Maxillofacial Prosthetics: Multidisciplinary Practice.* Baltimore: The Williams and Wilkins Co.; 1971.

14. Sandeep K, Gupta S, Nayan P. Reconstruction of cranial defect with an alloplastic implant. *JIPS.* July 2007;7(3): 150–152.

15. Bulbulian AH. *Facial Prosthetics.* Springfield: Charls C Thomas Publisher; 1973.

16. Shah Farhan K, Himanshu A. Prosthetic management of ocular defect: esthetics for social acceptance. *JIPS.* 2008; 8(2):66–70.

17. Khaidem D, Nadeem Y, Amit Kumar T. Oral & maxillofacial prosthetics I: objectives & history. *Heal Talk.* 2012; 4(5):18–20.

18. Dostalova T, Kozak J, Hubacek M, Holakovsky J, Pavel akubS, Seydlova ichaela. In: Turkyilmaz I, ed. *Facial Prosthesis, Implant Dentistry - A Rapidly Evolving Practice.* InTech; 2011. ISBN: 978-953-307-658-4.

19. Paprocki Gregory J. Maxillofacial prosthetics: history to modern applications. Part 1 – obturators. *CCED.* 2013; 34(8):e84–e86.

20. Paprocki Gregory J. Maxillofacial prosthetics: history to modern applications. Part 1I – speech and swallow prostheses. *CCED.* 2013;34(9):e91–e95.

21. Beumer J, Curtis TA, Marunick MT. *Maxillofacial Rehabilitation: Prosthetic and Surgical Considerations.* 1st ed. St. Louis: The C. V. Mosby Company; 1996.

22. Olin William H. *Cleft Lip and Palate Rehabilitation.* Springfield, Illinois, U. S. A.: C. C. Thomas Publisher; 1960.

23. Platt JH. The history of obturator principles and design. *J Speech Hear Disord.* 1947;12(1):111–123.

24. Anand F, Chethan H, Krishnaprasad D. A simplified technique to make an immediate surgical obturator for a maxillectomy patient. *J Int Dent.* 2013;3(2):125–128.

CHAPTER 2

Anatomical Considerations in Maxillofacial Surgery and Rehabilitation

VITHAL SHENDGE, MD, MRCSED

INTRODUCTION

The knowledge of head and neck anatomy is crucial not only to optimize surgical resections in head and neck cancer but also to plan for accurate prosthetic fitting. This improves both esthetic and functional outcomes, leading to better patient satisfaction.

This chapter is structured to enable this process in mind, and hence, details of embryological development, brain, and spinal cord neuroanatomy have been deferred to dedicated textbooks of anatomy.

HEAD AND NECK ANATOMY SUBDIVISIONS

Head is defined as a craniofacial complex structural region where functions of vision, hearing, smell, taste, mastication with digestion and swallowing, breathing, and neural integration are carried out.

Skeleton of the head is called the **skull,** which also includes the **mandible** (lower jaw) (Figs. 2.1 and 2.2).

Parts of skull are as follows:

1) **Calvarium (brain box)**: upper part of the cranium enclosing the brain.
2) **Facial Skeleton**: rest of the skull and mandible. Skull has total 28 bones (calvarium = 14 bones, facial skeleton = 14 bones).
   Calvarium is composed of the 14 bones including the three paired ear ossicles.
a) Paired: (1) parietal, (2) temporal, (3) malleus (4), incus, (5) stapes
b) Unpaired: (1) frontal, (2) occipital, (4) sphenoid, (5) ethmoid
   Facial skeleton includes 14 bones.
a) Paired: (1) maxilla, (2) zygomatic, (3) nasal, (4) lacrimal, (5) palatine, (6) inferior nasal concha
b) Unpaired: (1) mandible, (2) vomer
   Detailed anatomy of each bone is beyond the scope of this chapter. General anatomy can be revised by an overview of the cranial vault in different views as mentioned in the following.

These bones and their anatomical structures can be best studied in the following views of skull and face:

a) Norma frontalis (frontal view of skull) Fig. 2.1
b) Norma occipitalis (hind view skull) Fig. 2.3
c) Norma lateralis (right lateral view skull) Fig. 2.2
d) Norma basalis (basal view of skull) Fig. 2.4
e) Mandible Figs. 2.5 and 2.6
f) Neck/cervical spine
g) Norma verticalis (head superior view) Fig. 2.7

Anatomical points of reference are used not only in anthropological and forensic studies, but also in analyzing an individual head and neck dimensions for prosthetic reconstruction.

The definition of anatomic points or landmarks on the soft tissue or bony landmarks of the head and neck enables this process. Different methods to measure distances between these points help measure the deficiencies as well as plan for prosthetic rehabilitation in head and neck congenital deformities as well as postsurgical resection deficiencies.

Methods of measurements can be as follows:

A) Direct methods: (1) sliding calipers, e.g., Vernier calipers, Mitutoyo digital sliding caliper, (2) hinged/spreading calipers, (3) coordinate calipers, (4) Todd's craniostat/head spanner, (5) osteometric board/stadiometer, (6) soft metric tapes/digital tapes.
B) Indirect methods: (1) surface scanners, (2) cephalometric landmarks or craniometric points are recognizable points on cephalometric radiographs or tracing representing certain hard or soft tissue anatomic structures.

These are depicted in Fig. 2.8, starting from the highest point in the skull. The facial soft tissue points are shown in the facial profiles (Fig. 2.9).

Prosthetic Rehabilitation of Head and Neck Cancer Patients. https://doi.org/10.1016/B978-0-323-82394-4.00014-8

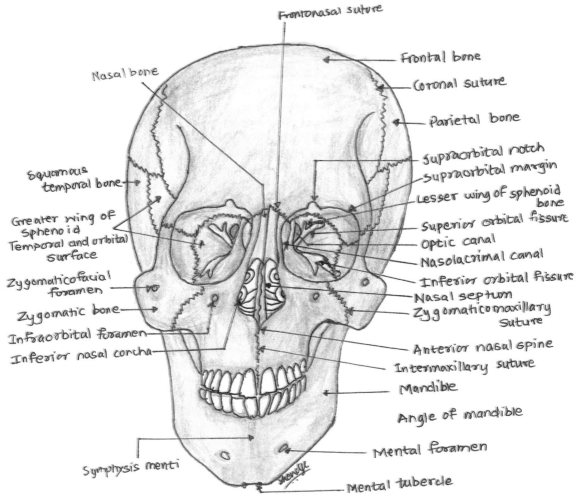

FIG. 2.1 Norma frontalis.

1) **Vertex:** Midline highest point on the skull in the sagittal plane in anatomic position.
2) **Bregma:** Intersection of the coronal and sagittal sutures, landmark of the anterior fontanelle.
3) **Ophryon:** Point just above the optic foramina.
4) **Trichion:** Midsagittal point of anterior hairline on forehead.
5) **Glabella (G):** Point in between the eyebrows—glabrous = hairless.
6) **Exocanthion (Eo):** Lateral-most point on the lateral canthus of eye.
7) **Endocanthion (En):** Innermost point in the medial canthus of eye.
8) **Nasion(N):** Midsagittal point base of nose, between the nasal bones and the frontal bone.
9) **Radix:** Base of nose.
10) **Rhinon:** Highest and anterior most point on the bony nasal bones.
11) **Tip defining point:** Anterior most projection of nasal tip.
12) **Columella point (Cm):** The most anterior point on columella of the nose.
13) **Alare (Al):** Lateral point on nasal alae.
14) **Cheilion:** Outermost point on the angle of mouth.
15) **Akanthion:** Midline nasal spine over maxilla.
16) **Prosthion (alveolar point):** midpoint of the maxillary alveolar point.
17) **Pogonion (P, Pg, Pog):** The most anterior point on the contour of bony chin in midsagittal plane, or point.

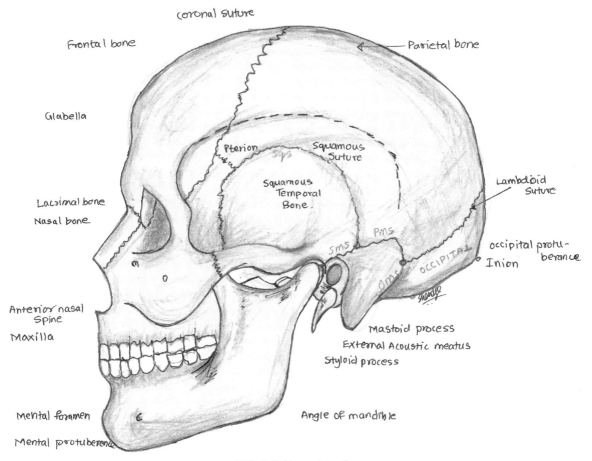

FIG. 2.2 Norma lateralis.

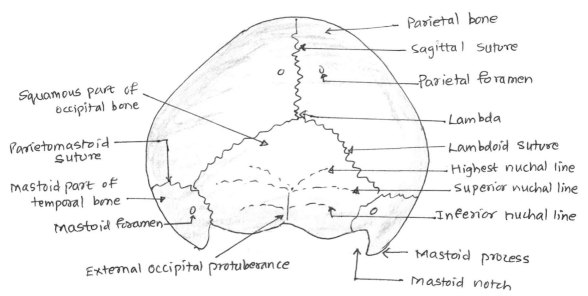

FIG. 2.3 Norma occipitalis.

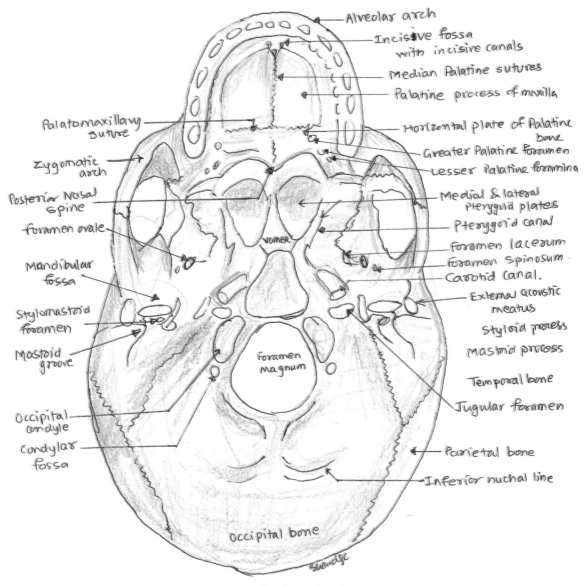

FIG. 2.4 Norma basalis.

18) **Sella Point (S):** Geometric center of sella turcica.
19) **Porion (Po):** Most superior point on the outline of external auditory meatus.
20) **Gonion (Go):** The point of intersection of the mandible plane and the ramus of the mandible and is the most prominent point of the angle of mandible.
21) **Suprapogonion/protuberance Menti (Pm):** Point at which the shape of the symphysis changes from convex to concave.
22) **Stomion:** Points where the lips meet.
23) **Jugal point:** The point of union of the frontal and the temporal processes of the zygomatic bone.
24) **Frontotemporale point:** Most anterior point of the temporal line on the frontal bone.
25) **Alveolare:** Most anterior point in midline on the alveolar process of maxilla.
26) **Alveolon:** Point of intersection of the midsagittal line of the palate and the tangent to the posterior margin of the alveolar arch.

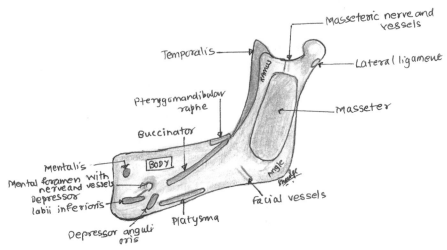

FIG. 2.5 Left half mandible (outer surface).

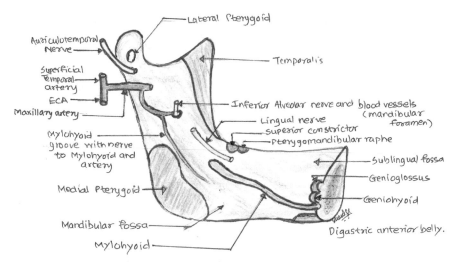

FIG. 2.6 Left half of mandible (inner surface).

27) **Articulare (Ar):** Point of intersection of sphenoid and posterior border of condyle of mandible at the TM joint.

28) **Anterior nasal spine (ANS):**

29) **Posterior nasal spine (PNS):** Most posterior point on the contour of palate.

30) **Basion (Ba):** Median(midline) point of the anterior margin of the foramen magnum.

31) **Gnathion (Gn):** Point of intersection of the facial plane and the tangent to lower border of the mandible.

32) **Infradentale:**

33) **Inion:** Tip of external occipital protuberance (EOP), midline bony prominence in occipital bone for attachment of the ligamentum nuchae and trapezius.

34) **Lambda:** The point of confluence of the lambdoid and sagittal sutures.

35) **Menton (Me):** Most inferior point on the chin's inferior contour.

36) **Nasospinale:**

37) **Obelion:** The point of intersection of the imaginary line between the two parietal foramina and the sagittal suture.

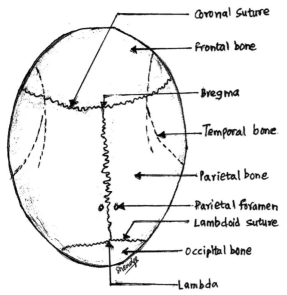

FIG. 2.7 Landmarks: Norma verticalis (superior view of skull).

38) **Opisthion:** The median (midline) point on the posterior margin of the foramen magnum.
39) **Opisthocranion:** posterior most point in midsagittal plane of the occiput.
40) **Orale:** The opening point of the oral cavity.
41) **Orbitale (Or):** The lowest point in the inferior margin of the orbit.
42) **Staphylion:** The median point on the posterior edge of the hard palate.
43) **Subnasale (Sn):** The lowest point on columella where it merges with upper lip in midsagittal plane.
44) **Labrale superius (Ls):** A point indicating mucocutaneous border of the upper lip.
45) **Labrale inferius (Li):** A point indicating the mucocutaneous border of lower lip.
46) **Stomion superius (Stms):** The lowermost point on the vermillion border of upper lip.
47) **Stomion Inferius (Stmi):** The uppermost point on the vermillion border of lower lip.
48) **Mentolabial sulcus (Ms):** The point of greatest concavity in midline between Li and Pg.

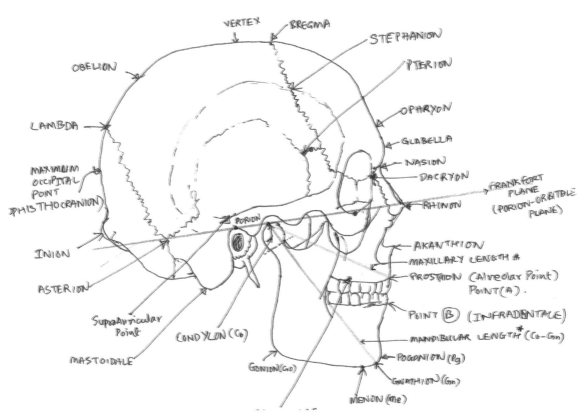

FIG. 2.8 Norma lateralis with craniometric points.

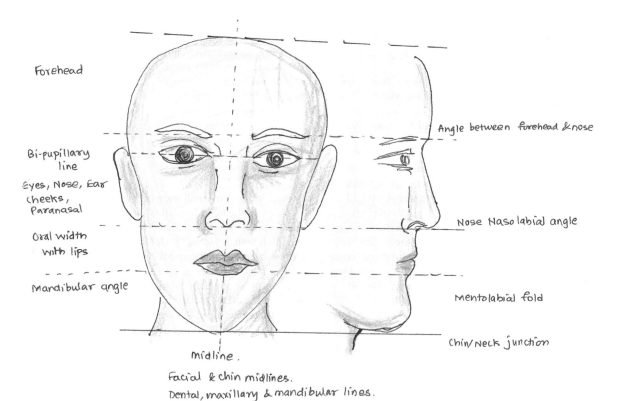

Forehead

Bi-pupillary line

Eyes, Nose, Ear cheeks, Paranasal

Oral width with lips

Mandibular angle

midline.

Angle between forehead & nose

Nose Nasolabial angle

Mentolabial fold

Chin/Neck junction

Facial & chin midlines.
Dental, maxillary & mandibular lines.

FIG. 2.9 Facial soft tissue landmarks and facial profile.

49) **Subspinale:** Point at the base of the nasal spine.
50) **Symphysion:** Most forward point on the alveolar point of mandible.
51) **Tragion:** The uppermost point on the tragus in anterior facial profile.
52) **A point:** Anterior point of the base of alveolus in lateral view over maxilla.
53) **B point:** Anterior point on the base of alveolus in lateral view over the mandible.
54) **Zygion (Zy):** Lateral most point in the zygomatic bones, the width of face measured between the left and right points.
55) **Cervical point:** The innermost point between the submental area and neck or point of intersection of the anterior border of neck and midsagittal plane where the neck meets the floor of mouth posteriorly.
56) **T1 Point:** Point of intersection of the facial and occlusal plane.

Important Craniometric Lines and Planes (Fig. 2.8)

A) Horizontal planes:
   1) **Frankfort plane:** orbitale (Or) to porion (Po) through.
   2) **Reid's base line:** Line/plane joining the mid-auricular point and the orbitale and extending backward to the center of occipital bone.
   3) **Anterior cranial base plane (S–N):** Line joining the sella (S) point to the nasion (N).
   4) **Mandibular plane:** Plane between the gonion (Go) and gnathion (Gn) also called Steiner line.
   5) **Nasal floor plane (N–F):** Plane joining the ANS and PNS points.
   6) **Functional occlusal plane:** Plane bisecting posterior occlusion.

7) **Palatal plane:**
8) **Down's line:** Gonion to menton.
9) **Bimler's line:** Line joining menton to antegonial notch.
10) **Tweed and Rickett line:** Straight line tangent to the lowermost border of mandible.

A) **Vertical Planes:**
   1) A-Pog plane: Point A on maxilla to pogonion on mandible.
   2) Facial plane: Nasion to pogonion.
   3) Facial axis: PTM point to gnathion.

Cephalometric analysis (Columbia analysis) enables measurements of important craniometric angles (Fig. 2.8):

1) **Frankfort's** mandibular plane angle: Angle between the mandibular plane (Go-Gn) and the anterior cranial base plane (S–N). Mean value = 32°.
2) **Y growth axis** is the measure of the acute angle formed between the sella turcica line to gnathion and the Frankfort plane. Normal range: 53–66°
3) **R angle:** Angle between N, Co, and Me.

Important Craniometric Measurements

1) Cranial circumference: circumferential measurement
2) Maximal cranial breadth/width: distance between left and right eurion
3) Minimal frontal breadth
4) Bigonial breadth
5) Upper facial height: distance between
6) Basion–prosthion length
7) Nasal breadth (maximum)
8) Lower nasal breadth
9) Orbital breadth
10) Biorbital breadth
11) Foramen magnum breadth
12) Cranial height
13) Maximum cranial length
14) Bizygomatic breadth
15) Total facial height
16) Basion–nasion length
17) Basal height
18) Upper nasal breadth
19) Orbital height
20) Interorbital breadth
21) Palate-external breadth and length
22) Palate-internal breadth and length
23) Condylosymphyseal length
24) Bicondylar width
25) Minimum ramus breadth
26) Mandibular body height
27) Symphyseal height
28) Mastoid length
29) Ascending ramus height
30) Mandibular body breadth
31) Mandibular body length
32) Total facial angle
33) Midfacial angle
34) Alveolar angle
35) Nasion–opisthion
36) Transverse arc, sagittal cord, coronal cord

Indices

Cranial index—dry skull measurements, dolichocranic

Shape of the head (cephalus), cephalic index/cranial ratio/cephalic ratio: calculated as CI = cranial width/cranial length × 100. (1) Dolichocephalic: long and narrow head. (2) Mesocephalic/mesaticephalic: moderate size head. (3) Brachycephalic: short head.

Face (prosopon), morphological facial index = morphological total facial height/bizygomatic width/breadth classification: (1) hypereuryprosopy, (2) euryprosopy, (3) mesoprosopy: average or medium, (4) leptoprosopy, (5) hyperleptoprosopy.

External palatal index or palatomaxillary index/palatal index: ratio of the palatomaxillary width (distance between the outer borders of the palate just above the second molar) and palatomaxillary length (distance between the alveolar point to the midpoint of the line at the posterior borders of the two maxillae) × 100.

Orbital index: Ratio of the orbital maximal vertical height to maximal orbital breadth × 100.

Classification: (1) chamaeconchy (wide orbits), (2) mesoconchy (average/medium orbits), (3) hypsioconchy: narrow or square orbits.

SCALP (FIGS. 2.10 AND 2.11)

The soft tissues covering the calvarium is called scalp.

Extent: (1) Anteriorly: supraorbital margins. (2) Posteriorly: external occipital protuberance and superior nuchal lines. (3) Laterally: superior temporal lines on each side.

Hairline does not correspond to boundaries of scalp as hair is deficient over front part of scalp and overlaps upper part of back of neck.

Structure consists of five layers, the first three of which are intimately connected and move as a unit. The layers of the scalp (Fig. 2.10) can be remembered by the mnemonic **SCALP:**

1) **S**kin thick, hair-bearing and contains sebaceous glands

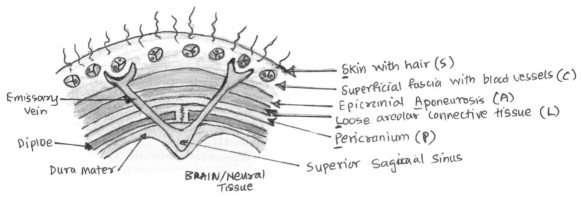

Emissary Vein

Diploe

Dura mater

BRAIN/Neural Tissue

Skin with hair (S)
Superficial fascia with blood vessels (C)
Epicranial Aponeurosis (A)
Loose areolar connective tissue (L)
Pericranium (P)
Superior Sagittaal Sinus

FIG. 2.10 Layers of scalp.

2) Connective tissue fibro-fatty layer containing anastomoses of arteries and veins
3) Aponeurosis (epicranial): galea of occipitofrontalis muscle
4) Loose areolar connective tissue contains emissary veins
5) Pericranium (periosteum of skull bones)

Blood supply (Fig. 2.11): Scalp has rich blood supply, and hence, small cuts tend to bleed profusely.

Arterial supply: In front of the auricle, is supplied anterior to posterior by (1) supratrochlear and (2) supraorbital branches of ophthalmic artery, branch of internal carotid artery (ICA), (3) superficial temporal terminal branch of external carotid artery (ECA). Behind the auricle, it is supplied from before backward by (4) postauricular branches of ECA, (5) occipital branches of ECA.

Venous drainage: (1) supratrochlear veins and (2) supraorbital veins unite at medial margin of orbit to

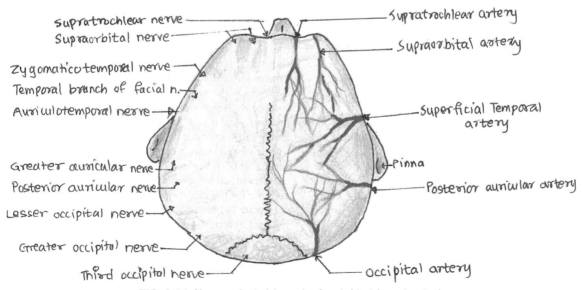

supratrochlear nerve
Supraorbital nerve
Zygomaticotemporal nerve
Temporal branch of facial n.
Auriculotemporal nerve
Greater auricular nerve
Posterior auricular nerve
Lesser occipital nerve
Greater occipital nerve
Third occipital nerve

Supratrochlear artery
Supraorbital artery
Superficial Temporal artery
Pinna
Posterior auricular artery
Occipital artery

FIG. 2.11 Nerve and arterial supply of scalp/skull (superior view).

form facial vein, (3) superficial temporal vein, (4) posterior auricular vein, (5) occipital vein suboccipital venous plexuses. The veins of the scalp anastomose with diploic veins. They are connected to the intracranial venous sinuses by emissary veins.

Lymphatic drainage: Anterior part of scalp drains into preauricular (parotid) lymph nodes, and posterior part of scalp into mastoid and occipital lymph nodes.

Nerve supply (Fig. 2.11):

(a) Sensory innervation of the scalp from anterior to posterior by branches of (1) ophthalmic nerve division of the fifth cranial nerve, (2) maxillary nerve division of the fifth cranial nerve, (3) mandibular nerve division of the fifth cranial nerve, (4) cervical plexus, (5) dorsal rami of cervical spinal nerve.

(b) Motor innervation is from branches of facial nerve, temporal branch to frontal belly, and posterior auricular branch to occipital belly.

Applied anatomy: (1) scalp bleeds profusely when injured due to rich blood supply, (2) emissary veins in loose areolar tissue (subaponeurotic) enable spread of infection from scalp and face to intracranial regions. The perioral philtrum area is thus called **"danger area"** of face. (3) Craniotomy flaps and the prosthetic mesh heal well and serve as watertight enclosure to maintain the pressures of the cranium and the CSF flow and intracranial pressure.

FACE

Landmarks and points utilized in measurements are mentioned before. For convenience of measurements, the face is divided into the following parts enabling plastic surgical and prosthetic measurements in reconstruction called as palatoplasty.

Subdivisions of the face (Fig. 2.9):

Facial Skin and Muscles

The skin overlying the face is modified with subcutaneous muscles inserted to enable facial expression, which are part of **panniculus carnosus**. Face has no deep fascia. Mainly the fascia under the skin is made up of variable amount of fat, blood vessels, and muscles of the second arch mesoderm equivalent of panniculus carnosus of animals arranged into sphincter, dilators, and expressors.

Facial muscles are mainly classified as constrictors or dilators of the orifices on the face: mouth, nose, and the eyes. The platysma is a flat sheet of muscle blending from the neck to the facial muscles inferiorly, and the frontalis blends the facial muscles via the scalp to the posterior neck muscles.

The facial muscles are (Fig. 2.12) classified as follows:

A) **Facial Expression:** Origin is the viscerocranium and insert into the facial skin. They are grouped according to the orifices governed. Functions are closing and opening these orifices.

Mouth: (1) buccinator, (2) depressor anguli oris, (3) depressor labii inferioris, (4) levator anguli oris, (5) levator labii superioris, (6) mentalis, (7) orbicularis oris, (8) risorius, (9) zygomaticus major, (10) zygomaticus minor.

Nose: (1) compressor narium minor, (2) dilator naris anterior, (3) levator labii superioris alaeque nasii (LLSAN), (4) nasalis, (5) procerus.

Eyes/orbital: (1) orbicularis oculi, (2) corrugator supercili.

B) **Masticatory muscles:** (1) medial pterygoid, (2) lateral pterygoid, (3) masseter, (4) temporalis.

C) **Calvaria muscle:** occipitofrontalis muscle.

EYES

These are paired specialized sensory organs of vision, located in bony orbits of the skull.

Eyeball

Fig. 2.13 These are pairs of important organs of sight. These are almost spherical in shape, with outer diameter of about 2.5 cm. These are lodged in the orbits and are made of three concentric coats: (1) outer fibrous coat or **sclera**, (2) middle or vascular coat also called the **uveal tract**, which consists of choroid, ciliary body, and the iris, (3) the inner most or nervous coat is the **retina**.

Sclera is the posterior opaque 5/6th of the eyeball, covered by **Tenon's capsule**, and anteriorly by the **conjunctiva**. Anterior 1/6th of the eyeball is transparent and is called **cornea**.

Muscles of the orbit, called as musculi externi bulbi oculi (MEBO), are set of seven muscles, six for the movement of the eyeball (four recti+ two obliques) and one for the elevation of the upper eyelid.

a) **Recti:** (1) superior rectus, (2) inferior rectus, (3) medial rectus, (4) lateral rectus.

b) **Obliques:** (1) superior oblique, (2) inferior oblique.

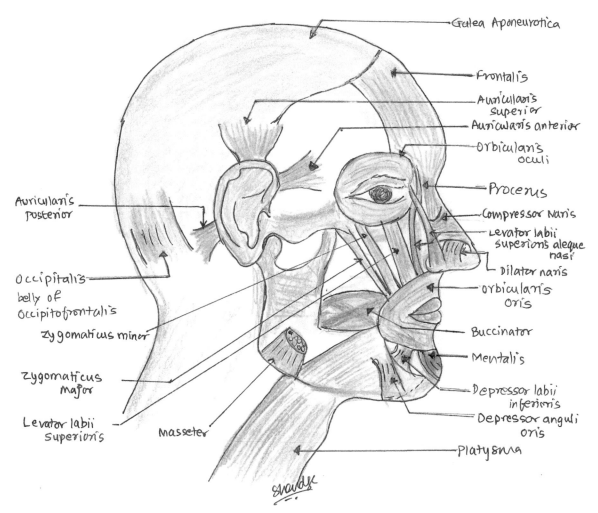

FIG. 2.12 Muscles of skull and facial expression (right lateral).

Nerve supply: Motor: All recti, inferior oblique, and levator palpebrae superioris are supplied by the oculomotor nerve (third cranial nerve), except lateral rectus (LR) supplied by sixth cranial nerve (abducens nerve) = LR6, and SO4: Superior oblique is supplied by the trochlear nerve. Ocular muscles and structures placed in the bony orbit are shown in Fig. 2.14.

The eyeball consists of three coats: (1) external, protective fibrous coat, (2) middle, vascular pigmented coat, and (3) internal nervous coat. It contains the aqueous humor, lens, and vitreous body.

Coats of the eyeball

Fig. 2.15 shows cross section of the eyeball.

a) **External fibrous coat:** It is made up of anterior transparent part: the cornea and a posterior opaque part, the sclera.

Cornea is mainly responsible for refraction of light. It is avascular, and transparency depends on its hydration. It is nourished by permeation. It is innervated by ophthalmic nerve via ciliary branches. Sclera is white-colored part of eyeball composed of dense fibrous tissue pierced by ciliary arteries and nerves, and posteriorly, pierced by optic nerve at **lamina cribosa**. Sclera receives tendons of muscles of the eyeball.

b) **Middle vascular coat:** This comprises, from behind forward, the choroid, ciliary body, and iris. Choroid

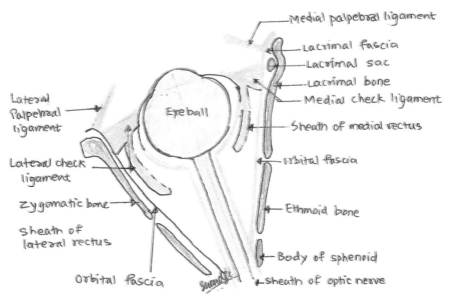

FIG. 2.13 Eyeball in the orbit, with fascia.

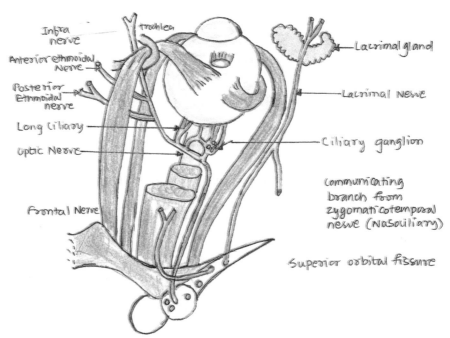

FIG. 2.14 Ocular structures and nerve supply.

is a brown coat lining the greater part of sclera, which consists of outer pigmented layer and inner vascular layer. Ciliary body connects the choroid to iris and is composed of (1) ciliary ring, (2) ciliary muscles, (3) ciliary processes Note: ciliary muscles are supplied by parasympathetic fibers from ciliary ganglion. Contraction of ciliary muscles results in the lens becoming more convex, increasing its

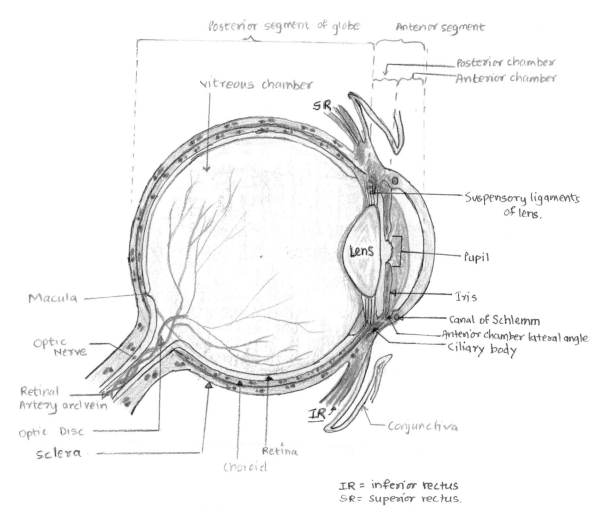

FIG. 2.15 Anatomy of cross section of eyeball.

refractive power. Iris is the circular pigmented diaphragm with a central opening just anterior to the lens, called the **pupil.** The iris divides space between cornea and lens into anterior and posterior chambers, both filled with aqueous humor. It contains muscles fibers forming (1) sphincter pupillae, which is supplied by parasympathetic fibers from oculomotor nerve, and (2) dilator pupillae, which is supplied by sympathetic fibers.

c) **Internal nervous coat** is also called retina. This consists of outer pigmented layer and inner nervous layer. The anterior nonreceptive portion is separated from posterior receptive part by the ora serrata. The posterior receptive part has the following features: (1) macula lutea (yellow spot), (2) fovea centralis is a central pit in the macula lutea, (3) blind spot is

part of optic disc where the optic nerve leaves the retina, due to of lack of receptors. The optic disc is pierced by the central artery of the retina.

Contents of the eyeball

This consists of the aqueous humor, lens, and vitreous body.

Aqueous humor fills anterior and posterior chambers of eye. Composition is close to that of protein-free plasma and is produced by ciliary processes. Functions: (1) supports wall of eyeball by exerting pressure and (2) nourishes lens and remove products of metabolism.

Human lens is a transparent, biconvex structure situated behind iris and anterior to vitreous body. It consists of (1) elastic capsule, (2) cuboidal epithelium, and (3) lens fibers.

Capsule is attached to ciliary body by suspensory ligaments of the lens. The contraction of ciliary muscles of ciliary body will alter the shape of the lens.

Vitreous body is a transparent gelatinous mass enclosed by vitreous membrane, which fills the eyeball behind the lens. Functions: (1) supports posterior surface of lens and (2) contributes to magnifying power of eye. Sensory nerve supply: short and long ciliary nerves from nasociliary nerve.

Blood supply: Ophthalmic artery. Venous drainage is into cavernous sinus.

Movements of the eyeball

Resolution of movements of the eyeball is around three primary axes: (1) vertical axis, (2) transverse axis, and (3) anteroposterior axis. The neutral position or primary position of rest is that in which the gaze is straight ahead. Equilibrium is maintained by all the eyeball muscles, which always act as a group. Movements of the eyes are brought about by increase in tone in one set of muscles and decrease in tone of the antagonistic muscles.

Movement around vertical axis: The reference point is the **center of the cornea**, and the movements are abduction and adduction, both are rotatory movements of the eyeball.

Abduction is where center of cornea moves laterally, enabled by (1) lateral rectus, (2) superior oblique, (3) inferior oblique.

Adduction is where center of cornea moves medially brought about by (1) medial rectus, (2) superior rectus, (3) inferior rectus.

Movement around transverse axis: The reference point is the **center of the cornea,** and the movements are elevation and depression, both also rotatory movements.

Elevation is where corner of cornea moves upward and caused by (1) superior rectus and (2) inferior oblique. Depression is where center of cornea moves downward and is by (1) inferior rectus and (2) superior oblique.

Movement around anteroposterior axis: The reference point is now the top part of the cornea, and the movements are intorsion and extorsion, both are also rotatory movements.

Extorsion is where top part of cornea moves, and **intorsion** is where the lower part of cornea moves.

Applied anatomy: Paralysis of a muscle of the eyeball is noted by (1) limitation of eye movement in the field of action of paralyzed muscle and (2) diplopia that is separated maximally when an attempt is made to use the paralyzed muscle.

Innervation: Oculomotor nerve supplies all extraocular muscles except LR and SO. Lesion of the oculomotor nerve results in (1) ptosis (paralysis of levator palpebrae superioris), (2) abduction (unopposed action of LR and SO), (3) limitation of movement, (4) diplopia, (5) dilatation of pupil called mydriasis (paralysis of sphincter pupillae), (6) loss of accommodation (paralysis of ciliary muscles).

Trochlear nerve supplies superior oblique (SO4). Damage results in limitation of movement and diplopia when the subject is asked to look downward with eye adducted.

Abducent nerve supplies the lateral rectus (LR). Damage results in inability to abduct the eye beyond the middle of the palpebral fissure.

Ophthalmic Artery

Origin: Branch of cerebral part of ICA and is given off medial to anterior clinoid process.

Course and relations: The artery enters orbit through orbital canal and is inferolateral to optic nerve. It then runs forward at first lateral to optic nerve, then crosses the nerve from above together with nasociliary nerve, then runs along med wall of orbit, and terminates near medial angle of eye by dividing into supratrochlear and dorsal nasal branches.

Branches: central artery of the retina, posterior ciliary arteries to the ciliary body and iris muscular branches (gives rise to anterior ciliary arteries) iris and ciliary body. Lacrimal artery to lacrimal gland, supraorbital artery supplies upper eyelid and scalp. Supratrochlear artery supplies forehead and scalp and lacrimal sac via dorsal nasal artery root and lacrimal.

Applied anatomy: Occlusion of ophthalmic artery/central artery of retina leads to blindness.

Lacrimal Apparatus (Fig. 2.16)

The structures concerned with secretion and drainage of tears constitute the lacrimal apparatus. Parts: (1) lacrimal gland and ducts, (2) lacrimal canaliculi, (3) lacrimal sac, (4) nasolacrimal duct.

Lacrimal gland located in the lacrimal fossa on anterolateral angle of roof of orbit. It rests on lateral rectus and levator palpebrae superioris muscles.

Parts of lacrimal gland: (1) orbital part, (2) palpebral part, both are continuous with each other around the lateral border of aponeurosis of the levator palpebrae superioris (LPS). It is drained by approximately 12 lacrimal ducts, which open into the superior fornix of the conjunctiva.

Nerve supply: Parasympathetic supply is via preganglionic fibers derived from lacrimal nucleus of facial

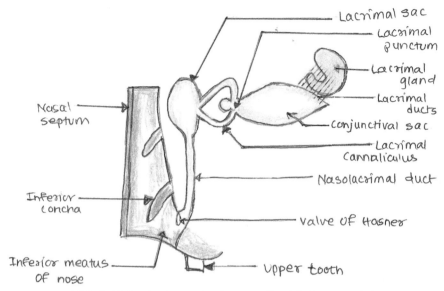

FIG. 2.16 Lacrimal apparatus (cross section; left diagrammatic.).

nerve, which travel in petrosal nerve—synapse in ptery-gopalatine ganglion, postganglionic fibers join maxillary nerve to pass into zygomatic and zygomaticotemporal nerve—reach the lacrimal gland within lacrimal nerve. Sympathetic supply fibers from superior cervical ganglion reach the gland via lacrimal nerve.

Lacrimal canaliculi: One in each eyelid, and is about 1 cm long, begins as lacrimal punctum and passes medially to open into lateral wall of lacrimal sac.

Lacrimal sac is in a fossa at medial margin of orbit, between the anterior and posterior lacrimal crests. Measures about 1 to 1 1/2 cm in length and is related anteriorly to medial palpebral ligament posteriorly to lacrimal part of orbicularis oculi laterally to ethmoidal air cells and middle meatus.

Nasolacrimal duct measures ~2 cm long, which extends from lower end of lacrimal sac to inferior meatus of nose, which is situated in a bony canal. Its opening is guarded by a fold of mucous membrane called as **lacrimal valve of Hasner**.

Applied anatomy: A **prosthetic eye** or **"ocular" prosthesis** or **indwelling eye** is provided when the eyeball has been lost. This is made of acrylic and is custom made to fit into an individual's eye socket or as a thin shell over an unseeing cloudy eye. An ocular prosthesis is colored to match the opposing eye exactly.

If the eyeball along with surrounding eyelids and skin are missing, a larger prosthesis called an **orbital prosthesis** can be manufactured. Although these prostheses do not move or blink, they are realistic as they often incorporate lashes and eyebrows. This is attached using a variety of different methods using magnetic inserts.

BASE OF SKULL (FIGS. 2.4 AND 2.17)
Interior of the base of the skull is divided into three cranial fossae: anterior, middle, and posterior cranial fossa.

Boundaries Anterior Cranial Fossa
Anteriorly and on sides: Inner surface of frontal bone (with falx cerebri in midline) lesser wings of sphenoid superior border of petrous part of temporal bone.

Posteriorly: Free border sharp lesser wing of sphenoid, anterior clinoid process, and anterior margin of sulcus chiasmaticus.

Floor: In median planes, cribriform plate of ethmoid, superior surface of anterior part of sphenoid body called jugum sphenoidale. On each side, floor is formed by orbital plate of frontal bone and posteriorly by lesser wing of sphenoid.

Boundaries of Middle Cranial Fossa
Anterior: (1) posterior border of lesser wing of sphenoid, (2) anterior clinoid process, (3) anterior margin of sulcus chiasmaticus.

Posterior: (1) superior border of petrous temporal bone, (2) dorsum sellae of sphenoid.

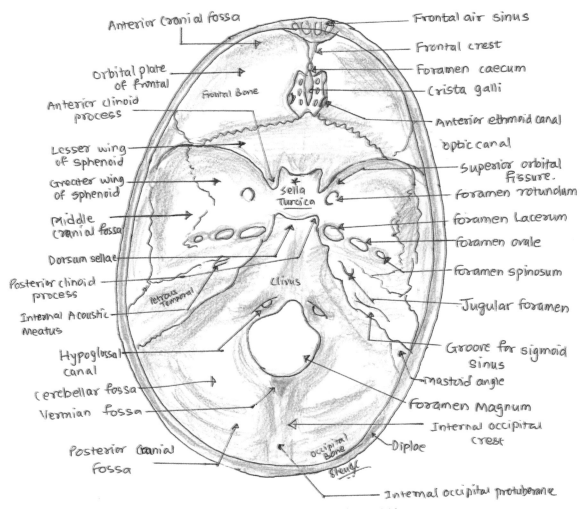

FIG. 2.17 Anterior, middle, and posterior cranial fossa.

Lateral: (1) greater wing of sphenoid, (2) anteroinferior angle of parietal bone, (3) squamous temporal bone in the middle.

Floor: body of sphenoid in median region and greater wing of sphenoid, squamous temporal bone, and anterior surface of petrous temporal bone on each side.

Boundaries of Posterior Cranial Fossa

Anterior: (1) superior border of petrous temporal bone, (2) dorsum sellae of sphenoid bone.

Posterior: squamous part of occipital bone. On each side, mastoid part of temporal bone and mastoid angle of the parietal bone.

Floor: median area is (1) sloping area behind dorsum sellae or **clivus** in front, (2) foramen magnum in the middle, (3) squamous occipital bone behind.

Lateral area: (1) condylar or lateral part of occipital bone, (2) posterior surface of petrous temporal bone, (3) mastoid temporal bone, (4) mastoid angle of parietal bone.

Major Foramina of the Cranial Fossae

These are openings in skull base bones, which transmit different structures.

a) Anterior cranial fossa perforations in cribriform plate of ethmoid transmit olfactory nerve. Foramen cecum is usually blind but occasionally transmits vein connecting nose to superior sagittal sinus.

b) Middle cranial fossa: (1) optic canal, (2) superior optic fissure, (3) foramen rotundum, (4) foramen ovale, (5) foramen spinosum, (6) foramen lacerum between lesser and greater wings of sphenoid.

c) Posterior cranial fossa: (1) foramen magnum transmits occipital medulla oblongata, spinal part of accessory nerve, right and left vertebral artery, (2) hypoglossal canal—hypoglossal nerve, (3) jugular foramen, (4) internal acoustic meatus between petrous part of temporal and condylar part of occipital petrous part of temporal glossopharyngeal, vagus and accessory nerve; sigmoid sinus contents IJV vestibulocochlear and facial nerve.

Neck is defined as the region between the head and the chest, which encompasses multiple tubular structures and glands supported by cervical vertebrae and muscles around.

Grossly the muscles of the neck help movements of the head in various directions for safety, food, and sensory perceptions. These muscles of the cervical spine (Fig. 2.18) are divided into anterior and posterior groups for ease of study. Anterior muscles are further divided into the following:

A) Superficial: (1) platysma and (2) sternocleidomastoid

B) Deep: (1) suprahyoid muscles that help elevate the hyoid bone: (i) digastric, (ii) mylohyoid, (iii) stylohyoid; (2) infrahyoid muscles that depress the hyoid bone: (i) sternohyoid, (ii) omohyoid, (iii) sternothyroid, (iv) thyrohyoid

C) Scalene muscles: lateral part: (1) anterior, (2) middle, and (3) posterior scalene

D) Prevertebral muscles anterior to cervical vertebra: (1) longus colli, (2) longus capitis, (3) rectus capitis lateral, (4) rectus capitis medial

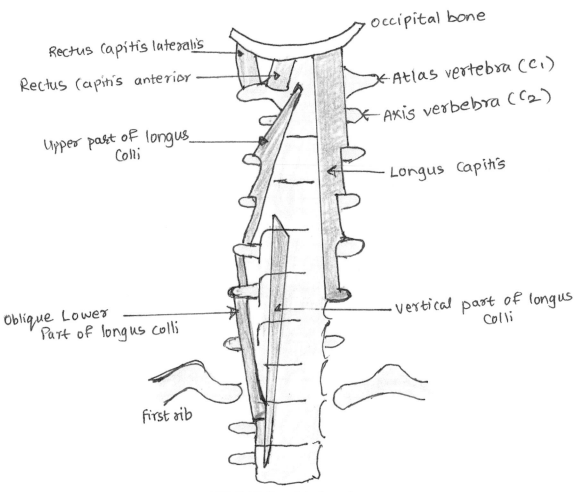

FIG. 2.18 Prevertebral muscles.

Posterior vertebral muscles are divided into upper and lower groups as follows:
a) Upper paired muscle group suboccipital: (1) obliquus capitis superior, (2) rectus capitis posterior minor, (3) rectus capitis posterior major, (4) obliquus capitis inferior
b) Lower posterior vertebral muscles: (1) trapezius, (2) levator scapulae, (3) splenius, (4) iliocostalis longissimus coli, (5) rotatores, (6) semispinalis, (7) interspinalis, (8) intertransversii

These important relevant muscles will be discussed, and they divide the neck into different triangles as mentioned in the following.

Anterior Triangle of the Neck
The sternocleidomastoid muscle divides the neck into anterior and posterior triangles (Fig. 2.19).
Boundaries:
Anterior: Anterior median line of neck.
Posterior: Anterior border of sternocleidomastoid.

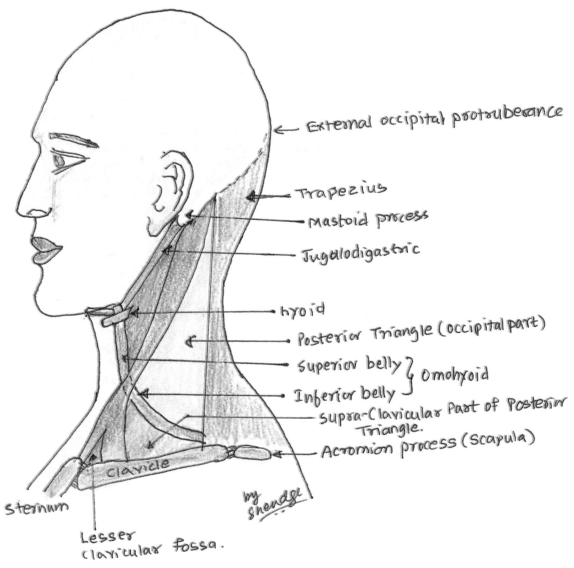

FIG. 2.19 Sternocleidomastoid, trapezius, omohyoid muscles, and posterior triangle of neck.

Superior: Inferior border of mandible and line drawn from angle of mandible to mastoid process.

Inferior: Apex of the triangle lies at the manubrium sterni.

Subdivision: Subdivided by digastric and superior belly of omohyoid into (1) submental, (2) digastric, (3) carotid, (4) muscular triangles (Fig. 2.19).
a) **Submental triangle:** base hyoid core on each side anterior belly of digastric.
b) **Digastric triangle:** anteroinferiorly: anterior belly of digastric; posteroinferiorly: posterior belly of digastric; superiorly: base of triangle by inferior border of mandible.
c) **Carotid triangle**: anteriorly: superior belly of omohyoid; posteriorly: anterior border of sternocleidomastoid; superiorly: posterior belly of digastric.
d) **Muscular triangle:** anteriorly: anterior median line of neck; posteriorsuperior: superior belly of omohyoid; posterior inferiorly: anterior border of sternocleidomastoid.
Roof: (1) skin, (2) fascia (3) platysma.
Floor: submental mylohyoid muscles. Digastric: (1) mylohyoid, (2) hyoglossus. Carotid: (1) thyrohyoid, (2) hyoglossus, (3) inferior and middle constrictors of pharynx. Muscular: (1) sternohyoid, (2) sternothyroid, (3) thyrohyoid, i.e., infrahyoid muscles.
Contents of neck triangles:
1) Submental triangle: (1) submental lymph nodes, (2) veins.

2) Digastric triangle: (1) submandibular gland, (2) facial artery and vein, (3) part of parotid gland, (4) external carotid artery deep, (5) internal carotid artery, (6) internal jugular vein, (7) glossopharyngeal nerve, (8) vagus nerve.
3) Carotid triangle: (1) common carotid artery (CCA), external carotid artery (ECA), and internal carotid artery (ICA), (2) branches of ECA, (3) internal jugular vein and some of its tributaries, (4) parts of X, XI, and XII cranial nerves, (5) larynx and pharynx, (6) internal and external laryngeal nerves.
4) Muscular triangle: (1) thyroid gland, (2) trachea and larynx, (3) esophagus.

Posterior Triangle of the Neck (Figs. 2.20 and 2.21)
Boundaries:
Anterior: posterior border of sternocleidomastoid.
Posterior: anterior border of trapezius.
Inferior: upper surface of middle 1/3 of clavicle.
Superior: apex at superior nuchal line where the sternocleidomastoid and trapezius meet.
Subdivisions: inferior belly of the omohyoid divides it into (1) Occipital triangle superiorly and (2) supraclavicular (subclavian) triangle, inferiorly.
Roof: (1) skin, (2) fascia, (3) platysma. The fascia is pierced by the EJV and supraclavicular nerve. Floor: (1) semispinalis capitis (inconstant), (2) splenius capitis, (3) levator scapulae, (4) scalenus post, (5) scalenus

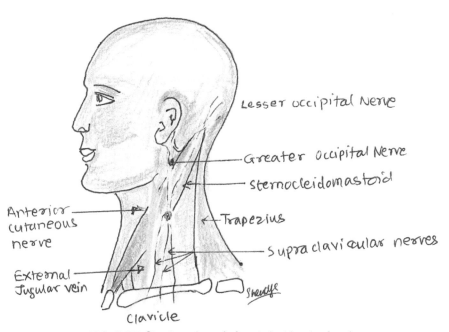
FIG. 2.20 Structures in roof of posterior triangle of neck.

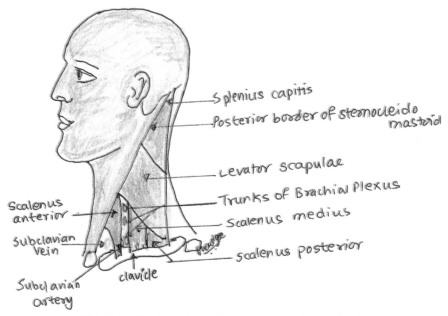

FIG. 2.21   Structures in the floor of posterior triangle of neck.

medius, (6) scalenus anterior (inconstant), (7) First digitations of serratus anterior. All these muscles are covered by prevertebral layer of fascia.

Contents of occipital triangle (Fig. 2.22): (1) spinal part of accessory nerve, (2) four cutaneous branches of cervical plexus: (i) lesser occipital nerve (C2), (ii) great

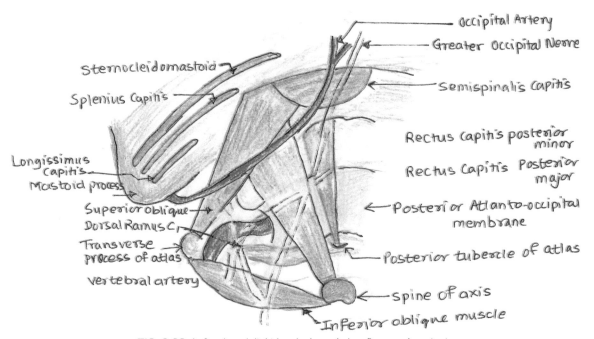

FIG. 2.22   Left suboccipital triangle: boundaries, floor, and contents.

auricular nerve (C2, C3), (iii) transverse or anterior cervical nerve (C2, C3), (iv) supraclavicular nerve (C3, C4), (3) dorsal scapular nerve (to rhomboids), (4) upper part of brachial plexus, (5) transverse cervical artery and vein, (6) occipital artery from ECA, (7) lymph nodes: along posterior border of sternocleidomastoid: supraclavicular nodes and occipital nodes.

Suboccipital Triangle (Fig. 2.22)

Deep to semispinalis capitis and splenius capitis.

Boundaries: Superomedial: Rectus capitis posterior major muscle supplemented by rectus capitis posterior minor. Superolateral: Superior oblique muscle. Inferior: Inferior oblique muscle.

Roof: Medially dense fibrous tissue covered by semispinalis capitis. Laterally longissimus capitis and occasionally splenius capitis.

Floor: (1) posterior arch of atlas, (2) posterior atlantooccipital membrane.

Contents: (1) vertebral venous plexus, (2) third part of vertebral artery (in groove of posterior arch of atlas), (3) suboccipital nerve (beneath vertebral artery). Greater occipital nerve lies on roof of triangle before piercing semispinalis capitis to be distributed to skin of occipital region.

Contents of subclavian triangle: (1) Three trunks of brachial plexus, (2) long thoracic **nerve of Bell** (to serratus anterior C5, C6, C7), (3) nerve to subclavius, (4) suprascapular nerve, (5) third part of subclavian artery and subclavian vein, (6) suprascapular artery and vein, (7) transverse cervical artery and vein, (8) lower part of external jugular vein, (9) supraclavicular lymph nodes.

Applied anatomy: (1) Metastatic enlargement of supraclavicular lymph nodes of Virchow (called **Troisier sign**). (2) Scalene brachial plexus anesthetic block between first rib and skin above clavicle.

Sternocleidomastoid muscles are large, paired superficial muscles of the neck.

Origin: (1) sternal head tendinous part arises from superior aspect of manubrium sterni, (2) musculotendinous clavicular head and arises from medial 1/3 of upper surface of clavicle.

Insertion: (1) Tendinous into mastoid process of the temporal bone. (2) Thin aponeurotic into lateral part of superior nuchal line of occipital bone.

Nerve supply: Spinal part of accessory and motor ventral rami of C2 and C3 sensory (proprioceptive).

Blood supply: Branches from occipital artery.

Actions: (1) Simultaneous contraction of bilateral muscles enables extension of head at atlantooccipital joint, and flexion of cervical vertebral column. (2) Single muscle contraction causes head tilting toward ipsilateral shoulder and contralateral head rotation. (3) Together, they help as accessory muscles of inspiration.

Relations:

a) Superficial: (1) Skin, (2) fascia with subcutaneous platysma, (3) external jugular vein (EJV), (4) great auricular nerve and medial supraclavicular nerves, (5) superficial cervical lymph nodes along EJV, (6) parotid gland.

b) Deep: (1) Carotid sheath with its contents: common carotid artery, internal carotid artery, internal jugular vein (IJV), and vagus nerve. (2) Muscles: sternohyoid, sternothyroid, omohyoid, anterior, medial, and posterior scaleni, levator scapulae, splenius capitis and posterior belly of digastric. (3) Common carotid artery (CCA) and internal carotid artery (ICA): (i) external carotid artery (ECA), (ii) occipital artery, (iii) subclavian artery and suprascapular artery. (4) Veins: (i) internal jugular vein (IJV), (ii) anterior jugular vein, (iii) facial vein, (iv) lingual vein. (5) Nerves: (i) vagus nerve, (ii) accessory nerve (iii) cervical plexus, (iv) upper part of brachial plexus, (v) phrenic nerve, (vi) ansa cervicalis. (6) Lymph nodes: deep cervical.

Applied anatomy: (1) the sternocleidomastoid divides the neck into anterior and posterior triangles, (2) congenital torticollis, (3) spasmodic torticollis: helmet therapy for wry neck or torticollis.

Static rotational control with cervical orthosis for treatment of congenital muscular torticollis and associated plagiocephaly and hemihypoplasia enabling stretching of the sternomastoid fibrosis.

Scalenus Anterior Muscle

Origin: Anterior tubercles of transverse processes of cervical vertebrae C3, C4, C5, C6. Insertion: (1) scalene tubercle on inner border of first rib, (2) ridge on upper surface of first rib. Nerve supply: ventral rami of C4, C5, C6.

Action: (1) Elevation of first rib (from above), (2) Lateral flexion and rotation of cervical vertebrae (action from below).

Relations: Anterior: (1) prevertebral layer of deep cervical fascia, (2) phrenic nerve, (3) superficial cervical and suprascapular artery, (4) internal jugular vein and subclavian vein.

Posterior: (1) subclavian artery, (2) brachial plexus, (3) cervical dome of pleura.

Medial: (1) vertebral artery and vein, (2) inferior thyroid artery, (3) thyrocervical trunk, (4) sympathetic trunk, (5) thoracic duct (left side).

Lateral: (1) roots of brachial plexus, (2) subclavian artery, (3) roots of phrenic nerve.

Thyroid Gland: (Greek: Thyros—Shield) (Figs. 2.23 and 2.24)

Shield or H-shaped endocrine gland regulates basal metabolic rate and growth.

Parts: Two lobes: Right and left lobes with connecting isthmus. Pyramidal lobe is occasionally present.

Position: Lies at the level of cervical vertebrae: C5, C6, C7, and T1, each lobe extending anteriorly from middle of thyroid cartilage to fourth or fifth tracheal ring. The isthmus extends from second to fourth tracheal ring. True capsule is condensation of the glandular connective tissue, and false external fibrous capsule adherent to underlying gland is pretracheal layer of deep cervical fascia, which form suspensory ligament of Berry, which anchor the gland to trachea, thyroid, and cricoid cartilages.

Note in total thyroidectomy gland is removed along with its true capsule to prevent bleeding.

Relations of the lobes

Anterolateral: (1) sternothyroid, (2) sternohyoid, (3) superior belly of omohyoid, (4) anterior border of sternocleidomastoid.

Posterolateral: carotid sheath and its contents: (1) CCA, (2) IJV, (3) vagus nerve.

Medially: (1) larynx, (2) trachea, (3) inferior constrictor of pharynx, (4) esophagus. Associated with these structures are (5) cricothyroid, (6) external laryngeal nerve, (7) recurrent laryngeal nerve (in tracheaesophageal groove).

Posterior borders of two lobes are rounded and related to (1) superior and inferior parathyroid glands, (2) anastomosis between superior and inferior thyroid artery, (3) thoracic duct (left side).

Relations of the isthmus:

Anteriorly: (1) sternothyroid, (2) sternohyoid, (3) anterior jugular vein, (4) fascia and skin.

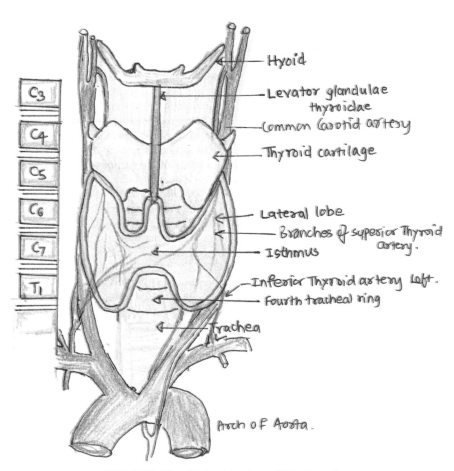

FIG. 2.23 Thyroid gland, levels, and blood supply.

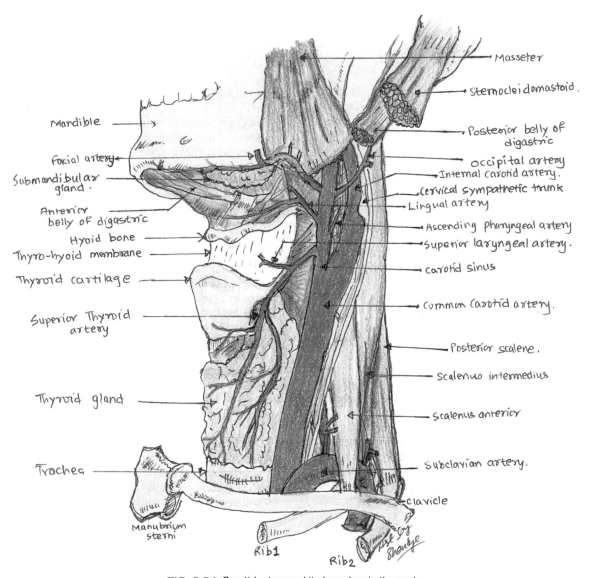

FIG. 2.24 Carotid artery and its branches in the neck.

Posteriorly: 2nd, 3rd, and 4th tracheal rings.

Superiorly: terminal branches of superior thyroid artery anastomose along upper border.

Arterial supply: superior thyroid artery from ECA, inferior thyroid art from thyrocervical trunk, and thyroidea ima artery from brachiocephalic artery or arch of aorta.

Venous drainage: superior thyroid vein and middle thyroid vein into IJV, inferior thyroid vein anastomoses with left brachiocephalic vein. Fourth thyroid vein of Kocher between middle and inferior veins drains into IJV.

Lymphatic drainage: follows arteries and drains mainly into (1) deep cervical lymph nodes and (2) a few lymph vessels pass to paratracheal nodes.

Nerve supply: vasoconstrictor nerves mainly from middle cervical ganglion, partly from superior and inferior cervical ganglia.

Applied anatomy: (1) important structures may be injured like the recurrent laryngeal nerve thyroidectomy may cause vocal cord paralysis.

Common Carotid Artery (CCA) (Fig. 2.24)

Origin: Right CCA is a branch of brachiocephalic trunk, and it begins in neck behind right sternoclavicular joint. Left CCA is a branch of aortic arch, which begins in thorax and passes behind left sternoclavicular joint.

Course: runs in carotid sheath along with IJV and vagus nerve and passes upward and backward in the neck, from sternoclavicular joint to upper border of thyroid cartilage and ends by dividing into external carotid artery (ECA) and internal carotid artery (ICA). Special Features: carotid sinus is a localized dilatation at terminal part of CCA or beginning of ICA.

Innervation: glossopharyngeal and sympathetic nerves act as baroreceptor to regulate blood pressure.

Carotid body is a small oval reddish-brown structure situated behind bifurcation of common carotid artery. It is innervated mainly by glossopharyngeal nerve and by vagus and sympathetic nerves.

Function: chemoreceptor responds to changes in concentration of O_2, CO_2, and pH of blood.

Relations:

Anterolateral: (1) trachea, skin, superficial fascia, platysma, investing layer of deep cervical fascia, (2) sternocleidomastoid overlaps it, (3) sternohyoid, (4) sternothyroid, (5) superior belly of omohyoid embedded in anterior wall of carotid sheath, (6) descendens hypoglossi, (7) ansa cervicalis crossing the artery, (8) superior and middle thyroid veins, (9) anterior jugular veins.

Posteriorly: (1) transverse processes of lower four cervical vertebral, (2) longus capitis and longus colli, (3) origin of scalenus anterior, (4) sympathetic trunk in the lower part of the neck, (5) vertebral vessels, (6) inferior thyroid artery (left side), (7) thoracic duct behind termination of CCA, carotid body.

Medially: (1) larynx and pharynx, (2) trachea, (3) esophagus, (4) lobe of thyroid gland, (5) inferior thyroid gland, (6) recurrent laryngeal nerve.

Laterally: (1) internal jugular vein, (2) vagus lies posterolateral.

Applied anatomy: (1) After ligature of CCA on one side, collateral circulation is established between (i) superior and inferior thyroid arteries (inferior thyroid and deep cervical from subclavian), (ii) descending branches of occipital and deep cervical artery and (iii) vertebral artery; (2) carotid pulse is felt at anterior tubercle of transverse process of C6 (**carotid tubercle of Chassaignac**), can be massaged to treat supraventricular tachycardia.

External Carotid Artery (ECA)

The ECA is one of the two terminal branches of the CCA and is the chief arterial supply to anterior structures in the neck and face.

Origin: carotid triangle at level of upper border of thyroid cartilage (C3 and C4).

Course: runs upward, slightly backward and laterally, and enters substance of parotid gland, terminating behind neck of mandible by dividing into the maxillary and superficial temporal artery.

Note: At first lies medial to ICA. It then passes backward and laterally to lie lateral to ICA.

Branches: eight branches: (1) superior thyroid, (2) ascending pharyngeal, (3) lingual, (4) facial, (5) occipital, (6) posterior auricular, (7) superficial temporal, (8) maxillary.

Relations:

Anterolateral: (1) sternocleidomastoid overlaps at its beginning above this level, it is relatively superficial and is covered by (2) skin and superficial fascia, (3) cervical branch of facial nerve, (4) transverse cutaneous nerve, (5) investing layer of deep cervical fascia, it is crossed by (6) hypoglossal nerve, (7) facial and lingual veins, (8) posterior belly of digastric, (9) stylohyoid muscles. Within parotid gland, it is crossed by (10) facial nerve and retromandibular vein.

Note: The IJV first lies lateral to the artery, then posterior.

Medially: (1) wall of pharynx, (2) styloid process, (3) ICA passing between the ECA and ICA, (4) stylopharyngeus, (5) glossopharyngeal nerve, (6) pharyngeal branch of vagus nerve, (7) portion of parotid gland.

Applied anatomy: Ligature of artery of one side enables collateral circulation between branches of ECA with those of the opposite side.

Internal Carotid Artery (Cervical Part)

The ICA is one of the two terminal branches of the CCA and is the principal artery to the brain and eyes. Course of ICA is divided into four parts: (1) cervical part, (2) petrous part, (3) cavernous part, (4) cerebral part.

Cervical part of carotid artery:

Origin: It begins in the carotid triangle at level of upper border of thyroid cartilage (i.e., between C3 and C4).

Course: It is enclosed in carotid sheath with IJV and vagus nerve, ascending vertically in the neck to lower end of carotid canal in petrous temporal bone. In the lower part (in carotid triangle) is comparatively superficial, after ascending deep to posterior belly of digastric, it lies deep to parotid gland, styloid process, and adjacent structures. It has no branches in the neck.

Special features: The ICA has two structures at its commencement: (1) carotid sinus, which is localized dilatation at terminal part of CCA (or beginning of ICA) and is innervated by glossopharyngeal and sympathetic nerves. Carotid sinus acts as baroreceptor (regulate blood pressure). (2) Carotid body is a small reddish-brown structure behind bifurcation of CCA and innervated mainly by glossopharyngeal nerve, acts as chemoreceptor (detect changes in blood O_2 and CO_2).

Relations:

Anterolateral (superficial):
a) Below digastric: (1) skin, superficial fascia, platysma, investing layer of deep cervical fascia, (2) transverse cutaneous nerve, (3) anterior border of sternocleidomastoid, (4) lingual and facial nerves, (5) hypoglossal nerve and its descending branch, (6) occipital artery.
b) Above digastric: (7) posterior auricular artery, (8) stylohyoid and stylopharyngeus, (9) styloid process, (10) glossopharyngeal nerve, (11) pharyngeal branch of vagus nerve, (12) parotid gland and its contents: facial nerve, retromandibular vein, and ECA.

Posteriorly: (1) superior laryngeal nerve, (2) cervical part of sympathetic trunk and superior cervical ganglion, (3) longus capitis and prevertebral layer of deep cervical fascia, (4) transverse processes of C1, C2, and C3.

Medially: (1) pharynx, (2) superior laryngeal nerve, (3) external and internal laryngeal nerves, (4) ascending pharyngeal artery.

Laterally: (1) IJV and (2) vagus.

Subclavian artery:

Principal artery of the upper limb supplies part of the neck and brain through its branches.

Origin: Right subclavian artery arises from brachiocephalic trunk behind right sternoclavicular joint. Left subclavian artery arises from arch of aorta behind left CCA and ascends to back of left sternoclavicular joint.

Course: The subclavian artery is divided into three parts by presence of the scalenus anterior muscle. First part arches upward and laterally from behind sternoclavicular joint to medial border of scalenus anterior. Second part lies behind scalenus anterior muscle. Third part extends from lateral border of scalenus anterior to outer border of first rib where it continues as axillary artery.

Branches:

First part: (1) vertebral artery, (2) thyrocervical trunk which divides into (i) inferior thyroid, (ii) transverse cervical, (iii) suprascapular, (3) internal thoracic artery.

Second part: costocervical trunk divides into (1) superior intercostal artery and (2) deep cervical artery.

Third part: descending (dorsal) scapular artery.

Relations of the first part:

Anteriorly: From medial to lateral: (1) CCA, (2) vagus, (3) internal jugular vein (IJV), (4) more superficial sternohyoid and sternohyoid muscles, (5) sternocleidomastoid, (6) vertebral veins, (7) thoracic duct (left side), (8) cardiac branches of vagus and sympathetic nerves.

Posterior (posterior–inferior): (1) dome of cervical pleura and suprapleural membrane (Sibson's), (2) apex of lung, (3) ansa subclavia that encircles the artery, (4) sympathetic trunk and inferior cervical ganglion, (5) right recurrent laryngeal nerve on right side.

Relations of the second part:

Anteriorly: (1) scalenus anterior, (2) sternocleidomastoid, (3) subclavian vein (separated by scalenus anterior), (4) right phrenic nerve on right side, deep to prevertebral fascia.

Posteriorly: (1) dome of cervical pleura and suprapleural membrane, (2) apex of lung, (3) scalenus medius.

Superiorly: upper and middle trunks of brachial plexus.

Relations of the third part:

Anteriorly: (1) skin, superficial fascia, platysma, investing layer of deep cervical fascia, (2) supraclavicular nerve, (3) EJV and tributaries, (4) middle 1/3rd clavicle and subclavius.

Posteriorly: (1) scalenus medius, (2) lower trunk of brachial plexus, (3) suprapleural membrane (Sibson's fascia), (4) cervical pleura, (5) apex of lung.

Superiorly upper and middle trunks of brachial plexus.

Inferiorly upper surface of first rib.

Applied anatomy: (1) third part of subclavian artery may be compressed against first rib to stop bleeding in upper arm, (2) aneurysms in third part of artery causing compressive brachial plexopathy causing pain, weakness, and numbness in upper limb, (3) cervical rib—artery is kinked as it passes over rib, causing occlusion.

VERTEBRAL ARTERY

Major arterial blood supply to brain, spinal cord, meninges, surrounding muscles, and bones.

Origin: Branch of first part of subclavian artery.

Course and relations: The course divided into four parts:

Cervical (1st) part extends from its origin to transverse process of C7 and enters foramen in transverse process of C6.

Anterior relations: (1) carotid sheath, and common carotid artery (CCA), (2) vertebral vein, (3) inferior thyroid artery, (4) thoracic duct (left side).

Posterior relation: (1) transverse process of C7, (2) stellate ganglion, (3) ventral rami of C7.

Vertebral (2nd) part extends from transverse processes of C6 to C1, i.e., runs through the foramina of the upper six cervical vertebrae and emerge from transverse process of atlas.

Suboccipital (3rd) part winds medially behind lateral mass of atlas and enters vertebral canal after piercing dura and arachnoid maters. It then passes through foramen magnum and then makes a sharp loop.

Intracranial (4th) part ascends medially in front of medulla oblongata, at lower border of pons, both vertebral arteries unite to form the basilar artery.

Branches: (1) Cervical branches: (i) spinal and (ii) muscular. (2) Cranial branches: (i) meningeal branches, (ii) posterior spinal artery, and (iii) medullary arteries.

Applied anatomy: (1) Thrombosis of vertebral artery (occlusion), (2) lesion of anterior spinal artery.

Internal Jugular Veins (IJVs)

Drains the brain, neck, and face.

Origin: It begins at jugular foramen at base of skull as a continuation of sigmoid sinus.

Course: IJV descends in carotid sheath and passes downward and anteriorly ends behind medial end of clavicle by joining with subclavian vein to form brachiocephalic vein.

Special features: (1) superior bulb: dilatation at its origin, (2) inferior bulb: dilatation near its termination and possesses one bicuspid valve directly above inferior bulb.

Relations:

Anterolateral: (1) skin, superficial fascia, platysma, investing layer of deep cervical fascia, (2) sternocleidomastoid, (3) posterior belly of digastric, (4) parotid salivary gland separated from it by styloid process and stylopharyngeus. Its lower part is covered by (5) sternohyoid, sternothyroid, and omohyoid. Crossing the vein: (6) ansa cervicalis, (7) stylohyoid, (8) posterior auricular and occipital artery, (9) spinal part of accessory nerve. Other superficial structures: (10) facial nerve, (11) anterior jugular vein, (12) the deep cervical lymph nodes run alongside the IJV.

Posteriorly: (1) transverse processes of cervical vertebrae, (2) levator scapulae, (3) scalenus anterior and medius, (4) cervical plexus, (5) phrenic nerve, (6) thyrocervical trunk, (7) vertebral vein, (8) first part of subclavian artery, (9) dome of cervical pleura, (10) thoracic duct (left side).

Medially: Below: (1) vagus nerve, (2) CCA at base of skull, (3) ICA, (4) IXth, Xth, Xth, and XIIth cranial nerves.

Tributaries: (1) inferior petrosal sinus, (2) facial vein, (3) lingual vein, (4) pharyngeal veins, (5) superior thyroid vein, (6) middle thyroid vein, (7) sometimes, occipital vein.

Note: Thoracic duct opens into angle of union between left IJV and left subclavian vein. The right lymphatic duct opens similarly on the right side.

Applied anatomy: (1) congestive heart failure or any disease where venous pressure is raised, the IJV is markedly dilated, engorged. (2) Deep cervical lymph nodes lie along the IJV. In malignancies involving these nodes, vein is usually removed along with nodes during surgical block dissection of neck.

CERVICAL PLEXUS

The cervical plexus supplies skin at the back of the head, neck, and shoulder as well as certain muscles of neck and the diaphragm.

It is formed by ventral rami of C1 to C4, which are joined by connecting branches to form a series of three loops from which branches arise.

Position and Relations

Anteriorly: (1) It is covered by prevertebral layer of deep cervical fascia. (2) IJV in carotid sheath. (3) Sternocleidomastoid.

Posteriorly: Origins of (1) levator scapulae and (2) scalenus medius.

Branches: (1) Superficial cutaneous branches: (i) lesser occipital (C2), (ii) great auricular (C2, 3), (iii) transverse cutaneous (cervical) (C2, 3), (iv) medial, intermediate, and lateral supraclavicular (C3, 4). The cutaneous branches emerge near middle of posterior border of sternocleidomastoid. (2) Deep and communicating branches: (i) each of the four rami receive gray rami communicans (GRC) from the superior cervical ganglion of the sympathetic trunk, (ii) branch from C1 to hypoglossal nerve, (iii) other branches to vagus and accessory nerve. (3) Muscular branches to (i) prevertebral muscles, (ii) sternocleidomastoid, (iii) levator scapulae, (iv) scaleni anterior medius and posterior, (v) trapezius, (vi) diaphragm via phrenic nerve, (vii) infrahyoid muscles (except thyrohyoid) via ansa cervicalis.

Ansa cervicalis lies superficial to (or inside) the carotid sheath (Fig. 2.28).

Formed by (1) descending branch of hypoglossal nerve (C1) (2.) descending cervical nerve (C2, 3), which unite to form a loop and supply omohyoid, sternohyoid, and sternothyroid (thyrohyoid is supplied directly via C1 fibers within hypoglossal nerve).

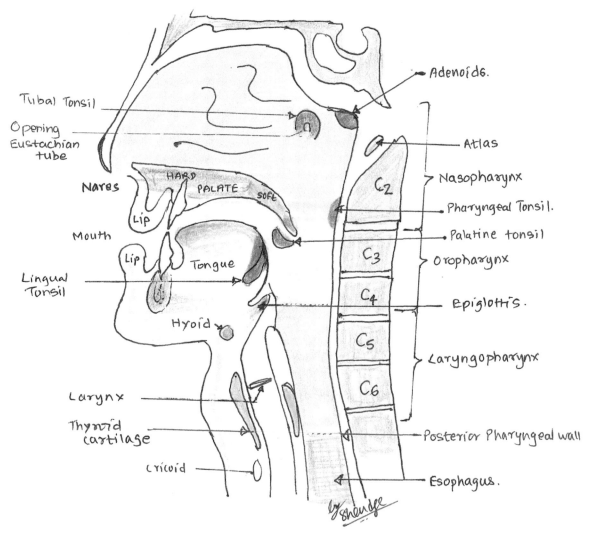

FIG. 2.25 Regions of pharynx, Waldeyer's ring of tonsils.

Phrenic Nerve (Cervical Part)

Mixed nerve with motor fibers to the ipsilateral hemidiaphragm (exclusively) and sensory fibers from the pleura, fibrous pericardium, peritoneum and diaphragm, and sympathetic fibers.

Origin: from ventral rami of C3, C4, C5 (mainly C4), at lateral border of scalenus anterior at level of cricoid cartilage. Contribution from C5 via nerve to subclavius is called **accessory phrenic nerve**.

Course: Runs downward vertically on anterior surface of scalenus anterior, behind prevertebral fascia, and crosses it from lateral to medial border. It then crosses internal thoracic artery from lateral to medial side and enters thorax by passing in front of subclavian artery and behind beginning of brachiocephalic vein. No branches in the neck.

Relations:

Anterior: (1) prevertebral layer of deep fascia, (2) IJV, (3) superficial fascia, cervical, and suprascapular artery, (4) beginning of brachiocephalic vein, (5) thoracic duct (left side).

Posterior: (1) scalenus anterior, (2) subclavian artery, (3) cervical dome of pleura.

Applied anatomy: Surgical interruption of the phrenic nerve on the scalenus anterior is sometimes performed to aid in collapse of a lung. Diaphragm on

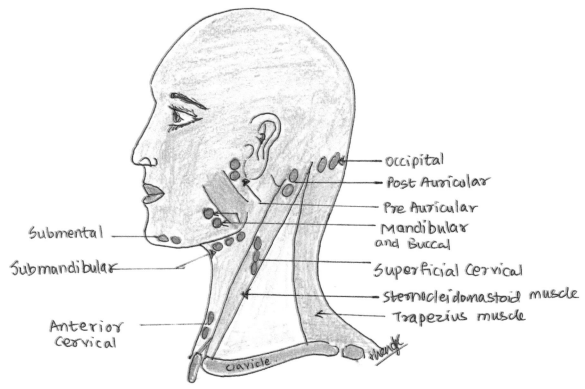

FIG. 2.26 Superficial lymph nodes of neck.

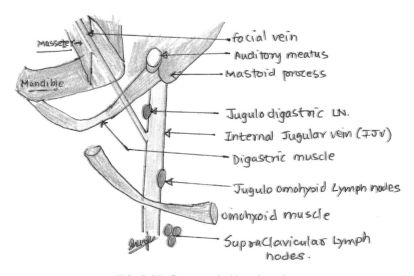

FIG. 2.27 Deep cervical lymph nodes.

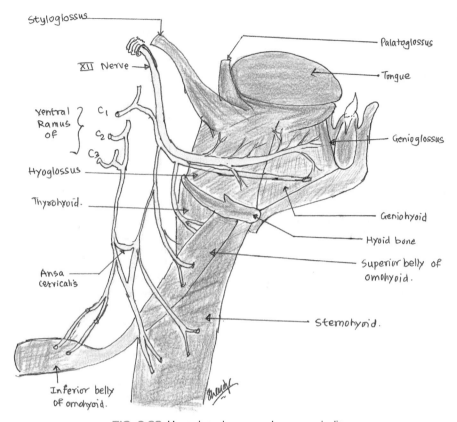

FIG. 2.28 Hypoglossal nerve and ansa cervicalis.

affected side is paralyzed and is therefore elevated, leading to collapse of the diseased lung for resting and promotion of healing.

Sympathetic Trunk (Cervical Part)

This is a ganglionated chain located one on each side of the cervical part of vertebral column. This provides sympathetic nerve supply to various head and neck structures.

Formation: Preganglionic fibers arising from thoracic segments; T1 to T4 of spinal cord pass to thoracic part of sympathetic trunk and then ascend into the neck.

Extent: Located prevertebral, extends upward to base of skull and downward to neck of first rib where it becomes continuous with thoracic part of sympathetic trunk.

Relations:

Anterior: (1) carotid sheath, (2) CCA and ICA, (3) inferior thyroid artery.

Posterior: (1) prevertebral fascia, (2) longus capitis and cervicis, (3) transverse processes of lower six cervical vertebrae.

Cervical Sympathetic Ganglia (CSG): Superior, Middle, and Inferior

The ascending preganglionic fibers synapse in these ganglia, from which postganglionic fibers arise to supply the submandibular, blood vessels, and glands of head and neck.

Superior cervical ganglion is largest of the three ganglia and is formed by the fusion of the upper four sympathetic ganglia.

Location: Base of skull at level of C1 to C3 behind ICA and in front of longus capitis. (1) Gray rami communicans (GRC) to C1 to C4 (ventral rami). (2) Branches to 9th, 10th, and 12th cranial nerves. (3) Internal carotid arterial (internal carotid plexus). (4) Arterial branches to CCA and ECA. (5) Pharyngeal branches and plexus (with branches of 9th and 10th cranial nerves). (6) Superior cervical branch supplies cardiac plexus in thorax.

Middle cervical ganglion is small and formed by fusion of fifth and sixth cervical ganglia lies in lower part of neck in front of C6 above arch formed by inferior thyroid artery. (1) GRC to ventral rami of C5 and C6. (2) Thyroid branches to thyroid gland. (3) Middle cardiac branch to cardiac plexus in thorax.

Inferior cervical ganglion is large, irregular, and star-shaped **(stellate ganglion)** formed by fusion of 7th and 8th cervical ganglia, and often with 1st thoracic ganglia. It lies between transverse process of C7 and neck of 1st rib behind vertebral artery. (1) GRC to anterior rami of C7 and C8. (2) Arterial branches of subclavian and vertebral arteries. (3) Inferior cardiac branch to cardiac plexus.

Applied anatomy: (1) Injury to cervical sympathetic trunk produces Horner's syndrome, (2) stellate ganglion block used in anesthesia.

Trachea (cervical part) (Figs. 2.23–2.25):

Trachea is a mobile, noncollapsible tube forming the beginning of the lower respiratory passages. It is kept patent by C-shaped cartilaginous rings. Cartilage is deficient posteriorly where membranous part permits expansion of the esophagus during passage of food, which has **trachealis** muscle.

Origin: It begins at lower border of cricoid cartilage of larynx (lower border of C6) in the midline.

Course: It runs downward and slightly backward in the midline and enters thorax in median plane.

Relations:

Anteriorly: (1) skin and fascia, (2) isthmus of thyroid gland (in front of 2nd, 3rd, and 4th rings), (3) inferior thyroid veins, (4) jugular arch, (5) thyroidea ima artery (if present), (6) sternothyroid and sternohyoids, (7) left brachiocephalic vein in children.

Posteriorly: (1) right and left recurrent laryngeal nerve, (2) esophagus, (3) vertebral column and some prevertebral muscles.

Laterally: (on each side) (1) lobes of thyroid gland, (2) carotid sheath and CCA. Blood supply mainly from inferior thyroid arteries.

Venous drainage: left brachiocephalic vein.

Lymphatic drainage: (1) pretracheal nodes, (2) paratracheal nodes.

Nerve supply: (1) parasympathetic: vagus and recurrent laryngeal nerve are sensory and secretomotor to mucous membrane motor to trachealis muscle, (2) sympathetic: from middle cervical ganglion of sympathetic trunks are vasomotor.

Applied anatomy: (1) trachea may be compressed by pathological enlargement of thyroid, thymus, lymph nodes, and aortic arch; (2) tracheostomy is usually done after cutting the isthmus of thyroid gland.

LYMPHATIC DRAINAGE OF HEAD AND NECK (FIGS. 2.26 AND 2.27)

The lymphatic system of head and neck consists of (1) lymph nodes and (2) lymph vessels.

Lymph nodes are made up of several peripheral groups and a terminal group. The terminal group receives all the lymphatics of head and neck, directly or indirectly via one of the peripheral groups.

Peripheral groups of lymph nodes are arranged in two groups: superficial and deep groups.

a) **Superficial group** consist of nodes, namely, (1) **occipital lymph nodes** located over occipital bone at apex of posterior triangle of neck. They receive lymph from back of scalp and efferent to deep cervical nodes. (2) **Retroauricular (mastoid) nodes** are located over lateral surface of mastoid process of temporal bone. These receive lymph from scalp above auricle and from posterior wall of external auditory meatus. (3) **Parotid nodes** that are located on or within parotid gland, which receive lymph from scalp, auricle, face, external acoustic meatus, and middle ear. (4) **Buccal nodes** that are located over buccinator muscle close to facial vein. These lie along course of lymph vessels, i.e., receive from several nodes. (5) **Submandibular nodes** are located on surface of submandibular gland receive lymph from wide area. (6) **Submental nodes** are in submental triangle between anterior bellies of digastric and receive lymph from lower lip, tongue, and superficial neck, and are efferent to submandibular and deep cervical nodes. These six groups of lymph nodes form a collar at the junction of the head with the neck called "pericervical collar." The superficial tissues of the head and neck drain into these nodes, as well as two other groups. (7) **Anterior cervical nodes** located along course of anterior jugular vein receive lymph from superficial tissue of front of neck and are efferent to deep cervical nodes. (8) **Superficial cervical nodes** that are located along the course of EJV and receive lymph from small part of face and external ear are efferent to deep cervical nodes.

b) **Deep group of peripheral lymph nodes** are (9) **retropharyngeal nodes** found in interval between pharyngeal wall and prevertebral fascia, i.e., retropharyngeal space, (10) **laryngeal nodes** found in front of larynx on cricothyroid ligament, (11) **paratracheal nodes** found lateral to trachea, (12) **pretracheal nodes** located in front of trachea.

Terminal group of lymph nodes are the deep cervical nodes found in a chain along the course of IJV, embedded in fascia of carotid sheath, receive all lymph of head and neck efferent join to form jugular lymph trunks, which drains into the thoracic duct or the right lymphatic duct.

Note: Clinically important ones: (1) jugulodigastric node, (2) juguloomohyoid node. Superficial vessels follow superficial veins, whereas deep vessels follow arteries and deep veins.

Applied anatomy: (1) enlargement of nodes may indicate infection in drainage area, (2) spread of cancer through the lymphatics, (3) block dissection of cervical nodes, i.e., removal of cervical nodes, IJV, submandibular gland and fascia may be performed in some cases of cancer.

MAXILLA (UPPER JAW) (FIGS. 2.29 AND 2.30)

This is second largest bone of the face. Upper jaw is the combined left and right maxillae fused in midline, with formation of face, nose, mouth, orbit, infratemporal and pterygopalatine fossae.

Each maxilla has a body and four processes: frontal, zygomatic, alveolar, and palatine processes.

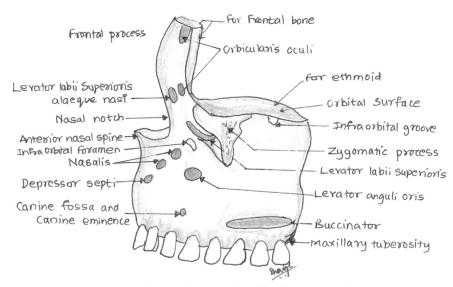

FIG. 2.29 Lateral aspect of maxilla with muscle origin.

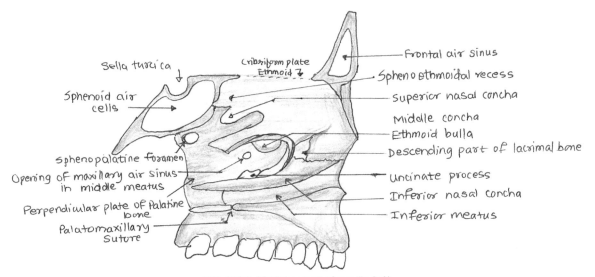

FIG. 2.30 Medial aspect of maxilla (left).

Body of maxilla is pyramidal shaped, with its base directed medially at the nasal surface and apex laterally at the zygomatic process. The body has four surfaces enclosing the maxillary sinus.

The four surfaces are as follows:

1) Anterior or facial surface: This has multiple foramina and areas for facial muscles. The **incisive fossa** is a depression above the incisor teeth, origin for depressor septi muscle. The origin of the other muscles, namely, incisivus and nasalis are shown in Fig. 2.29. The canine fossa is small depression lateral to the canine eminence, where levator anguli oris muscle originates (Fig. 2.29).
2) Superior or orbital surface.
3) Medial or nasal surface.
4) Posterior or the infratemporal surface.

Oral cavity or mouth is divided into outer smaller vestibule of mouth (space between the teeth and cheek) and inner larger part the oral cavity proper (Fig. 2.31).

Lips are fleshy folds lined externally by skin and internal mucous membrane. The mucocutaneous junction or the vermillion border lines the edge of the lips and is used landmark for surgical reconstruction. They have the orbicularis muscle, which needs to be repaired. Inner surface of each lip is supported by frenulum. Upper lip has the philtrum, which is deficient in cleft lip and palate, which needs plastic surgical and prosthetic reconstruction and rehabilitation.

Palate: Parts of palate: hard and soft palate (Figs. 2.32 and 2.33):

Hard palate: It is the partition between the nose and the oral cavity. The anterior margins are continuous with alveolar arch and gums. Posterior margins give attachment to the soft palate. Superior surface is the floor of the nose and inferior surface roof of the oral cavity.

Blood supply: Arteries are greater palatine branch of the maxillary artery and veins that drain into the pterygoid plexus.

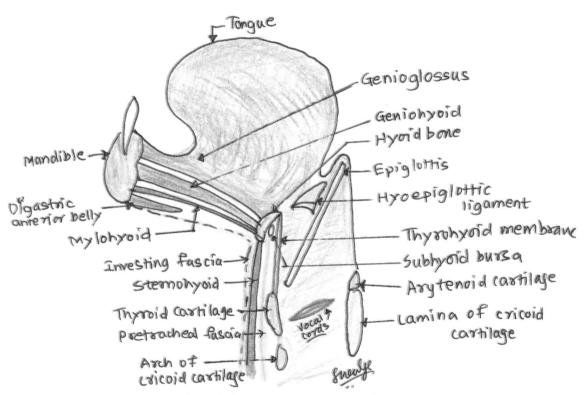

FIG. 2.31 Sagittal section through floor of mouth.

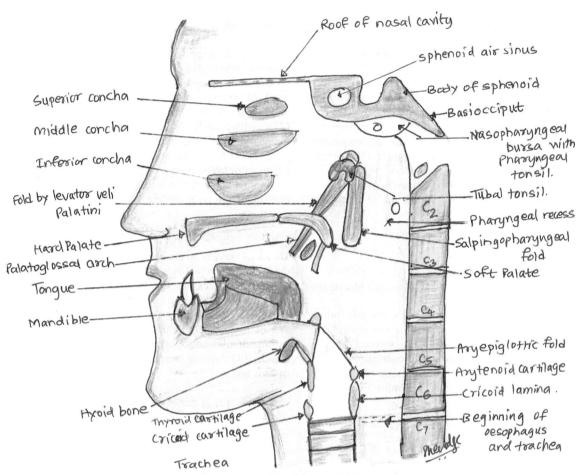

Roof of nasal cavity

sphenoid air sinus

Body of sphenoid

Basiocciput

Nasopharyngeal bursa with Pharyngeal tonsil.

Superior concha

middle concha

Inferior concha

Fold by levator veli Palatini

Hard Palate

Palatoglossal arch

Tongue

Mandible

Hyoid bone

Thyroid cartilage

Cricoid cartilage

Trachea

Tubal tonsil.

Pharyngeal recess

Salpingopharyngeal fold

Soft Palate

Aryepiglottic fold

Arytenoid cartilage

Cricoid lamina.

Beginning of oesophagus and trachea

C2

C3

C4

C5

C6

C7

FIG. 2.32 Sagittal section through face, head neck, palate, and larynx.

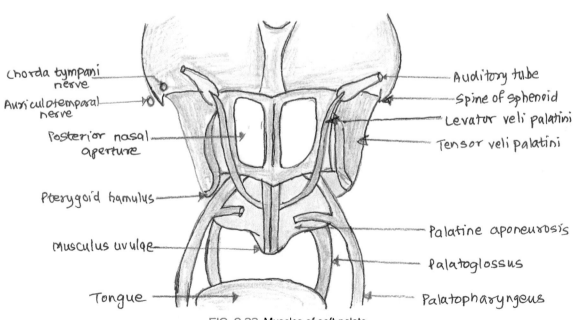

Chorda tympani nerve

Auriculotemporal nerve

Posterior nasal aperture

Pterygoid hamulus

musculus uvulae

Tongue

Auditory tube

Spine of sphenoid

Levator veli palatini

Tensor veli palatini

Palatine aponeurosis

Palatoglossus

Palatopharyngeus

FIG. 2.33 Muscles of soft palate.

Nerves: Greater palatine and nasopalatine branches of the pterygopalatine ganglion suspended by maxillary nerve.

Lymphatics: They drain into upper deep cervical nodes and partly into retropharyngeal nodes.

Soft palate: It is the movable muscular fold suspended from the posterior border of the hard palate. It separates the nasopharynx form the oropharynx and behaves as the controller between the air and food passages.

Palatal measurements: They are used in prosthetic reconstructions as mentioned before in craniometric measurements.

FACIAL ARTERY (FIG. 2.34)

Chief artery of the face.

Origin: branch of ECA is given off in carotid triangle in the neck.

Course: Brief course in the neck then winds round lower border of mandible at anterior margin of masseter and proceeds upward and forward on the face, ending with anastomosis with ophthalmic artery at medial canthus of eye. The tortuous course with numerous anastomoses permits free movement of the mandible, lips, and cheeks.

Venous drainage facial area. Fig. 2.36 shows facial veins—connects to cavernous sinus and pterygoid plexus, thus spreading infection from face (danger area) into cranial cavity.

Branches in the neck: (1) ascending palatine artery, (2) tonsillar branch, (3) glandular branch to submandibular gland. In the face, it supplies the lips and extending nose via (1) submental artery, (2) inferior labial artery, (3) superior labial artery, (4) Lateral nasal artery.

Applied anatomy: Rich anastomosis enables collateral circulation great healing.

FACIAL NERVE (FIGS. 2.37 AND 2.38)

The facial nerve is the seventh cranial nerve and nerve of the second branchial arch.

Facial nerve carries four modalities: (1) Motor to muscles of facial expression, stylohyoid, digastric, and stapedius. (2) Special senses taste fibers to anterior 2/3 of tongue. (3) Parasympathetic secretomotor to submandibular, sublingual, lacrimal, and parotid glands. (4) Sensory small area of external auditory meatus and auricle.

Nuclei and functional components: (1) motor nucleus SVE, (2) superior salivatory nucleus GVE, (3)

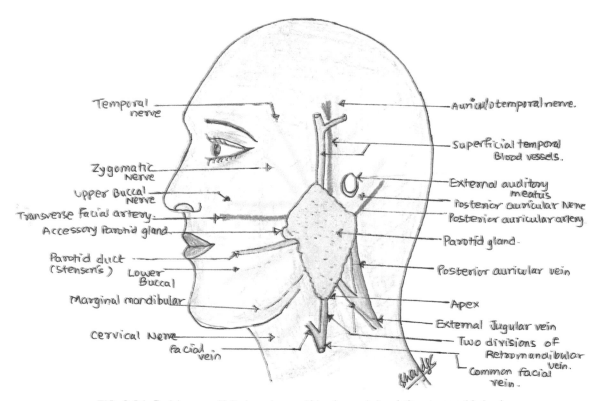

FIG. 2.34 Facial nerve with its branches and blood vessels in relations to parotid gland.

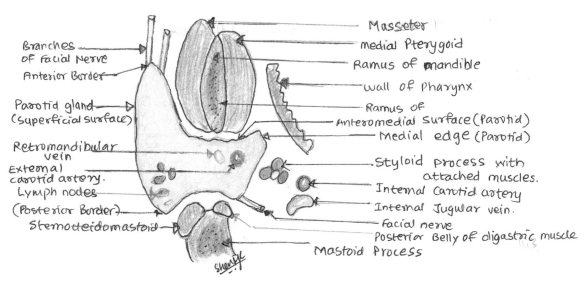

FIG. 2.35 Horizontal section through parotid gland.

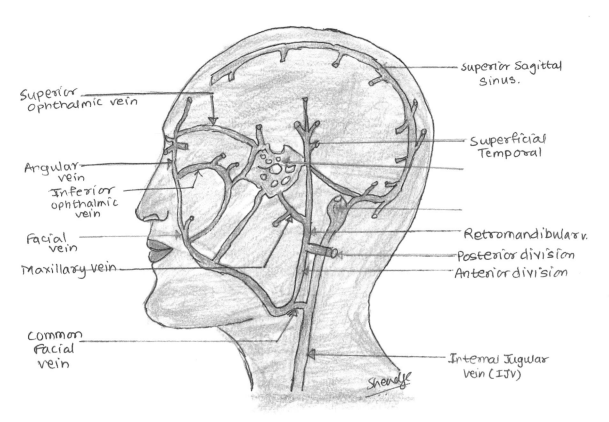

FIG. 2.36 Veins of face, head, and neck and deep connections.

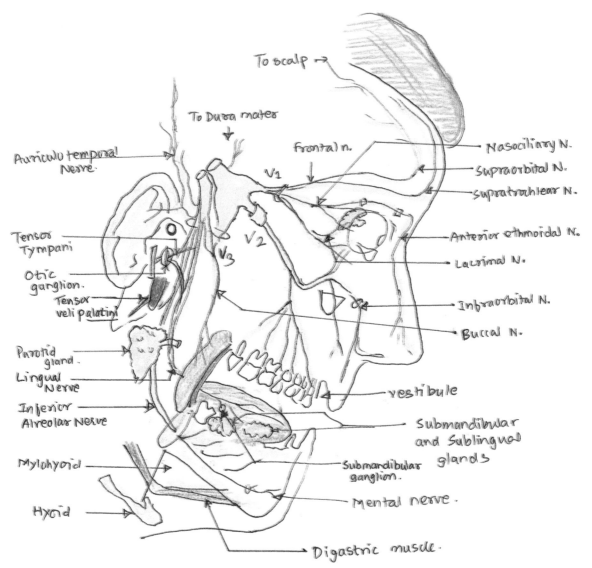

FIG. 2.37 Distribution of three branches of trigeminal nerve and facial nerve.

lacrimatory nucleus GVE, (4) nucleus of solitary tract SVA, (5) spinal nucleus of vagus GSA.

Course: **Intracranial course** starts off as two roots—motor–sensory (nervus-intermedius) and secretomotor to leave brain at lower border of pons and enters internal acoustic meatus. It then enters facial canal of temporal bone—above promontory of medial wall of middle ear, it forms geniculate ganglion (containing cells of taste fibers) and then emerges from skull at stylomastoid foramen. **Extracranial course**: The nerve crosses laterally at base of styloid process, enters posteromedial surface of

parotid gland, and runs forward within the gland, superficial to retromandibular vein, and ECA. It divides into five terminal branches just behind neck of mandible, which emerge at the anterior border of the gland.

Branches:
a) Intracranial branches within facial canal: (1) greater petrosal nerve, (2) nerve to stapedius, (3) chorda tympani (joins lingual nerve).
b) Extracranial branches at exit from stylomastoid foramen: (1) posterior auricular, (2) muscular branches to digastric and stylohyoid muscles.

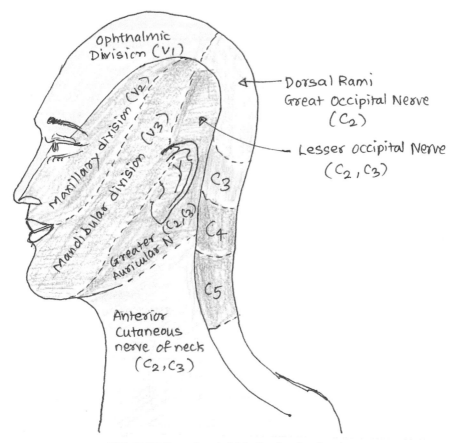

Ophthalmic Division (V1)

Maxillary division (V2)

Mandibular division (V3)

Greater Auricular N (C2,C3)

Dorsal Rami Great Occipital Nerve (C2)

Lesser Occipital Nerve (C2,C3)

C3

C4

C5

Anterior Cutaneous nerve of neck (C2,C3)

FIG. 2.38 Dermatomal distribution head and neck.

c) Terminal branches at the anterior border of parotid gland: (1) temporal, (2) zygomatic, (3) buccal, (4) mandibular, (5) cervical. The facial nerve supplies all the muscles of facial expression, except the skin.

d) Communicating branches: communicate with adjacent cranial and spinal nerves.

Applied anatomy:

1. Lesions of the facial nerve below or at the level of the motor nucleus result in lower motor-neuron lesion. This leads to paralysis of entire facial musculature on affected side seen as displacement of mouth, drooping, and ptosis with inability to close eyes, no wrinkles on forehead.

2. Lesions of the facial nerve above level of the motor nucleus result in upper motor-neuron lesion, leading to contralateral lower half of facial paralysis as orbicularis oculi and frontalis muscles spared because they receive dual side cerebral cortical nerve fibers. This is seen as displacement and drooping of mouth contralaterally, with retained ability to wrinkle forehead and close eyes.

3. **Maxillofacial prostheses** replace anatomy inside the mouth (**intraoral**), or a part of the face such as the eye, ear, nose, or cheek (known as **extraoral prostheses**). These removable prostheses are usually put on and taken off daily much like a pair of dentures. Other prostheses such as cranial plates that restore a missing part of the skull may be permanently implanted into the body.

External facial prostheses are used to simulate important facial features such as the nose, ear, or eye and lids. In addition to function, these types of prostheses are important tools for restoring social confidence after treatment for illness that results in a major facial deformity.

EAR: AURIS (LATIN)

Paired sensory organ for hearing and balance, and hence called the **vestibulocochlear apparatus** (VCA), which is in the temporal bone.

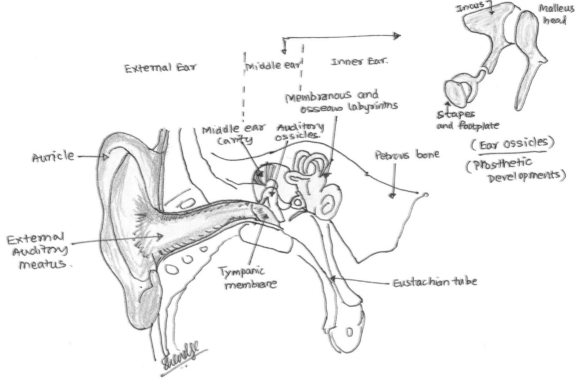

FIG. 2.39 Parts of the ear and cross section.

Ear: Fig. 2.39: Three parts: conductor system: (1) external ear, (2) middle ear, (3) receptor system: inner ear.

External ear consists of the auricle (pinna), external auditory meatus.

Pinnae/auricle is the external receptacle, which collects the sound waves and is made up of a single crumpled plate of elastic cartilage, which is lined on both sides by skin.

The parts of the pinna are shown in Fig. 2.40. The lowest part of the auricle is soft and consists only of fibro-fatty tissue covered by skin. This is called as the lobule where piercings for earrings are made. The large

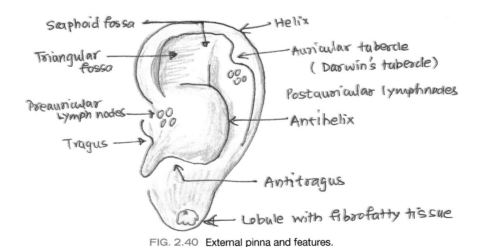

FIG. 2.40 External pinna and features.

depression in the center that leads to external auditory meatus is the concha. Muscles of the external ear are vestigial.

Blood supply is from posterior auricular and superficial temporal arteries. Lymphatics drain to the preauricular, postauricular, and superficial cervical lymph nodes.

Nerve supply to upper 2/3 of the lateral surface by or auriculo temporal nerve (ATN) and lower 1/3 by greater auricular nerve. The upper 2/3 of the medial surface is supplied by lesser occipital nerve and lower 1/3 by great auricular nerve.

External acoustic meatus is an opening with the tube, which is S-shaped, outer most part is directed medially forward, and upward, middle part is directed medially backward and upward, and the inner most part is directed medially, forward and downward. This is approximately 24 mm long of which medial 2/3(16 mm) his bony and the lateral 1/3 (8 mm) is cartilaginous. The canal is oval in cross section.

Bony part is formed by tympanic plate of the temporal bone, which is C-shaped. Cartilaginous part is also C-shaped in cross section and is adherent to the perichondrium and contains hair, sebaceous glands, sweat glands, and modified sweat glands called ceruminous glands.

Blood supply of the outer part of the canal is by superficial temporal and posterior auricular arteries and the inner part by deep auricular branch of maxillary artery.

Lymphatics drainage to preauricular, postauricular, and superficial cervical lymph nodes.

Nerve supply: Skin lining the anterior half of the meatus is supplied by auriculotemporal nerve(ATN) and posterior 1/2 by auricular branch of vagus nerve.

Absence of pinna: Bleeding in boxers causes crumpled appearance called cauliflower ear. This condition and loss of external ear due to cancer can be replaced by **silicone ear prosthesis**, which can be very realistic.

External ear prosthetic components: Fig. 2.41.

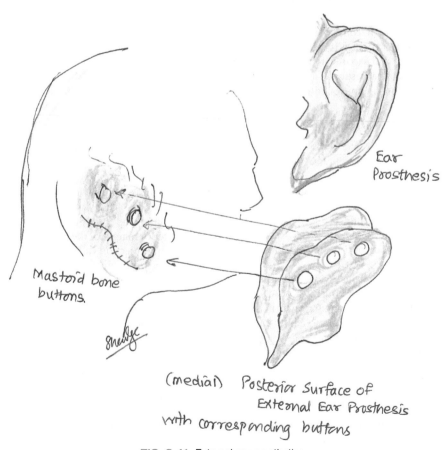

FIG. 2.41 External ear prosthetics.

They help to keep glasses on and assist to capture sound by duplicating the lost anatomy of the external ear. An ear prosthesis is attached using adhesive or bone anchored implants. Prosthetic replacement of the stapes to the oval window is used in otosclerosis. Implantable bone conduction and bone-anchored hearing prosthetic devices can be used in combinations after manufacturing these using 3D printing and computer-assisted designing.

Middle ear: Contents: (1) Three ossicles, namely, malleus (hammer), incus (anvil), and stapes (stirrup). (2) Ligaments of the ossicles. (3) Two muscles—tensor tympani and stapedius. (4) Blood vessels supplying and draining the middle ear. (5) Nerves—chorda tympani and tympanic plexus. (6) Air.

Internal ear: Mainly located in petrous part of the temporal bone. It consists of bony labyrinth, within which is located the membranous labyrinth, which is filled with endolymph and is surrounded by perilymph (Fig. 2.39).

A) Bony labyrinth consists of three parts, namely, cochlea anteriorly, vestibule in the middle, and semicircular canals posteriorly.

B) Membranous labyrinth: It consists of three main parts: (1) spiral duct of cochlea (organ of hearing) anteriorly, (2) utricle and saccule are the organs of static balance within the vestibule, (3) the semicircular ducts are the organs of kinetic balance posteriorly.

MANDIBLE: LOWER JAW (FIGS. 2.5 AND 2.6)

This is the strongest and largest bone of the face. Horseshoe-shaped body that lodges the teeth and pair of rami, which project upward for attachment of muscles of mastication.

Parts of the mandible include (1) body and (2) ramus.

A) Outer surface of the body of the mandible has the following features:
   1. Midline symphysis menti is a ridge connecting right and left halves of the bone.
   2. Mental protuberans is a triangular area in the lower part of the midline inferolateral parts, which are called mental tubercles.
   3. Oblique line is in continuation with the sharp anterior border of the ramus, and it runs toward the mental tubercle.
   4. Incisive fossa is a small depression just below the incisor teeth.
   5. Mental foramen on each side lies below the interval between the premolar teeth.

B) Inner surface of the mandible (Fig. 2.6):
   1. Mylohyoid line is a prominent ridge that runs downward and forward obliquely from the third molar tooth to the median area below the genial tubercles.
   2. Below the mylohyoid line is the hollow surface for lodging the submandibular gland called as the submandibular fossa.
   3. Above this line is the sublingual fossa for sublingual gland.
   4. The posterior surface of the symphysis menti has small four elevations called the superior and inferior genial tubercles. The superior tubercles are origin for genioglossus and inferior for genohyoid muscles.
   5. The mylohyoid groove on the ramus extends onto the body below the posterior and of the mylohyoid line.

C) Upper border/alveolar border bears the sockets for teeth. Fig. 2.42 shows cross section the teeth and socket which is similar for maxillary and mandibular side.

D) Lower border/base of the mandible in the midline has a small depression called the digastric fossa.

Ramus of the Mandible

This is a quadrilateral-shaped extension from the body that has medial and lateral surfaces and four borders, mainly, upper, lower, anterior, and posterior borders. This also has two processes: the coronoid and the condyloid processes.

A) Lateral surfaces are flat and bear multiple ridges.

B) Medial surface has the following features:
   1) Mandibular foramen is just above the center of the ramus at the level of occlusal surface of the teeth. This leads into the mandibular canal, which opens anteriorly to the mental foramen.
   2) Anterior margin of the mandibular foramen has sharp projection called lingula.
   3) Mylohyoid groove begins just below the mandibular foramen.

C) Upper border of the ramus is thin and has the mandibular notch.

D) The lower border is continuation of the base of the mandible and ends to the angle of the mandible. The anterior border is thin, and the posterior border is thick.

E) The coronoid process is flattened and continues with anterior border of the ramus. The posterior border bounds the mandibular notch.

F) The condyloid process has an upward expanded portion forming the head of the mandible, which is

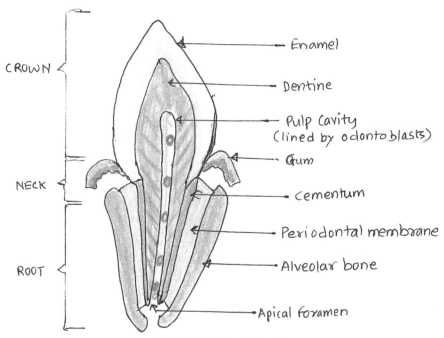

CROWN

NECK

ROOT

Enamel

Dentine

Pulp Cavity
(lined by odontoblasts)

Gum

Cementum

Periodontal membrane

Alveolar bone

Apical foramen

FIG. 2.42 Parts of a tooth.

covered with fibrocartilage and articulates with the temporal bone to form the temporomandibular joint. The mandibular neck is a small constriction just below the head. The neck has small depression on anterior surface called pterygoid fovea.

Structures related to the mandible: Figs. 2.5, 2.6, and 2.43.

1. Salivary glands (bilateral): Parotid gland, submandibular gland, and sublingual.
2. Lymph nodes: Parotid, submandibular, and submental.
3. Blood vessels: Maxillary, superficial temporal, masseteric, inferior alveolar, mylohyoid, mental, and facial.
4. Nerves: Lingual, auriculotemporal, masseteric, inferior alveolar, mylohyoid, and mental.
5. Muscles of mastication: Temporalis, masseter, medial, and lateral pterygoid.
6. Ligaments: Lateral ligament of temporomandibular joint, stylomandibular ligament, sphenomandibular ligament, pterygomandibular raphe.

Temporomandibular Joint (TM Joint) (Fig. 2.44)

Type: synovial joint of condylar variety.

Articulation: Between (1) articular tubercle and anterior part of mandibular fossa of temporal bone above,

(2) head of mandible (mandibular condyles) below. Glenoid fossa and articular eminence are covered by thin fibrocartilage layer with 60° posterior slope.

The joint cavity is divided into upper ginglymoarthrodial or hinge joint and lower parts by the intraarticular disc.

Articular disc is an oval fibrous plate that divided the joint to upper and lower compartments. Upper compartment enables gliding movement, whereas lower compartment for rotatory and gliding movements. The disc has concavoconvex superior surface and a concave inferior surface. The periphery of the disc is attached to the fibrous capsule of the joint.

The articular disc/meniscus has three zones of thickness: posterior band (3 mm), intermediate zone (1 mm), and anterior band (2 mm) and is made of mixed avascular connective tissue.

Functions of articular disc: (1) increase surface area, (2) fluid distribution, (3) load absorption, (4) compartmentalize the joint for complex movements (rotation + translation).

Synovial membrane lines all loaded surfaces in both compartments with an intimal layer of 1–24 cells thick. It has two types of cells: type A phagocytic and type B secretory cells.

Functions lubrication and nutrition as well as maintenance of the articular cartilage.

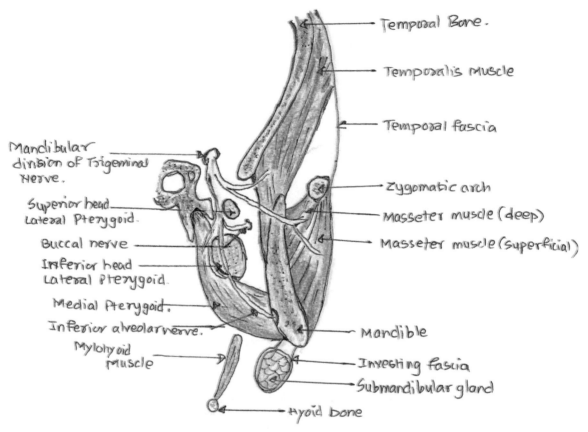

FIG. 2.43 Muscles of mastication.

Intraarticular pressures are maintained to (1) resting (−4 mm of Hg), opening (−54 mm of Hg), and closing (+64 mm of Hg).

Capsule surrounds the joint and attachments: above—to articular tubercle and margin of mandibular fossa; below—to neck of mandible.

Ligaments: (1) lateral temporomandibular ligament, (2) lateral sphenomandibular ligament, (3) medial stylomandibular ligament.

Blood supply: (1) superficial temporal artery; (2) maxillary artery (both from ECA).

Nerve supply branches of mandibular nerve: (1) auriculotemporal, (2) masseteric, (3) deep temporal.

Relations:

Anteriorly: (1) lateral pterygoid, (2) masseteric nerve and artery.

Posteriorly: (1) tympanic plate of external auditory meatus, (2) parotid gland, (3) superficial temporal vessels, (4) auriculotemporal nerve.

Medially: (1) tympanic plate between joint and ICA. (2) Spine of sphenoid and sphenomandibular ligament. (3) Middle meningeal artery. (4) Auriculotemporal and chorda tympani nerves.

Laterally: (1) parotid gland, (2) fascia and skin, (3) temporal branches of facial nerve.

Superiorly: (1) middle cranial fossa and (2) middle meningeal vessels.

Inferiorly: (1) maxillary artery and veins.

Movements of the mandible/temporomandibular joint

The movements of the mandible and TM joints are controlled mainly by different **muscles of mastication** (Fig. 2.43) and shape of the articular surfaces or the ligaments. In the position of rest, the teeth of the upper and lower jaws slightly apart. On closure of the jaws, the teeth come into contact.

The chief movements of the mandible are (1) depression, (2) elevation, (3) protrusion, (4) retraction, (5) lateral.

Mechanism and muscles involved:

1) Depression causes opening of the mouth, where head of mandible rotates around horizontal axis under the articular disc. Both head and disc are then pulled forward so that the disc now moves onto articular tubercle. The head now articulates with most anterior part of disc. Muscles causing depression are (1) lateral pterygoids, (2) digastrics, (3) geniohyoids and mylohyoids.
2) Elevation enables closing of the mouth, during which head of mandible and articular disc moves backward and head then rotates under articular disc. Muscles causing elevation: (1) masseter, (2) temporalis, (3) medial pterygoids.
3) Protrusion: Lower teeth drawn forward beyond upper teeth during which articular disc is pulled forward onto anterior tubercle together with head of mandible, movement occurring in upper compartment of joint. Muscles causing this are (1) lateral pterygoids and (2) medial pterygoids. ·
4) Retraction: Mandible drawn backward to position of rest, because articular disc and head of mandible are pulled backward into mandibular fossa. This is enabled by (1) posterior fibers of temporalis and (2) may be assisted by masseter.
5) Lateral movement or chewing is due to alternate protrusion and retraction of the mandible on each side. Muscles on both sides work alternately to enable a certain amount of rotation that helps this complex motion. These are (1) medial pterygoids and (2) lateral pterygoids.

Force transmission of the masticatory process involves following structures of the facial and head skeleton, which serve as pillar-like struts to reinforce and dissipate forces:
1) Frontonasal pillar
2) Zygomatic arch pillar with vertical and horizontal branches
3) Basal arch in upper jaw
4) Basal arch in lower jaw
5) Occipital Pillar
6) Pterygoid-palatine pillars

Applied anatomy: (1) Dislocation of the mandible sometimes occurs when the mandible is depressed the head of the mandible on one or both sides slips anteriorly into infratemporal fossa causing inability to close mouth. (2) Detachment of articular disc causes clicking sounds with jaw movements.

Bilateral TM joints behave as single unit, and their movements can be palpated just anterior to the preauricular point.

Dental articulation is defined as the contact relationships of maxillary and mandibular teeth as they move against each other in a dynamic process.

Anatomical articulation is an occlusal arrangement where the posterior artificial teeth have masticatory surfaces (can make normal masticatory movements with comfort and efficiency) that closely resemble those of the natural healthy dentition and articulate with similar natural or artificial surfaces.

Occlusion is the static relationship (process of closure) between the incising or masticating (occluding) surfaces of the maxillary and mandibular teeth when they are in contact.

Centric occlusion is the relation of opposing occlusal surfaces which provides the maximum planned contact and/or intercuspation.

Centric relations are relations of the mandible to maxilla when the condyles are in uppermost and rearmost position in the glenoid fossa at a given degree of vertical dimension (jaw separation).

Centric occluding relation is a term sometimes used to describe the condition in which the jaws are in centric relation and the teeth or occlusal surfaces in centric occlusion.

Balanced occlusion means that artificial teeth are set up so that as many teeth as possible are in occlusion in any occlusal relationship.

Balanced articulation is bilateral, simultaneous, anterior, and posterior occlusal contact of teeth in centric and eccentric positions. It means an arrangement of the teeth so that in any occlusal relationship as many teeth as possible are in occlusion, and when changing from one relationship to another, they move with a smooth, sliding motion, free from cuspal interference and maintaining even contact.

These occlusal and articulation concepts are used when measuring for maxillary or mandibular reconstruction and prosthetic rehabilitation.

Curve of Spee (anteroposterior curve) is the anatomic curve established by the occlusal alignment of the teeth, as projected onto the median plane, beginning with the cusp tip of the mandibular canine and following the buccal cusp tips of premolar and molar teeth, continuing through the anterior border of the mandibular ramus, ending with the anterior most portion of the mandibular condyle.

Curve of Menson is the curve of occlusion in which each cusp and incisal edge touches or conforms to a segment of the surface of a sphere 8 inches in diameter with its center in the region of the glabella.

Curve of Wilson (mediolateral curve) means in mandibular arch, that curve, as viewed in frontal plane, which is concave inferiorly and contacts the buccal and lingual cusps of the mandibular molars. In the maxillary arch, that curve, as viewed in frontal plane, which is convex superiorly and contacts the lingual and buccal cusps of the maxillary molars. The curve is formed by the facial and lingual cusp tips on both sides of dental arch.

Compensating curve is anteroposterior curvature (in the median plane) and the mediolateral curvature (in frontal plane) in the alignment of occluding surfaces and incisal edges of artificial teeth that are used to develop balance articulation.

These curves introduced in the construction of complete dentures to compensate for the opening influences produced by the condylar and incisal guidance during lateral and protrusive mandibular excursive movements; these curves are artificial counterparts of the curve of Spee and Menson, which are found in the natural dentition.

Face-Bow is a caliper-like device that is used to record the relationship of the jaws to the temporomandibular joints or the opening axis of the jaws and to orient the casts in this same relationship to the opening axis of the articulator.

Microvascular grafts enable sensate tissue, where impossible to reconstruct alloplastic material helps reproduce anatomic base. Mandibular reconstruction—osteomyocutaneous flap reconstruction for discontinuity. Newer technology using 3-D CT-guided jaw and prosthetic reconstruction done accurately and bone grafting done to enable osteogenesis. Implant bone and then place the implants in new jawbone and restore teeth. Bone donor sites from fibula, scapula used to rebuild cheek bones, eye sockets, and palate (maxillary reconstruction).

Competent tongue is essential for bolus manipulation and will not improve after mandibular discontinuity.

Intrastructural maxillectomy—osteomyocutaneous flap reconstruction of maxillectomy cavity can obstruct paranasal sinus, immobilize the upper lip and tethering the free end of palate and restricting the mandibular motion.

Submandibular region: Figs. 2.28, 2.31, 2.37, 2.43 and 2.45 include deep structures between the mandible and the hyoid bones including the floor of the mouth and root of the tongue. This contains the suprahyoid muscles, submandibular and sublingual salivary glands, and submandibular ganglion.

a) Suprahyoid muscles: arranged in four layers: (1) first layer is the digastric and stylohyoid, (2) second layers formed by mylohyoid, (3) third layer is genioglossus and hyoglossus, (4) fourth layer is formed by genioglossus.

b) Submandibular salivary gland situated in anterior part of the digastric triangle.

PAROTID (PARA—AROUND; OTIC—EAR) REGION AND PAROTID GLAND (FIGS. 2.34 AND 2.35)

Lodges are the largest of the salivary glands called the parotid gland, which is almost entirely serous. The region is just below the external acoustic meatus between ramus of the mandible and the sternocleidomastoid. The parotid gland is covered by the investing layer of the deep cervical fascia forming its capsule.

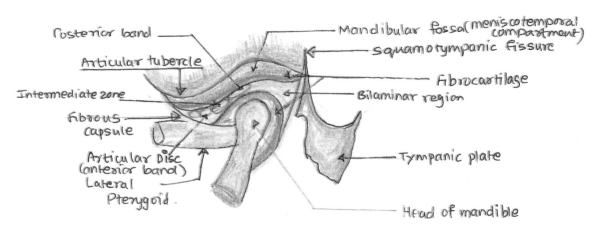

FIG. 2.44 Structure of left temporomandibular joint.

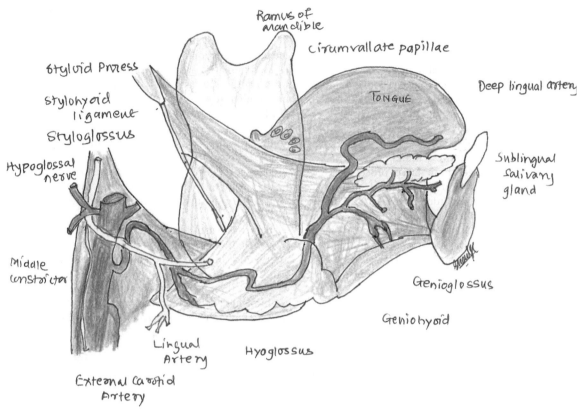

FIG. 2.45 Muscles at floor of mouth, blood supply.

Parotid is three-sided pyramid-shaped, with superior base of the pyramid and superficial and anteromedial as well as posterior medial surfaces. Figs. 2.34 and 2.35 shows the relationship of the parotid gland and structures at the head–neck junction. Parotid (**Stenson's**) duct runs obliquely between buccinators and oral mucosa before turning medially and opening to the gingivobuccal vestibule of the mouth, opposite the crown of the upper second molar tooth.

Shape and Parts of the Gland

Shape: roughly wedge-shaped, with the base above and apex behind angle of the mandible.

Parts: facial nerve divides the gland into (1) superficial lobe and (2) deep lobe.

Processes: (1) glenoid process, (2) facial process, (3) pterygoid process.

Capsules: Two capsules: inner fibrous capsule and outer capsule derived from investing layer of deep cervical fascia. A portion of fascia between styloid process and mandible is thickened to form the stylomandibular ligament,

Relations: The surface of parotid gland is divided into superficial, superior, posteromedial, and anteromedial surfaces.

Superficial: (1) parotid lymph nodes, (2) great auricular nerve, (3) superficial fascia and skin.

Superior: (1) external auditory meatus, (2) posterior surface of temporomandibular joint. Glenoid process is related to auriculotemporal nerve.

Posteromedial: (1) mastoid process, (2) sternocleidomastoid, (3) posterior belly of digastric, (4) styloid process and attached muscles—stylohyoid, stylopharyngeus, and styloglossus, (5) carotid sheath with ICA, IJV, and vagus, (6) IX, XI, and XII cranial nerves, (7) facial nerve.

Anteromedial: (1) posterior border of ramus of mandible, (2) temporomandibular joint, (3) masseter, (4) medial pterygoid, (5) terminal branches of facial nerve, (6) stylomandibular ligament.

The gland lies in close contact with pharyngeal wall at the union of anteromedial and posteromedial surfaces. The anterior border of the gland is formed by union of superficial and anteromedial surfaces, from which several structures emerge: (1) parotid duct, (2) terminal branches of facial nerve, (3) transverse facial vessels.

Structures within the gland (lateral to medial) (Fig. 2.35)

1. Facial nerve and its terminal branches.
2. Retromandibular vein—anterior division with facial vein joins IJV posterior division, which joins posterior auricular vein drains into EJV.
3. ECA along with branches—superficial temporal artery, maxillary artery.
4. Parotid group of lymph vessels and nodes.
5. Parotid duct emerges from facial process of the gland and passes forward over lateral surface of masseter. At anterior border of masseter, it turns medially to pierce buccal pad of fat and buccinator, then runs forward briefly between buccinator and oral mucous membrane, and opens into vestibule of mouth opposite upper second molar tooth.

Note: Its oblique course acts as a valve to prevent infection of the duct during chewing as well as buccinator fibers.

Blood supply: ECA and its terminal branches mainly superficial temporal artery and maxillary artery. Venous drainage into retromandibular vein and then into facial and EJV.

Lymphatic drainage into parotid lymph nodes and deep cervical nodes.

Nerve Supply:

a) Parasympathetic is secretomotor. Preganglionic fibers that arise from inferior salivatory nucleus travel via IXth cranial nerve to synapse in **otic ganglion**. Postganglionic fibers pass through auriculotemporal nerve to reach the gland.

b) Sympathetic is vasomotor and is derived from plexus around ECA.

c) Sensory—from auriculotemporal nerve, and parotid fascia is supplied by sensory fibers from great auricular nerve.

Applied anatomy: (1) parotid fascia is unyielding; therefore, parotid swellings are painful; (2) viral infection, e.g., mumps, (3) inflammation of retrograde bacterial infection from parotid duct, (4) malignant parotid involving the facial nerve leads to unilateral facial paralysis, (5) Frey's syndrome is sweating over parotid region while eating. This is caused by cross-innervation after penetrating wounds of parotid that damage auriculotemporal and great auricular nerve.

Maxillary artery:

The maxillary artery distributes the upper and lower jaws including teeth, muscles of mastication, external and middle ears and eustachian tube, dura mater, root of pharynx, palate, nose and paranasal sinuses.

Origin: Larger terminal branch of ECA, arises in parotid gland behind neck of mandible.

Course and relations: It is divided into three parts by the lateral pterygoid:

Mandibular (1st) part: From its origin, it runs forward and lies between neck of mandible and sphenomandibular ligament reaches and runs along lower border of lateral pterygoid.

Pterygoid (2nd) part: From lower border of pterygoid, it runs upward and forward superficial to lower head of lateral pterygoid.

Pterygopalatine (3rd) part passes between two heads of lateral pterygoid and then through pterygomaxillary fissure to enter the pterygopalatine fossa.

Branches: From the 1st part gives off five branches of which the most important is middle meningeal artery and inferior alveolar artery. From the 2nd part, five branches supply the muscles of mastication as well as the buccinator. From the 3rd part gives off six branches: (1) infraorbital artery, (2) greater palatine, (3) pharyngeal, (4) sphenopalatine, (5) artery of pterygoid canal, (6) posterior superior alveolar artery.

Applied anatomy: (1) middle meningeal artery involved in intracranial hemorrhages, (2) sphenopalatine artery involved in nose bleeds(epistaxis).

Maxillary nerve: Fig. 2.46.

The maxillary nerve is 2nd division of the trigeminal nerve.

Origin: It arises from trigeminal ganglion and lies in dura lateral to cavernous sinus.

Course and relations: From origin, it passes through foramen rotundum to enter pterygopalatine fossa, where it continues as infraorbital nerve, and enters orbit through inferior orbital fissure. Here it runs in infraorbital groove then canal, to pass through infraorbital foramen to emerge onto the face where it ends by dividing into several branches.

Branches: (1) meningeal branch in middle cranial fossa, (2) three posterior superior alveolar branches zygomatic nerve in pterygopalatine fossa, (3) middle and (4) anterior superior alveolar branches in infraorbital canal, (5) inferior palpebral branches, (6) nasal branches, (7) superior labial branches on face.

Mandibular nerve:

It is the 3rd and largest division of trigeminal nerve having both sensory and motor fibers.

Origin: It begins in the middle cranial fossa as a large sensory root and small motor root. The sensory root arises from trigeminal ganglion, and motor root arises from motor nucleus of Vth nerve in pons.

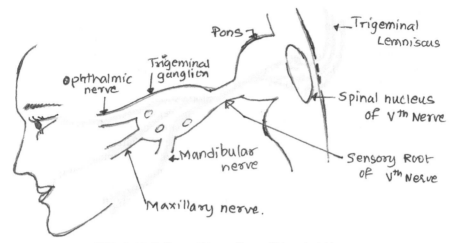

FIG. 2.46 Pathway of nerve fibers of trigeminal (v) nerve.

Course and relations:

Sensory root lies above motor root, and both pass out of the skull through foramen ovale to enter infratemporal fossa. Both roots unite just below the foramen to form a single main trunk—lies on tensor palatini, deep to lateral pterygoid. This soon divides into a small anterior and large posterior division.

Branches:

a. Main trunk: (1) meningeal branch and (2) nerve to medial pterygoid.
b. Anterior trunk: (1) buccal nerve (sensory) and motor branches are (1) masseteric nerve, (2) deep temporal nerve, (3) nerve to lateral pterygoid.
c. Posterior trunk: (1) auriculotemporal nerve, (2) lingual nerve, (3) inferior alveolar nerve.

Applied anatomy: (1) mandibular nerve block carried out intraorally for extraction of teeth, (2) pain from disease of the tooth sometimes gets referred along the auriculotemporal nerve to the ear.

Pterygopalatine ganglion:

Larger parasympathetic peripheral ganglion is a relay station for secretomotor fibers to the lacrimal and mucous glands of nose, paranasal sinuses, palate, and pharynx, located in pterygopalatine fossa near the sphenopalatine foramen.

Connections (roots): (1) Motor (parasympathetic) root is secretomotor formed by (i) greater petrosal nerve and (ii) nerve of pterygoid canal. Preganglionic fibers arise from lacrimal nucleus and pass through nervous intermedius of facial nerve, and synapse in the ganglion. Postganglionic fibers pass to lacrimal, nasal, and palatine glands via maxillary, zygomatic, and lacrimal nerves. (2) Sympathetic root is vasomotor and is formed by (i) deep petrosal nerve, (ii) nerve of pterygoid canal, fibers derived from ICA plexus and they are postganglionic fibers having come from superior cervical ganglion. (a) Sensory from maxillary nerve.

Branches of maxillary nerve are both parasympathetic and sympathetic: (1) orbital branches, (2) palatine branches (greater and lesser), (3) nasal branches, (4) pharyngeal branches.

Applied anatomy: Ganglion block injections at mandibular notch and pterygopalatine fossa.

Submandibular gland: Figs. 2.37 and 2.45.

Large salivary gland with mixture of serous and mucous acini, located in the anterior part of digastric triangle, partly under cover of body of mandible.

Structure: It is J-shaped and divided into (1) large superficial part (superficial to mylohyoid) and (2) small deep part (deep to mylohyoid). The two parts are continuous with each other around posterior border of mylohyoid. Double capsular layer covers the gland: (1) internal fibrous capsule and (2) external capsule derived from investing layer of deep cervical fascia, extending between styloid process and angle of mandible and stylomandibular ligament.

Superficial part of gland lies in digastric triangle, partly under cover of mandible. Posteriorly, it is separated from parotid gland by stylomandibular ligament.

Relations:

Anterior: anterior belly of digastric.

Posterior: (1) stylohyoid, (2) posterior belly of digastric, (3) stylomandibular ligament, which separates it from (4) parotid gland.

Medial: (1) mylohyoid, (2) mylohyoid nerve and vessels, (3) hyoglossus, (4) lingual and hypoglossal nerve.

Lateral: (1) submandibular fossa on medial surface of mandible, (2) cervical branch of facial nerve, (3) facial vein, (4) submandibular lymph nodes, (5) fascia, platysma, and skin inferolateral.

Deep part of the gland extends forward to interval between mylohyoid (inferolateral), and hyoglossus and styloglossus (medially) posterior end is continuous with superficial part of gland around posterior border of mylohyoid muscle. The anterior end reaches as far as sublingual gland.

Relations:

Anterior: sublingual gland.

Posterior: (1) stylohyoid, (2) posterior belly of digastric, (3) stylomandibular ligament, (4) parotid gland.

Superior: (1) lingual nerve, (2) submandibular ganglion, (3) it is covered by mucous membrane of floor of the mouth inferiorly hypoglossal nerve medially hyoglossus and styloglossus.

Lateral: (1) mylohyoid, (2) superficial part of the gland.

Submandibular duct emerges from anterior end of deep part of gland and passes forward alongside of the tongue, beneath mucous membrane of floor of mouth and opens into the mouth on the summit of a small papilla situated at the sides of the frenulum of the tongue.

Blood supply: (1) facial artery and vein; (2) lingual artery and vein.

Lymphatic drainage into submandibular nodes and then into deep cervical nodes.

Nerve supply: Parasympathetic secretomotor fibers from superior salivatory nucleus of VIIth cranial nerve, Preganglionic fibers pass via chorda tympani, through lingual nerve that synapses in submandibular ganglion. The postganglionic fibers reach gland directly from the ganglion. Sympathetic nerves from plexus on facial artery. Sensory from lingual nerve.

Sublingual gland:

It is roughly almond-shaped and smallest of the salivary glands, contains serous and mucous acini, with mucous predominating, lies beneath mucous membrane of floor of mouth close to midline.

Relations:

Anterior: gland on opposite side.

Posterior: deep part of submandibular gland.

Medially: (1) genioglossus, (2) lingual nerve, (3) submandibular duct. Laterally sublingual fossa on medial surface of mandible.

Superior: mucous membrane of floor of the mouth elevated to form sublingual fold.

Inferior: mylohyoid muscle. Sublingual ducts are 8–20 in number, which open into mouth on summit of sublingual fold, and some may open into submandibular duct.

Blood supply: (1) facial artery and vein, (2) lingual artery and vein.

Lymphatic: submandibular and deep cervical nodes.

Nerve supply: Parasympathetic preganglionic fibers from superior salivary nucleus of seventh cranial nerve via chorda tympani and lingual nerve and submandibular ganglion. Parasympathetic postganglionic fibers via lingual nerve supply the gland. Sympathetic from plexus around facial and lingual arteries. Sensory from lingual nerve.

Applied anatomy: (1) Sialadenitis is infection and enlargement of gland. (2) Floor of mouth prosthetics.

Lingual nerve:

The lingual nerve is sensory to anterior 2/3 tongue and fiber of the mouth. It also receives fibers from the chorda tympani branch of the facial nerve. (1) Secretomotor (parasympathetic) to submandibular and sublingual salivary glands. (2) Taste (gustatory) fibers to anterior 2/3 of tongue.

Origin: One of the two terminal branches of posterior division of mandibular nerve, which begins slightly below skull (stylomandibular ligament).

Course and relations: Runs downward on medial surface of lateral pterygoid, and then on lateral surface of medial pterygoid. It is joined by chorda tympani and emerges at lower border of lateral pterygoid and continues downward between ramus of mandible and medial pterygoid. Next it passes forward and medially beneath lower border of superior constrictor of pharynx, where it is related to styloglossus medially and to lower 3rd molar tooth laterally. It passes forward on lateral surface and anterior margin of hyoglossus, and winds round submandibular duct from lateral to medial and lies on genioglossus. Here, it divides into terminal branches.

Branches: Preganglionic parasympathetic nerve fibers passing to submandibular ganglion, arise from superior salivatory nucleus of facial nerve, and travel via chorda tympani and lingual nerve to give sensory branches to anterior 2/3 of the tongue, floor of mouth, and lingual surface of gums communicating branches to hypoglossal nerve.

Applied anatomy: Close relation of lingual nerve to third molar tooth, may cause injury during tooth extraction.

Nasal cavity: Figs. 2.47 and 2.48.

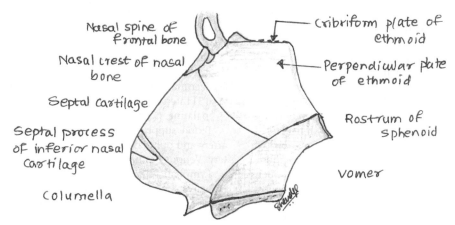

FIG. 2.47 Structure of nasal septum.

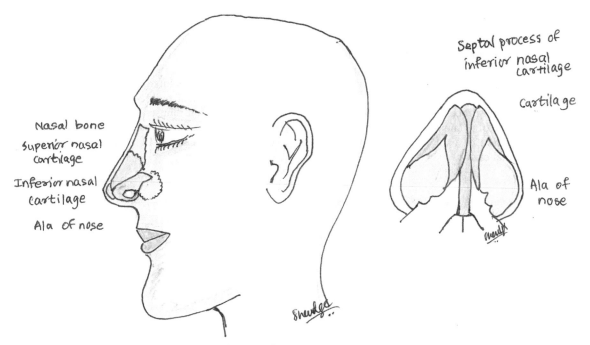

FIG. 2.48 External nose skeleton.

Relations, openings, and branches.

Extends from the nostrils (nares) in front to the choanae behind. It is divided into two halves by the nasal septum.

Relations:

Superior: (1) frontal sinus, (2) anterior cranial fossa, (3) sphenoidal sinus, (4) middle cranial fossa.

Inferior: (1) hard palate, which separates it from (2) oral cavity.

Posterior: communicates with nasopharynx, which can be regarded as the back of the cavity.

Lateral: (1) exterior (front part of cavity), (2) orbit, (3) maxillary and ethmoid sinuses, (4) pterygopalatine and pterygoid fossae.

Openings that lead into or out of the nasal cavity are (1) nostrils, (2) choanae, (3) openings of maxillary, frontal, sphenoidal and ethmoidal air sinuses, and opening of nasolacrimal duct.

Nostrils are anterior external apertures of the nose. They are bounded medially by nasal septum and laterally by ala of nose.

Choanae are the posterior apertures of the nose. They are larger than nostrils and communicate with nasopharynx. They are bounded, superiorly by body of sphenoid, inferiorly by horizontal plate of palatine bone, medially by vomer and laterally by medial pterygoid plate.

Openings of paranasal air sinuses: (1) Maxillary sinus opens into middle meatus of nasal cavity through hiatus semilunaris. (2) Frontal sinus opens into middle meatus via infundibulum. (3) Sphenoidal sinus opens into sphenoethmoidal recess. (4) Ethmoidal sinuses: anterior and middle groups open into middle meatus; posterior group opens into superior meatus. (5) Nasolacrimal duct opens into inferior meatus of nasal cavity; its opening is guarded by a fold of mucous membrane called lacrimal fold or imperfect **valve of Hasner**.

Boundaries: Each half of the nasal cavity has a roof, floor, medial and lateral walls (Fig. 2.49).
1) Roof: (1) nasal cartilages, (2) nasal bone, (3) frontal bone, (4) cribriform plate of ethmoid bone, (5) body of sphenoid (from anterior to posterior); the roof is narrow and slopes downward.
2) Floor: (1) palatine process of maxilla (anterior), (2) horizontal plate of palatine bone (posterior) forms the upper surface of hard palate separates nasal cavity from oral cavity.

3) Medial wall: (1) septal cartilage, (2) perpendicular plate of ethmoid, (3) vomer (from anterior to posterior) consists of nasal septum, commonly deviated to one side.
4) Lateral wall: (1) nasal bone, (2) maxilla bone, (3) lacrimal bone, (4) ethmoid (labyrinth and conchae), (5) inferior nasal concha, (6) perpendicular plate of palatine, (7) medial pterygoid plate sphenoid.

Blood supply: maxillary artery via sphenopalatine artery and ophthalmic artery via anterior ethmoidal artery. Venous drainage into veins that follow arteries.

Lymphatic: drainage deep cervical nodes.

Nerve supply: (1) parasympathetic from pterygopalatine ganglion and (2) sympathetic from superior cervical ganglion.

Medial nasal wall (Fig. 2.30) has three projections: **superior concha** and **middle concha** parts of ethmoid bone, and **inferior concha** is separate bone by itself. Area below each concha is called **meatus**:

A. **Superior meatus** lies inferolateral to superior concha and receives opening of posterior group of ethmoidal sinuses.
B. **Middle meatus** lies inferolateral to middle concha and has ethmoidal bulla which is an opening of middle ethmoidal sinuses. Hiatus semilunaris is an opening of maxillary sinus, and ethmoidal infundibulum is opening of frontal and anterior ethmoidal sinuses.

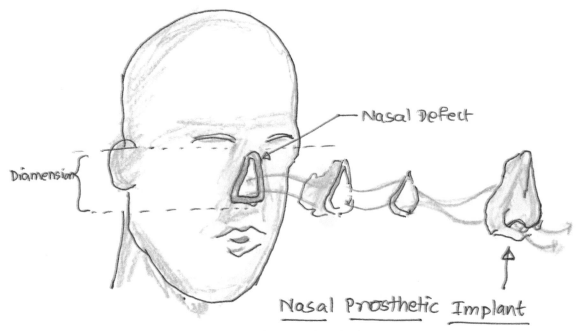

FIG. 2.49 Nasal prosthetic implant.

C. **Inferior meatus** lies inferolateral to inferior concha and receives openings of nasolacrimal duct.

Applied anatomy: (1) Fracture of nasal bones and septum due to frontal blows, causes saddle nose deformity. (2) Infection from nasal cavity spreads into intracranial region via cribriform plate of ethmoid. (3) Nasal bleeding or epistaxis due to sphenopalatine and facial vessels in the **Little's area.** (4) Drainage or lavage of the maxillary sinus can be carried by antral puncture. (5) **prosthetic nasal reconstruction** involves replacing a whole or part of the nose after excision in case of malignancy. These are used when surgical reconstruction is impossible. Realistic looking **silicone prosthetic nose** can be sculpted, and color matched to the surrounding skin, based on photographs of the patient prior to surgery. Nasal prostheses help humidify the nasal cavity during breathing and like a real nose protect the delicate mucosal tissue that lies below or proximally. A nasal prosthesis is removable and attached using spectacles, adhesive, or bone-anchored implants (Fig. 2.49).

TONGUE (FIGS. 2.50–2.52)
Muscular organ in the floor of the mouth responsible for taste, mastication swallowing, and speech. Muscles that form the tongue are attached to the hyoid bone, mandible, styloid processes, and pharynx.

Structure: composed chiefly of skeletal muscle and is covered by mucous membrane. The anterior 2/3 lies in the mouth and posterior 2/3 in the pharynx (Fig. 2.25).

The tongue has (1) tip and margin, (2) dorsum, (3) inferior surface, (4) root.
1) Tip and margin: Tip or apex of the tongue rests against the incisor teeth, and margins are related on each side to gums and teeth.
2) Dorsum/superior surface: It is situated mostly in oral cavity and partly in oropharynx. **Sulcus terminalis** is a V-shaped demarcation, which divides tongue into anterior 2/3 (oral part) in oral cavity posterior 1/3 (pharyngeal part) in oropharynx. Apex of sulcus terminalis that projects backward is marked by a small pit called **foramen cecum.**
   Oral part of tongue is divided into left and right halves by shallow median groove. This has lingual papillae of three types: (1) filiform papillae, (2) fungiform papillae, (3) vallate papillae. Pharyngeal part of tongue that forms the anterior wall of pharynx is devoid of papillae, and contains lymphatic nodules called lingual tonsils.
3) Inferior surface is smooth, devoid of papillae and attached to floor of mouth by a fold of mucous membrane called frenulum of tongue. The deep lingual vein can be seen beside frenulum. The fold of mucous membrane lateral to the vein is called **plica fimbriata.**

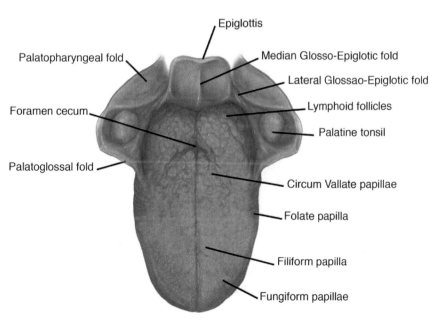

FIG. 2.50 Tongue anatomy dorsum.

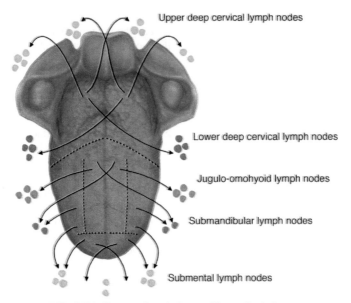

Upper deep cervical lymph nodes

Lower deep cervical lymph nodes

Jugulo-omohyoid lymph nodes

Submandibular lymph nodes

Submental lymph nodes

FIG. 2.51 Tongue dorsal view and lympatic drainage.

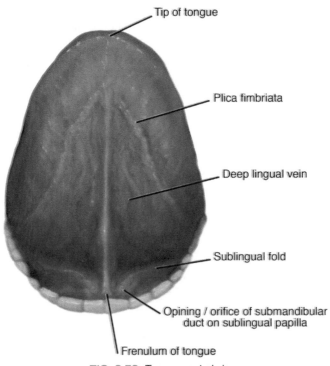

Tip of tongue

Plica fimbriata

Deep lingual vein

Sublingual fold

Opining / orifice of submandibular duct on sublingual papilla

Frenulum of tongue

FIG. 2.52 Tongue ventral view.

4) Root is formed by muscles attached to the mandible and hyoid bones mainly geniohyoid and mylohyoid along with nerves, vessels, and extrinsic muscles that enter or leave the tongue.

Muscles of the Tongue (Fig. 2.45)

Mainly: (1) intrinsic and (2) extrinsic. All the muscles are bilateral, those on one side being partially separated from those of opposite side by a median septum.

Intrinsic muscles are confined to the tongue without attachment to bone. Depending on the planar direction of their fibers, they are classified as (1) superior longitudinal, (2) inferior longitudinal, (2) transverse, (3) vertical.

Actions: Alter shape of tongue to enable chewing and swallowing.

Extrinsic muscles arise from nearby parts and inserted into the tongue: (1) genioglossus, (2) hyoglossus, (3) styloglossus, (4) palatoglossus.

Actions: Movements of the tongue: (1) Protrusion by bilateral genioglossus acting together. (2) Retraction by styloglossus and hyoglossus of both sides acting together. (3) Depression by hyoglossus and genioglossus of both sides acting together.

Blood supply: (1) lingual artery, (2) tonsillar branch of facial artery, (3) ascending pharyngeal artery.

Lymphatic drainage (Figs. 2.26 and 2.27): Tip drains into submental nodes. Anterior 2/3 tongue into submandibular and deep cervical nodes. Posterior 1/3 tongue drains into deep cervical nodes.

Nerve supply: Two-fold.

1) Motor supply mainly hypoglossal and accessory nerves: All intrinsic and extrinsic muscles of tongue are supplied by hypoglossal nerve, except palatoglossus which is supplied by cranial part of accessory nerve.

2) Sensory: (1) Anterior 2/3 of tongue: (i) supplied by lingual nerve (a branch of mandibular nerve) for general sensation, (ii) supplied by chorda tympani (a branch of facial nerve) for taste. Note: **chorda tympani** branches run in lingual nerve. (2) Posterior 1/3 of tongue: (i) supplied by lingual branch of glossopharyngeal nerve for both taste and general sensation, (ii) internal laryngeal nerve branch of vagus nerve for both taste and general sensation and taste.

Applied anatomy: Lesion of hypoglossal nerve cause ipsilateral tongue paralysis, whereas lesion of facial nerve causes loss of taste sensation on anterior 2/3 of tongue. **Tongue prosthetic application** is future direction as difficult to achieve functional benefits. Neo tongue and swallowing tube prosthetics can be measured for rehabilitation.

PHARYNX (FIGS. 2.25 AND 2.32)

Pharynx extends from base of skull to lower border of cricoid cartilage (C6) and continues as the esophagus.

Parts: (1) nasopharynx, (2) oropharynx, (3) laryngopharynx.

Nasopharynx: part behind nasal cavities and above soft palate and is continuous as posterior part of nasal cavity.

Structure: roof, floor, anterior and posterior, and left and right walls.

Roof: formed by (1) body of sphenoid and (2) basilar part of occipital bone.

Contains lymphoid tissue in mucosa called pharyngeal tonsil.

Floor: formed by sloping upper surface of soft palate. Pharyngeal isthmus is the opening between free edges of soft palate and posterior pharyngeal wall, serves as communication of nasopharynx to communicate with oropharynx—during swallowing, this opening is closed by raising the soft palate and forward the postpharyngeal wall.

Anterior wall: formed by posterior nasal apertures (choanae) and is separated by postedge of nasal septum. This communicates with nasal cavity anteriorly through the choanae.

Posterior wall: forms a continuous sloping surface with the roof of pharynx and is supported by anterior arch of atlas (C1).

Lateral wall: Bears the opening of auditory tube tubal elevation, and posterior margin of auditory tube forms an elevation salpingopharyngeal fold due to salpingopharyngeus muscle (attached to lower margin of tube) forms a vertical fold of mucous membrane. Pharyngeal recess behind tubal elevation is a small depression. Tubal tonsil behind opening of auditory tube is a collection of lymphoid tissue in the submucosa.

Blood supply: Ascending pharyngeal artery branch of ECA. Venous drainage into venous plexuses below mucosa.

Lymphatic drainage into deep cervical nodes.

Nerve supply: pharyngeal plexus.

Applied anatomy: (1) Adenoids is enlargement and hypertrophy of pharyngeal tonsil, removed by adenoidectomy. (2) Spread of infection to middle ear via auditory tube may cause deafness. 3. Indirect nasopharynx examination through the mouth (Figs. 2.53 and 2.54).

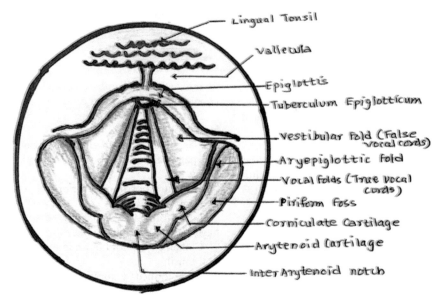

FIG. 2.53 Indirect Laryngoscopy.

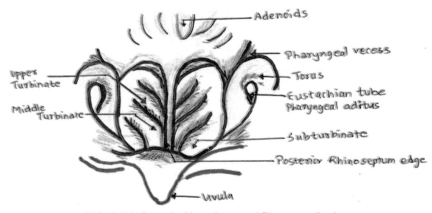

FIG. 2.54 Posterior Nasopharyngeal Diagrammatic view.

Constrictor Muscles of Pharynx (Figs. 2.55 and 2.56)

Pharyngeal wall is composed of two layers of muscles.

Inner longitudinal layer consists of two levator muscles: (1) palatopharyngeus and (2) stylopharyngeus.

Outer circular layer consists of three constrictors: (1) superior constrictor, (2) middle constrictor, (3) inferior constrictor. The constrictor muscles have their fixed points anteriorly as attachment to bones and cartilage. They expand posterior superiorly and overlap one another from below upward and end in a median tendinous raphe posteriorly (Figs. 2.55 and 2.56).

Pharyngeal Constrictors

Superior constrictor origin: (1) pterygomandibular raphe, (2) pterygoid hamulus, (3) posterior end of mylohyoid line on mandible, (4) side of posterior part of tongue.

Middle constrictor origin: (1) lower part of stylohyoid ligament, (2) lesser and upper border of greater cornu of hyoid bone. Fig. 2.57 shows the hyoid bone anatomy to which many muscles of the anterior neck are attached.

Inferior constrictor origin: (1) Thyropharyngeus: (i) oblique line on lamina on thyroid cartilage including inferior tubercle, (ii) tendinous band crossing

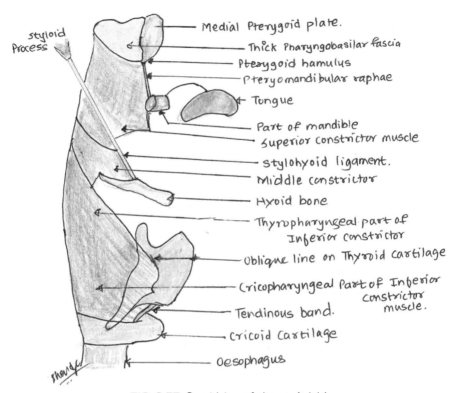

FIG. 2.55 Constrictors of pharynx (origin).

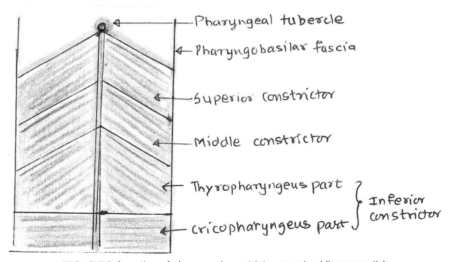

FIG. 2.56 Insertion of pharyngeal constrictor muscles (diagrammatic).

cricothyroid muscle and is attached to inferior tubercle of thyroid cartilage, (iii) inferior cornua of thyroid cartilage. (2) Cricopharyngeus from cricoid cartilage.

Insertion: (1) upper fiber curve medial and upward and pharyngeal tubercle of occipital bone, (2) middle fibers into median tendinous raphe, (3) lower fibers

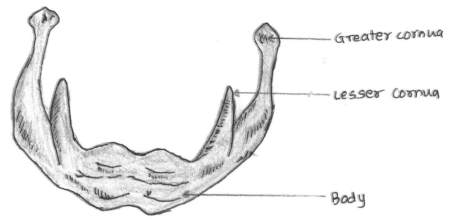

FIG. 2.57 Hyoid bone (anterior view).

curve medially and inferiorly into median tendinous raphe. They are overlapped by middle constrictors into median tendinous raphe. The fibers of superior constrictor overlap lateral surface of superior constrictor, and inferior fibers are overlapped laterally by inferior constrictor before insertion into median tendinous raphe. The superior fibers overlap lateral surface of middle constrictor muscle. The inferior fibers run horizontally medially and are continuous with circular fibers of esophagus below.

Nerve supply: Pharyngeal plexus.

Action of constrictor muscles: During process of swallowing, (1) upper fibers of superior constrictor contract and pull the posterior pharyngeal wall forward, which helps palate in closing off upper part of pharynx (nasopharynx), (2) successive contraction of the superior, middle, and inferior constrictor muscles propels bolus of food down into the esophagus, (3) the lowest fibers of inferior constrictor (sometimes called cricopharyngeus muscle) exert a sphincteric effect on lower end of pharynx, which prevent entry of air into esophagus between acts of swallowing.

Applied anatomy: The pharyngeal plexus is from pharyngeal branches of vagus nerve, which originate from cranial part of accessory nerve. Lesions of vagus nerve causes pharyngeal paralysis leading to dysphagia.

Mechanism of Swallowing

Food in mouth is broken down by grinding of teeth and is mixed with saliva. The resultant bolus on dorsum of the tongue triggers process of swallowing. Swallowing has voluntary and involuntary phases.

Voluntary phase: The anterior part of tongue is raised and pressed against hard palate by intrinsic muscles of the tongue, due to which bolus of food is pushed into posterior part of oral cavity. The contraction of styloglossus muscles and palatoglossus then pulls root of tongue upward and backward, leading to pushing the bolus of food into oropharynx.

Involuntary phase: Closure of nasopharyngeal isthmus is caused as the bolus enters oropharynx, due to elevation of soft palate pulling forward of posterior pharyngeal wall by contraction of superior constrictors and palatopharyngeus muscles. This prevents food regurgitation into nasopharynx. This is followed by elevation of the larynx and laryngopharynx, leading to closure of larynx as the bolus moves downward over the epiglottis. The food bolus reaches lower part of pharynx as a result of gravity and successive contraction of superior, middle, and inferior constrictor muscles.

Soft Palate Prosthesis Application

Speech and swallowing are enabled by the function of anatomically normal pharyngeal and tongue muscles. Their assessments are conducted in three phase anatomic issues: (1) oral phase: lip seal to oral preparatory mastication.

Prosthetic devices aid in overcoming alterations made to these muscles by birth, trauma, or treatment of disease.

Swallowing and speaking are result of complex movement of muscles at the back of the mouth and oropharynx. The soft palate forms the muscular back part of the roof of the mouth and vibrates to produce speech. The pharyngeal muscle along with soft palate in the front forms the **palatopharyngeal** or **velopharyngeal sphincter**. During swallowing and speaking, the valvular action of this sphincter prevents food/

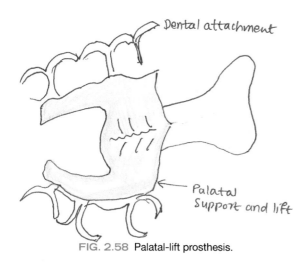

Dental attachment

Palatal Support and lift

FIG. 2.58 Palatal-lift prosthesis.

liquid from going into the nose (nasopharynx) during swallowing, and it prevents excessive air from escaping when speaking (**hypernasality**).

Palatopharyngeal inadequacy is a result of inadequate closure of velopharyngeal sphincter. This can be a result of the following:

A) Palatopharyngeal insufficiency: (1) Failure of development, e.g., cleft palate, and (2) altered due to trauma or surgery.
B) Palatopharyngeal incompetence: Muscles fail to move normally due to disease or trauma to the nerves (whiplash, stroke, blunt force to back head) or stiffening from radiation therapy.

Maxillofacial prosthetics help to plug the hole or pick up the soft palate. **Soft palate obturator** (also known as a speech and feeding aid/device) replaces the missing piece(s) of muscle(s) and fills the hole. A **palatal lift prosthesis** aids in repositioning the soft palate in raised closed position (Fig. 2.58).

Patients require some adjustments to the prosthesis, as this is an area that moves during speech or swallowing. Adjusting either of these prostheses is a fine balance between swallowing and speaking. If the valve is closed too tightly, then swallowing is particularly good but speaking will sound as if the patient has a cold or stuffy nose (**hyponasality**). If the valve is left more open, then speech will sound better but food/liquid leakage when swallowing may be increased. Healing from surgery or radiotherapy will alter this area and require frequent adjustments until all healing is completed.

These two prostheses aid in improving a complex muscular valve dysfunction. With patience and time, these prosthetic devices can be fine-tuned to be very functional and comfortable.

Intraoral obturator prosthesis may be temporary prosthesis at the time of surgery. Definitive **external facial prosthesis** can be fitted after completion of radiotherapy and complete healing without residual edema.

CREDITS

(1) Illustrations of the Tongue by Mr Roy Schneider, Department of Medical Illustrations, University of Toledo Medical Centre.

(2) Diagrams and figures source adapted from Human Anatomy: Head and Neck, Brain, Volume 3 BD Chaurasia, fifth Edition.

BIBLIOGRAPHY

1. Franco FCM, Araujo TM, Vogel CJ, Quintão CCA. Brachycephalic, dolichocephalic and mesocephalic: is it appropriate to describe the face using skull patterns? *Dental Press J Orthod.* 2013;18(3):159–163.
2. Glossary of prosthodontic terms. *J Pros Dent.* 2005;94(1): 1–104.
3. Standing S. *Head and Neck Gray's Anatomy: Anatomical Basis of Clinical Practice.* 42nd ed. Elsevier.
4. Garg K. *Human Anatomy: Head and Neck, Brain (Volume 3 BD Chaurasia's Human Anatomy).* 5th ed.
5. Anatomy of Head and Neck.

CHAPTER 3

Tumors of Head and Neck Region: An Overview

JYOTI SHARMA, MD • SUNITA BISHT, MS

Head and neck tumors are those that grow in oral cavity, pharynx, larynx, nasal cavity, paranasal sinuses, salivary glands, thyroid glands, and parathyroid glands. They are broadly categorized into benign, and malignant neoplasms.

Cancers of head and neck region are the sixth most common cancer worldwide with an increasing frequency in developing world,[1] and with worldwide incidence accounting for more than 650,000 cases annually. They constitute a major public health concern throughout the world and are an important cause of morbidity and mortality, interfering with vital functions such as breathing, swallowing, speech, hearing, vision, olfaction, and taste. Head and neck cancers are more common in men; accounting 66%–95% of cases. The incidence increases with age, with most patients between 50 and 70 years of age.[2]

More than 90% of head and neck cancers are squamous cell carcinomas. Other histological types include lymphoma, sarcoma, adenocarcinoma, melanoma, and neuroendocrine tumors. This chapter gives an overview of the tumors of head and neck region with an emphasis on tumors of oral cavity and oropharynx, being the most common sites of head and neck cancers.

ETIOLOGY AND RISK FACTORS

(a) Tobacco and alcohol are the two most important factors in the etiology of squamous cell carcinoma of the oral cavity, oropharynx, larynx, hypopharynx, and paranasal sinuses. There is a synergistic interaction between these two agents that is multiplicative for the mouth, additive for larynx, and between additive and multiplicative for esophagus. Smoking is also associated with salivary gland malignancy in males. Other than alcohol and tobacco, areca nut chewing in form of paan leads to development of submucous fibrosis of oral cavity, which is a premalignant condition.

(b) Dental factors such as poor oral hygiene leading to gingivitis, alteration of microbiological flora of oral cavity, and ill-fitting dentures/sharp teeth causing repeated trauma at same site leading to chronic inflammation are factors in oral cavity carcinoma.

(c) In cancer of oral cavity, oropharynx, several viruses have been implicated in carcinogenesis including human papilloma virus (HPV), human immunodeficiency virus (HIV), and herpes simplex virus (HSV). Nasopharyngeal carcinoma is specially associated with Epstein–Barr virus (EBV) infection. There is a strong association between undifferentiated nasopharyngeal cancer and positive serology for EBV antigens.

(d) Several studies suggest increased intake of antioxidants or free radical scavenging such as vitamin A, C, and E present in fresh fruits and vegetables is associated with decreased incidence of squamous cell carcinoma of upper aerodigestive tract.

(e) Several genetic conditions such as Li-Fraumeni syndrome involving mutation in p53 gene, Fanconi anemia, Bloom syndrome, and ataxia telangiectasia are associated with increased risk of head and neck cancer. Inherited conditions such as Gardner's syndrome, familial polyposis. MEN syndrome and Cowden disease have an increased incidence of thyroid cancer. People on immunosuppressant drugs are also susceptible for development of cancers of head and neck region.

(f) Occupational exposure to dust from wood, textiles and leather, glues, formaldehyde, solvents used in furniture and shoe production, nickel and chromium dust, mustard gas, isopropyl alcohol, and radium are risk factors for development of carcinoma of nasal cavity and paranasal sinuses.

Prosthetic Rehabilitation of Head and Neck Cancer Patients. https://doi.org/10.1016/B978-0-323-82394-4.00016-1

63

(g) A history of radiation treatment in childhood, exposure to radioactive fallout from nuclear power plant accidents or nuclear weapons also have increased incidence of thyroid cancer and salivary gland neoplasia.

(h) Exposure to UV light is a risk factor for the development of lip cancer.

(i) There is an increased risk of development of squamous cell carcinoma in background of premalignant conditions of oral cavity such as lichen planus, leukoplakia, erythroplakia, and oral submucosal fibrosis.

CLINICAL PRESENTATION

Head and neck cancers typically produce signs and symptoms depending on the anatomic site such as dysphagia, odynophagia, globus sensation, hoarseness, alteration in phonation, epistaxis, epiphora, otalgia, hemoptysis, stuffiness of the ears, and trismus. Most patients present with metastatic disease at the time of diagnosis (regional nodal involvement in 43% and distant metastasis in 10%).[2]

The malignancy of the oral cavity may present initially with very subtle signs such as nonhealing ulcer in the oral cavity, exophytic or an endophytic growth, loose tooth or an ill-fitting denture, ulcer in the hard palate leading to perforation of the palate. With advanced stage of the disease and involvement of underlying structures, there may be complaints of trismus, ankyloglossia, mandibular pain, dysphagia, change in voice, or respiratory distress due to extension of the tumor into oropharynx, referred otalgia from the tumors involving lateral border of tongue.

Presentation of squamous cell carcinoma of the oropharynx is varied. It can present as a nonhealing ulcer, exophytic or verrucous or papillary growth. Base of tongue malignancies can present as submucosal growth, which present late. In early disease, the symptoms can be mild like soreness in throat or globus sensation or painless cervical lymphadenopathy. Advanced lesions present with dysphagia, odynophagia, halitosis, respiratory distress and change in voice, referred otalgia (due to involvement of CN IX, X), and trismus (involvement of pterygoid muscles). There is high incidence of early cervical metastasis due to rich lymphovascular supply to the area. 15%–75% of all cases present with cervical nodal metastasis.[3]

Clinical presentation of tumors in larynx and hypopharynx depends on the anatomic site. The most common early symptom in glottic carcinoma is hoarseness.

Symptoms of supraglottic and hypopharyngeal tumors include dysphagia, change in quality of voice, foreign body sensation in the throat, hemoptysis, odynophagia, and neck mass. Symptoms of subglottic tumors include dysphagia and stridor.

The common signs and symptoms of tumors of nasal and paranasal cavities include epistaxis, nasal obstruction, nasal discharge, proptosis, facial swelling, alterations in phonation and olfaction, and headache. Blocking of the nasolacrimal duct may cause epiphora. Nasal polyps of the benign inflammatory type produced by vascular obstruction may be the first manifestation of a more deep-seated malignant growth. Endoscopic examination of the nasal cavities may reveal a mass or growth.[4]

Benign salivary gland neoplasms usually present as a painless slow-growing, solitary swellings. Malignant tumors usually present as solitary swelling and may be associated with pain, discomfort, skin ulceration, and facial nerve involvement. Sublingual and minor salivary gland tumors usually present as painless submucosal swelling.

Thyroid cancers can present with thyroid swelling, which is usually painless, difficulty swallowing, difficulty breathing, hoarseness, lateral cervical lymphadenopathy.

ORAL CAVITY

The oral cavity is the foremost part of the digestive tract starting from the mucocutaneous junction of the lips (vermillion border) and extending posteriorly up to the oropharyngeal isthmus. The superior border of the oropharyngeal isthmus is the junction of hard palate and soft palate. Laterally, it is bounded by the anterior tonsillar pillars and inferiorly by the circumvallate papillae. Oral cavity is a complex area lined by stratified squamous epithelium with varying degrees of keratinization interspersed with minor salivary glands and dentoalveolar structures. Primary tumors of the oral cavity may arise from the squamous epithelium, minor salivary glands, neurovascular structures, and bones or dental tissue. Squamous cell carcinoma constitutes over 80% of the oral cavity tumors.[5,6] Notably, the estimated incidence for lip/oral cavity cancer is highest for the Southeast Asia region (6.4 per 100,000) followed by Eastern European countries.[7] Incidence of oral cancer is more common in males, who usually present in the sixth or seventh decade, although an upward trend is seen in young adults in many European countries reason being increased consumption of alcohol in young population.[8]

Diverse histological types of tumors are found in the head and neck region. Leukoplakia and erythroplakia are the terms applied to clinically identifiable precancerous mucosal lesions that may undergo malignant transformation.[2] There is a sequence of disease progression from atypia/dysplasia through carcinoma in situ to frankly invasive cancer. Squamous dysplasia refers to neoplastic alterations of the surface epithelium prior to invasion of the subepithelial connective tissues. These changes include nuclear atypia, loss of polarity, increased mitotic activity, nuclear enlargement with pleomorphism. These alterations are typically graded as mild, moderate, and severe (carcinoma in situ) based on the degree of nuclear abnormality and increasing depth involvement of epithelium i.e., involvement of lower one-third, two-thirds, and full thickness of the epithelium, respectively. Severe dysplasia or carcinoma in situ may further progress and infiltrate through basement membrane into subepithelial connective tissue leading to invasive carcinoma. Tumor may further invade skeletal muscle, craniofacial bones, skin, lymphatic spaces or may extend along nerves. More than 90% of head and neck cancers are of epithelial origin, of which squamous cell carcinoma constitutes the greatest majority.[9] Histologic grades of prototypical HNSCC (head neck squamous cell carcinoma) is based on the degree of keratinization, i.e., well-differentiated tumor characterized by > 75% keratinization; a moderately differentiated tumor, by 25%–50%; and a poorly differentiated tumor, by < 25% keratinization.

Morphological variants of SCC include papillary, verrucous, and basaloid variant. Papillary SCC is typified by an exophytic growth pattern with fronds of fibrovascular tissue covered by severely dysplastic squamous epithelium with limited areas of invasive carcinoma. Verrucous carcinoma is seen clinically as an exophytic mass with a warty or papillary surface and is observed histologically as a markedly thickened squamous epithelium with minimal atypia and mounds of parakeratotic squamous cells. In contrast to conventional squamous cell carcinoma, verrucous carcinoma invades as a burrowing mass with broad pushing borders and has no potential to metastasize. The basaloid squamous variant shows histomorphologically solid lobules of cells with peripheral palisading, scant cytoplasm, and dark nuclei with highly aggressive behavior.[10,11]

Other oral mucosal malignancies include adenocarcinomas (surface epithelium of nose and sinuses), sinonasal undifferentiated (anaplastic) carcinoma, olfactory neuroblastoma (esthesioneuroblastoma), malignant melanoma (nasal cavity, sinuses), lymphomas (sinonasal tract and tonsils), and nasopharyngeal carcinoma.[11]

Anatomical Subsites

(a) **Lip:** Lip carcinoma accounts for 20% of all oral cavity carcinoma. Most common histology is squamous cell carcinoma. Most common site is lower lip, which is attributed to more sun exposure compared to upper lip. It usually presents early as an exophytic growth or a nonhealing ulcer. As the lymphatics from lip drain into level I, II, and III, these groups of nodes are involved in nodal extension of the disease. Lesions involving midline lip have high chance of bilateral nodal spread. Early lesions are treated with wide local excision or radiotherapy with local resolving rate of approximately 90%. Advanced lesions are managed with surgery along with advent radiotherapy. Lip defects less than half can be closed primarily. Defects involving more than half of the length require closure with the help of local or free flaps. Elective neck dissection (level I–III) is reserved in case of recurrent tumors, size of the tumor more than 4 cm, thickness more than 1 cm, perineural spread of the tumor, or involvement of bone. Midline lower lip lesions require bilateral neck dissection in view of drainage of lower lip.

(b) **Oral tongue:** It is the freely mobile anterior two-thirds of the tongue. The posterior margin is demarcated by the circumvallate papillae. Oral tongue is subdivided into the tip, dorsum, lateral borders, and the ventral surface. The tip and dorsum of tongue is lined by specialized gustatory mucosa with keratinized stratified squamous epithelium. The ventral surface is lined by nonkeratinized squamous epithelium. The lateral border and ventral surface of tongue are continuous with the floor of mouth. The lateral border is the most commonly involved site due to pooling of saliva containing carcinogens in that area. Squamous cell carcinoma of the tongue can present as a nonhealing ulcer, exophytic or an endophytic growth. Tongue lesions usually present early usually in stage I/II. Tumors of the tongue usually metastasize to level I and II, but skip metastasis to level IV is not unusual. Tumors crossing midline and tumors from tip may involve bilateral neck nodes. Occult nodal metastasis has been reported in up to 51% of cases and is most commonly to level II. Occult nodal metastasis is highly dependent on thickness of the lesion. Lesions with thickness more than 3–4 mm have higher chances of occult nodal metastasis.[12,13] For early T1/T2 lesions that can be approached perorally, wide local excision with a 1 cm margin in three dimensions is curative with the primary lesion and is allowed to heal by secondary intention, or primary closure of the defect is done. Advanced lesions require paramedian mandibulotomy with segmental or hemimandibulectomy with reconstruction by local or free flaps. Elective neck dissection (level I– IV) or elective neck radiotherapy should be considered N0 cases, where the primary tumor is thicker than 3–4 mm, T2 or greater in dimension and T1 tumor that demonstrates poor histological features.[14] Comprehensive neck dissection is done in disease with nodal metastasis.

(c) **Buccal mucosa:** The buccal mucosa is the mucosal lining on the inner side of the cheek and extends from the oral commissure to the retromolar trigone. The buccal mucosa is lined by nonkeratinizing stratified squamous epithelium. Buccal carcinoma usually develops in the background of premalignant lesions line leukoplakia, melanoplakia, lichen planus, and submucous fibrosis, and it is considered as an aggressive neoplasms in view of late presentation, early nodal spread, and difficulty to achieve poor locoregional control.[6,15,16] Advanced lesions may involve the lower or upper alveolus, skin of the cheek, buccinator muscle, buccal pad of fat, skin of mandible, or maxilla. The cervical nodes, which are most commonly involved, are level I, II, and III. Tumors, which are T2 or greater, are poorly differentiated, have a poor lymphocytic response, and have thickness greater than 5 mm, are more likely to present with cervical metastasis.[17,18] The mainstay of treatment is surgical excision with adequate margins (1 cm) or 2–3 cm if skin is involved with or without postoperative adjuvant therapy.[19–21] Small lesions can be approached per orally, whereas advanced lesions may require bony resection of maxilla or mandible or access. T1/T2 lesions can be left to heal by secondary intention or by a split skin graft supported with a silicone sheet. Larger defects will require microvascular free flaps. Trismus is a known complication postoperatively, which should be managed aggressively by physiotherapy. Patients with T2 or greater stage or tumor thickness more than 5 mm irrespective of size of the tumor should undergo elective neck dissection.[18,22] Patients with clinically or radiologically positive nodal disease should undergo comprehensive neck dissection with or with PORT.[23] Retromolar trigone

accounts for only 6%–7% of all squamous cell carcinoma of oral cavity. As the area is hidden behind the molars, carcinoma of retromolar trigone area reports very late with complaints of trismus. Other complaints are pain, referred otalgia, and lingual paresthesia. Due to proximity with ramus of mandible, lesions spread early to mandible. At the time of initial presentation, 12%–50% of all cases have involved the mandible. Nodal metastasis is to level III and HI. Treatment includes surgical excision with postoperative adjuvant therapy. Early lesions can be approached per orally, while advanced lesions will require a lip split. Marginal mandibulectomy is required for tumor-free margins. In case of small lesions, defeat is allowed to heal by secondary intention or split skin grafting. Larger lesions require distant free flaps. Like cancer of other subsites of oral cavity, elective neck dissection is required for N0 lesions. N + disease requires comprehensive neck dissection.

(d) **Floor of mouth:** The floor of mouth bounded anteriorly and laterally by the attached mucoperiosteum of the mandibular alveolus. Posteriorly, it is limited by the anterior tonsillar pillars. Medially the floor of mouth merges with the ventral aspect of the tongue. It is lined by nonkeratinizing stratified squamous epithelium with a less dense submucosa. Underlying the mucosa lie minor salivary glands, the sublingual glands. The paired mylohyoid muscles form the muscular floor for the oral cavity. Floor of mouth accounts for 18%–33% of oral cavity cancers, squamous cell carcinoma being most common. The higher incidence of cancer in this region can be attributed to pooling of saliva and lack of keratinized squamous epithelium. Early lesions present as nonhealing ulcers or small exophytic lesions. Advanced lesions may infiltrate deep into the genioglossus, hyoglossus, and mylohyoid muscles. Nodal metastasis is to level I, II, and III. There are high chances of bilateral nodal involvement in lesions approaching midline. There is 25%–30% incidence of clinical or occult nodal disease in floor of mouth cancer.[24] Early lesions are treated with surgery or radiotherapy. Advanced lesions require adjuvant treatment. Small lesions are approached per orally with primary closure of the defect or healing by secondary intention. Larger lesions involving lower alveolus require mandibulectomy with reconstruction by free composite flaps (radial artery free forearm flap, free fibula osteocutaneous flap). All N0 lesions with tumor thickness 4 mm undergo selective neck dissection (level I, II, and III). Advanced nodal disease requires comprehensive neck dissection. The only parameter that is a statistically significant predictor of recurrence is clinically positive lymph nodes.[25]

(e) **Maxillary alveolus and gingiva:** The maxilla comprises of the maxillary alveolus and the hard palate. It is lined by mucoperiostium and is lined by squamous epithelium, which merges with the buccal mucosa at the gingivobuccal sulcus. Maxillary alveolus accounts for 3.5%–6.5% of oral squamous cell carcinoma, whereas incidence of cancer in hard palate is rarer.[26–28] The hard palate also contains minor salivary glands in the submucosa, 33% of palatal tumors being derived from salivary glands.[29] These malignancies present as ulcer, falling tooth, or an ill-fitting denture. Malignancies of the hard palate usually present at an advanced stage, which spread to maxillary sinus, nasal cavity, or may include symptoms of infraorbital paresthesia due to involvement of infraorbital nerve. Nodal metastasis is to level I, II, and III. Approximately 8% of patients with carcinoma of the hard palate or maxillary alveolus present with cervical metastasis, a further 27% having occult metastasis.[30,31] Surgical excision is the treatment of choice. Early lesions can be easily accessed perorally. Larger lesions require access by upper cheek flap or midfacial degloving with T3/T4 lesions may require a partial or total maxillectomy. Cervical metastasis is present in 35% of hard palate and maxillary alveolar carcinoma; an elective neck dissection (level I–III) has been advocated for lesions of T2 size or greater.

(f) **Mandibular alveolus and gingiva:** Mandibular alveolus is the intraoral part of the mandible and is covered by mucoperiosteum and is lined by squamous epithelium. It merges with the buccal mucosa laterally and with the floor of the mouth medially. Squamous cell carcinoma of the mandible is approximately three times more common than maxillary alveolus and represents 7.5%–17.5% of all oral cavity SCC.[26] The most common symptom is pain, occurring in 54%–86% of cases. Other symptoms include a nonhealing ulcer, ill-fitting dentures, delayed healing of extracted socket, labial paresthesia due to involvement of inferior alveolar nerve. Carcinoma of the lower alveolus commonly involves the edentulous and free margin of gingiva. 30%–50% of cases have radiological or histological mandibular invasion at the time of initial presentation. Nodal

metastasis is to level I, II, and III. Lesions in the midline have higher chances of bilateral nodal involvement. Early lesions are managed surgically, advanced lesions require adjuvant therapy. Early lesions are approached perorally with marginal mandibulectomy. Advanced lesions with evidence of mandibular involvement require segmental mandibulectomy. For N0 lesions, elective neck dissection is done. With higher nodal diseases, comprehensive neck dissection is done. Reconstruction of the defect is done by prosthesis or distant composite flaps.

OROPHARYNX

The oropharynx is a four-dimensional space and is an important space in the respiratory and alimentary conduits and performs an important role in respiration, speech, and swallowing. Oropharyngeal malignancies consist of 11%–12% of all head and neck malignancies, and squamous cell carcinoma is the most common histology. There is a rapid increase in HPV-associated oropharyngeal squamous cell carcinoma in the younger population of affluent countries. This type of oropharyngeal malignancy is less associated with the habit of smoking, tobacco, or alcohol consumption compared with HPV-negative SCC and has better outcome.[32] For staging purpose, tumors of oropharynx are broadly divided into p16-negative cases or cases without a p16 immunohistochemistry performed and tumors that have positive p16 immunohistochemistry overexpression.

The oropharynx separates oral cavity from nasopharynx superiorly and supraglottis inferiorly. It is continuous with oral cavity anteriorly, the separation between these two anatomical spaces is marked by the oropharyngeal isthmus (superior border by junction of hard palate and soft palate, circumvallate papillae inferiorly and by anterior tonsillar pillar laterally on each side). The anterior wall (glossoepiglottic area) of the oropharynx is divided into base of tongue and vallecula. The tonsils along with tonsillar fossa, tonsillar pillars, and glossotonsillar sulci constitute the lateral wall of the oropharynx. Posterior limit of this space is the posterior pharyngeal wall, which extends from the level of hard palate to the level of floor of vallecula. The superior extent of the oropharynx is the level of hard palate. The inferior limit of oropharynx is the vallecula and the pharyngoepiglottic fold. The superior wall is formed by the inferior surface of the soft palate and uvula. The oropharynx is lined by nonkeratinized squamous epithelium. The oropharynx is the gateway to the aerodigestive tract, the primary defense of which is done by the lymphoid tissue of the Waldeyer's ring. The other common type of tissue present in the oropharynx is the minor salivary glands.

Anatomical Subsites

(a) **Tonsil:** 50% of the oropharyngeal tumors arise from the tonsils. Initial complaints are nonspecific such as irritation of throat, referred ipsilateral otalgia. Advanced lesions may present with odynophagia and respiratory distress. Tonsilar lesions spread early to nodes; commonest nodes involved are of level II. Lesions can extend superiorly to involve the soft palate and the pterygoid muscles, inferiorly into the BOT, PE fold, pyriform fossa (lateral wall) and anteriorly to involve the retromolar trigone, buccal mucosa. Advanced lesions can spread laterally to involve the parapharyngeal space.

(b) **Base of tongue**: Base of tongue makes up approximately 30% of oropharyngeal squamous cell carcinoma. Early lesions are usually submucosal, which may be asymptomatic or occult diagnosed only during workup for an enlarged cervical lymph node. Nodal metastasis is most commonly to level II followed by level III and IV. Advanced lesions lead to odynophagia, dysphagia, change in voice (hot potato voice), fixity of tongue musculature, and respiratory distress.

(c) **Soft palate**: Soft palate malignancy accounts for 10%–15% of oropharyngeal tumors. Oropharyngeal surface is most commonly involved, and these tumors present early. Nodal metastasis is late, and level II is involved most commonly followed by level III and IV. Bilateral nodal spread is common.

(d) **Pharyngeal wall**: It is the rarest site to be involved. Generally, patients present late with advanced lesions spreading to nasopharynx and hypopharynx. Parapharyngeal and retropharyngeal nodal metastasis is common. These tumors have a poor prognosis.

Immunocytochemistry plays an important role in the diagnosis of primary head and neck cancers, particularly for the less common entities, with current guidance recommending a combination of immunocytochemistry for p16 protein overexpression and in situ hybridization for high-risk HPV DNA. Poorly differentiated carcinomas arising in the oropharynx and nasopharynx, and their metastatic foci may be distinguished by the presence of HPV and Epstein–Barr virus DNA, respectively.[11] Oropharyngeal cancers caused by HPV have a significantly better prognosis compared with those caused by tobacco or alcohol;

hence, all oropharyngeal tumors should be routinely tested for HPV.[33]

The modality of choice for treatment of oropharyngeal malignancies is primarily nonsurgical with an aim for organ preservation. Moreover, it is an anatomically difficult to reach area for conventional surgical approach. Early lesions can be managed surgically via CO_2 laser or by robotic method.

LARYNX AND HYPOPHARYNX

The larynx extends from the tip of the epiglottis to the inferior border of the cricoid cartilage. The larynx is divided into three compartments—supraglottis, glottis, and subglottis. The hypopharynx lies behind the larynx and partially surrounds it on either side, commencing from a plane of the superior border of the hyoid bone (or floor of the vallecula) to the inferior border of the cricoid cartilage. It is continuous with the oropharynx above and with the cervical esophagus below. The most common benign tumor of the larynx is papilloma (85%). Other types include chondroma, hemangioma, lymphangioma, schwannoma, neurofibroma, adenoma, granular cell myoblastoma, leiomyoma, rhabdomyoma, fibroma, lipoma, and paraganglioma. Squamous cell carcinoma (SCC) comprises about 95% of laryngeal malignancies. Other types include adenocarcinoma, sarcoma, undifferentiated carcinoma, and neuroendocrine tumor. The majority of SCCs originate from the supraglottic and glottic regions. Laryngeal and hypopharyngeal SCCs occur most frequently in the sixth and seventh decades. They are more common in men. SCC in glottis, supraglottis, and hypopharynx is optimally treated with surgery and adjuvant RT. Prognosis is inversely related to TNM stage and extracapsular spread.[34]

NASAL CAVITY AND PARANASAL SINUSES

The nose opens into the nasal cavity, which is divided into two nasal passages. Air moves through these passages during breathing. The nasal cavity lies above the bone that forms the roof of the mouth and curves down at the back to join the throat. The area just inside the nostrils is called the nasal vestibule. A small area of special cells in the roof of each nasal passage sends signals to the brain to give the sense of smell.

Together the paranasal sinuses and the nasal cavity filter and warm the air, and make it moist before it goes into the lungs. The movement of air through the sinuses and other parts of the respiratory system help make sounds for speech. Paranasal sinuses are hollow, air-filled spaces around the nose, lined with mucus-secreting cells. These are namely frontal, maxillary, ethmoid, and sphenoid sinuses.

Papillomas, adenomas, and cystadenomas and rarely aberrant salivary tumors are among the benign epithelial growths of the nasal and paranasal cavities. Less common tumors include angioma, osteoma, ossifying fibroma, leiomyoma, myxoma, glioma, and schwannomas. Most of these growths appear in the nasal cavity, in the region of the septum or lower turbinate and in the vestibule. The majority of carcinomas of the nose arise in the region of the middle turbinate at the embryonic site of the outpouching of the sinuses, and are epidermal in type. Adults and more often males are usually affected.[4]

The most common malignant tumor of paranasal sinus and nasal cavity is SCC. Other neoplasms include melanoma, sarcoma, inverted papilloma, and midline granuloma.

Epidermal carcinomas of the maxilloethmoidal region may be divided into two major groups according to their clinical and pathological features, i.e., squamous or transitional cell carcinomas and lymphoepitheliomas. The majority comprises squamous cell or transitional cell cancer, which produce large local growths invading the adjoining structures, but distant metastases rarely occur. These tumors are more frequent in the fifth, sixth, and seventh decades of life. Lymphoepithelioma is most common in the nasopharynx, also observed in the nose and antrum. Contrary to the former, these tumors occur as small growths, but metastasis occurs early. Patients reporting early with T1 maxillary tumours may be cured with surgery alone. Majority of patients with sinonasal malignancy present with advanced disease and will require combination therapy.

SALIVARY GLANDS

Salivary glands are exocrine glands responsible for the production of saliva. They are comprised of three paired major glands (parotid, submandibular, and sublingual) and the minor salivary glands. Minor salivary glands are widely distributed throughout the oral cavity, oropharynx, upper respiratory and sinonasal tracts, and the paranasal sinuses. These are most numerous at the junction of the hard and soft palate, lips, and buccal mucosa. Between 64% and 80% of all primary epithelial salivary gland tumors occur in the parotid gland; 7%–11% occur in the submandibular glands; fewer than 1% occur in the sublingual glands; and 9%–23% occur in minor glands.[34] Majority of salivary gland tumors are benign, and only 20% are malignant. The annual incidence of salivary gland

cancers ranges from 0.5 to 2 per 100,000 in different parts of the world. The majority of the cases arise in the sixth decade.[35] Malignant tumors comprise 50% of minor gland tumors. Females are more frequently affected, but some gender variation is also seen according to the tumor type.[36] Benign neoplasms usually presents as a painless slow-growing, solitary swellings. Malignant tumors usually present as solitary swelling and may be associated with pain, discomfort, skin ulceration, and facial nerve involvement. Sublingual and minor salivary gland tumors usually present as painless submucosal swelling.

Among all patients, the most common tumor type is pleomorphic adenoma or benign mixed tumor, which accounts for about 50%–70% of all tumors, with majority (80%) of them located in the parotid gland. Warthin tumor is second most common benign salivary gland tumor, with nearly all arising in the parotid gland or periparotid lymph nodes.[34] These tumors usually present as slowly growing mass, show male predilection, and strong association with cigarette smoking. Both pleomorphic adenoma and Warthin tumor are well-encapsulated lesions.[36]

Mucoepidermoid carcinoma (MEC) is the most common primary salivary gland malignancy in both adults and children. Approximately half of tumors (53%) occur in the major salivary glands. The parotid glands predominate, representing 45%, with 7% for submandibular glands and 1% in sublingual glands. The most frequent intraoral sites are the palate and buccal mucosa. Most tumors present as firm, fixed, and painless swellings. Symptoms can include pain, otorrhea, paresthesia, facial nerve palsy, dysphagia, bleeding, and trismus.[34]

Adenoid cystic carcinomas comprise approximately 10% of all epithelial salivary neoplasms and most frequently involve the parotid, submandibular and minor salivary glands. They comprise 30% of epithelial minor salivary gland tumors with the highest frequency in the palate. The tumor occurs in all age groups with a high frequency in middle-aged and older patients. There is no apparent sex predilection except for a high incidence in women with submandibular tumors. The most common symptom is a slow-growing mass followed by pain due to the propensity of these tumors for perineural invasion. Facial nerve paralysis and extraparenchymal invasion may also occur. Histopathologically, these tumors show two main cell types: ductal and modified myoepithelial cells that typically have hyperchromatic, angular nuclei and frequently clear cytoplasm. There are three defined patterns: tubular, cribriform, and solid.[34,36]

Acinic cell carcinoma affects women more than men at all ages. The parotid gland is involved in >80% of cases (representing 2%–4% of all parotid tumors); the intraoral minor salivary glands, in 17%; and the submandibular gland, in 4%. Polymorphous low-grade adenocarcinoma (PLGA) is almost exclusively a minor SGN, but cases arising in the major salivary glands have also been reported. It has been estimated that PLGA constitutes 10%–20% of malignant intraoral malignancies, second only to MEC.[36]

Carcinoma ex-pleomorphic adenoma frequently presents as a painless mass in the parotid gland, and occasionally in the submandibular gland (82%) and in the palatal and intraoral minor salivary glands (18%). Salivary duct carcinoma is an aggressive neoplasm, typically found in older men and most often in the parotid. It accounts for up to 7%–10% of malignant SGNs. Adenocarcinoma (not otherwise specified) is usually the diagnosis of exclusion.[36]

Prognosis correlates most strongly with clinical stage, emphasizing the importance of early diagnosis of salivary gland malignancies. Fine needle aspiration cytology (FNAC) is a useful diagnostic modality for salivary gland neoplasms with sensitivity up to 85% and specificity up to 99%.[35] Surgery is the mainstay of treatment for salivary gland tumors.

THYROID AND PARATHYROID GLANDS

Thyroid gland is located at base of throat anterior to trachea. There are two types of cells located within the thyroid parenchyma: the follicular cells and the supporting cells (also called the C cells or parafollicular cells). Follicular cells secrete thyroxine hormone that regulates basal metabolic rate, heart rate, blood pressure, and body temperature. C cells produce calcitonin hormone, which, along with parathyroid hormone, (PTH) regulate calcium and phosphate levels in blood. Parathyroid glands are endocrine glands located in the neck behind the thyroid gland They are four in number with two behind each lobe of thyroid. Parathyroid adenoma is a benign tumor that can lead to hyperparathyroidism (raised PTH levels). The common symptoms include bony pain, bone fractures, renal stones, excessive urination, muscular pain, confusion, lethargy, etc. Parathyroid cancer is a rare disease.

Thyroid nodules are very common, and most of them are benign. These nodules can be palpable clinically or may be detected incidentally on imaging studies, such as ultrasound, computed tomography (CT), magnetic resonance imaging (MRI), and positron emission tomography (PET), performed for other reasons. The nodules detected on PET scans have 33% increased risk of malignancy compared with those detected with other methods, which is approximately 5%. Benign thyroid lesions include follicular adenoma, colloid goiter, adenomatous goiter, lymphocytic thyroiditis, Hürthle cell adenoma, thyrotoxicosis, or Grave's disease. Factors that raise suspicion for malignancy in any newly detected thyroid nodule include size more than 4 cm , history of radiation to the head and neck region, a family history of thyroid cancer or thyroid disease, suspicious ultrasound findings, cervical lymphadenopathy, and female gender (female to male ratio of 3:1).[37] Any thyroid nodule should be evaluated thoroughly to exclude malignancy.

The incidence of thyroid cancer has risen in recent years. They can occur in any age group but more so in adults aged 45–54 years, with a mean age of 50 years at diagnosis. Papillary thyroid carcinoma is the most common thyroid malignancy, accounting to 70%–80% of all thyroid malignancies. It grows and metastasizes slowly. Lymph node metastasis can be present in 20%–90% of patients. Follicular thyroid carcinoma accounts for approximately 14% of thyroid cancers and is more aggressive than papillary thyroid carcinoma. Hürthle cell carcinoma is a variant of follicular carcinoma. Medullary thyroid carcinoma represents approximately 3% of thyroid cancers and is often associated with multiple endocrine neoplasia 2 (MEN 2). Calcitonin is a useful tumor marker, which is secreted by tumor cells. Anaplastic thyroid carcinoma represents approximately 2% of thyroid cancers and has the worst prognosis because of early distant metastasis.[37] Other thyroid malignancies include lymphoma.

Fine needle aspiration cytology (FNAC) along with imaging studies is to be performed for diagnosis. Follicular neoplasms on FNAC that includes both follicular adenoma and follicular carcinoma can be distinguished on histopathology based on evidence of capsular or vascular invasion in latter.

Prognosis and treatment of thyroid cancers depends on tumor stage at the initial evaluation. Surgery is the mainstay of treatment. Therapeutic central compartment neck dissection should be performed along with the total thyroidectomy when lymph nodes are clinically involved. Radioactive iodine (I^{131}) plays an integral adjuvant role in the treatment of thyroid cancer.

Novel targeted therapies, such as tyrosine kinase inhibitors, have been approved recently with advanced thyroid cancer.[37] External beam radiation therapy is used for palliative treatment for inoperable cases.

DIAGNOSIS

The need for expeditious diagnosis of head and neck cancers cannot be overemphasized, as early diagnosis can lead to a reduction in mortality due to head and neck cancers. The diagnostic workup includes the following:

(a) History and physical evaluation: History of exposure to risk factors as outlined previously can be assessed. Physical examination includes appearance, size, site, extension into adjacent anatomical subsites, depth of the lesion (especially in tongue lesions), fixation to underlying structures, trismus, ankyloglossia, involvement of skin of cheek in case of buccal lesions, palpation of neck for cervical lymphadenopathy, and evaluation of upper aerodigestive tract by fibreoptic endoscopic assessment. A dental evaluation should be part of early assessment so that dental treatment can be instituted prior to surgery or radiotherapy.

(b) Radiological evaluation: Diagnostic imaging includes plain X-rays, contrast-enhanced computed tomography (CECT), PET, and MRI. CECT is done for evaluation of primary as well as nodal disease and bony invasion. MRI may be asked for evaluation in tongue carcinoma to measure depth of the lesion and involvement of intrinsic muscles of tongue, extension into parapharyngeal space and pterygoid space. USG is the investigation of choice in case of thyroid malignancy. CECT is only done in cases with retrosternal extension.

(c) Biopsy: Punch or incisional biopsy from the primary site is done for histological diagnosis. Biopsy site should be at the periphery of the lesion to include a part of normal mucosa, as it also allows the invasive front to be examined, which can yield useful prognostic information.[1,33] If the patient presents with a small primary with no nodal disease on neck palpation, it is judicious to conduct imaging prior to biopsy as reactive lymphadenopathy may upstage the disease on radiological evaluation. Similarly, small alveolar lesions should be evaluated radiologically prior to biopsy since increased marrow signal intensity may commit the patient to segmental resection.

(d) Fine needle aspiration cytology from suspected metastatic cervical lymph node or suspicious nodule of the thyroid can be a useful diagnostic modality.

(e) Fiber optic laryngoscopy is required to see completely the extent of the lesion and to rule out involvement of larynx in oropharyngeal cancer. Nasal endoscopy is essential in case of malignancies of soft palate and to rule out involvement of nasopharyngeal space.

(f) Examination under anesthesia is required to see extent and operability of the lesion and for taking biopsy from the primary site.

TREATMENT

The treatment of head and neck cancer involves a multidisciplinary approach. The various modalities include surgery, radiation alone or in combination and with or without chemotherapy and target drug therapy. The treatment of lymphatics is determined by the primary site, histologic criteria, and risk of lymph node metastasis. Radiation therapy may be used alone for debilitated patients with advanced disease who cannot tolerate the sequelae of chemotherapy and unfit for surgical intervention.[38] A stepwise approach to pain management plays a critical role in management. Tumor recurrence can be managed by radiation therapy, chemotherapy, or both but have limited effectiveness.

Post primary management, plastic and reconstructive surgery in head and neck cancer cases plays a key role with the advent of use of prostheses, grafts, regional pedicle flaps, and complex free flaps, for functional and cosmetic reconstruction of defects, which significantly improve a patient's quality of life.[38] Rehabilitation and supportive care is an important aspect of head and neck tumor care comprising of physiotherapy, occupational therapy, speech therapy, psychosocial counseling, and nutritional counseling.

PROGNOSIS

Prognosis in head and neck cancer varies greatly depending on the tumor size, primary site, etiology, and presence of regional or distant metastases. With appropriate treatment, 5-year survival can be as high as 90% for stage I, 75%–80% for stage II, 45%–75% for stage III, and up to 50% for some stage IV cancers.[38] The survival rates vary greatly depending on the primary site and etiology (Figs. 3.1–3.11).

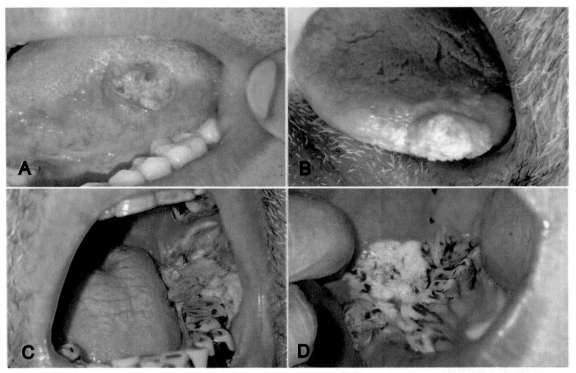

FIG. 3.1 Clinical photographs showing various presentation of squamous cell carcinoma in oral cavity. (a) Ulcerated growth at lateral border of tongue. (b) Verrucous/papillary growth at lateral border of tongue. (c) and (d) Indurated and ulcerated growth in the buccal mucosa.

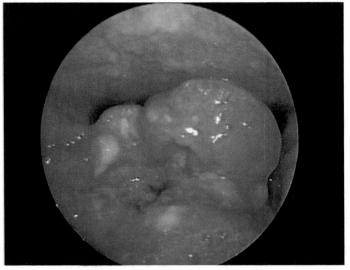

FIG. 3.2 Photograph showing endoscopic view of growth (SCC) at base of tongue.

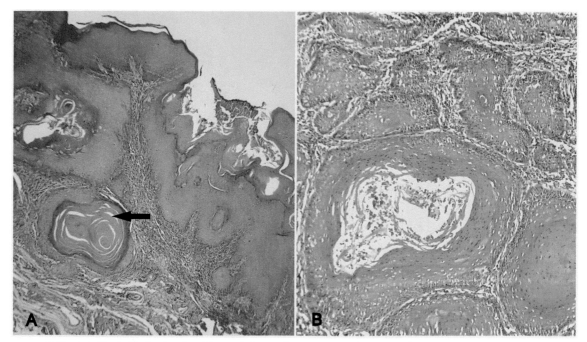

FIG. 3.3 Photograph showing histopathology of moderately differentiated squamous cell carcinoma. Hyperkeratotic and dysplastic stratified squamous epithelium with nests of atypical squamous cells in subepithelial tissue and keratin pearl formation (*arrow*). (a) H/E 200X, (b) H/E 400X.

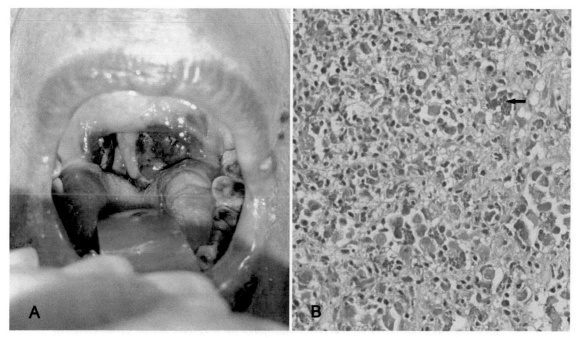

FIG. 3.4 Photograph showing malignant melanoma oropharynx. (a) Clinical presentation. (b) Microscopy showing nests of tumor cells with melanin pigments (*arrowhead*).

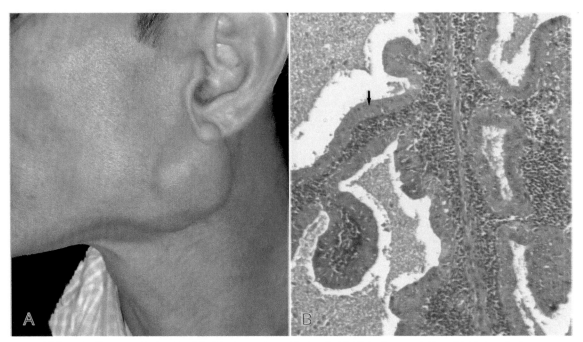

FIG. 3.5 Photograph showing Warthin tumor (parotid gland). (a) Clinical presentation. (b) Histopathology showing double-layered surface epithelium comprising of oncocytic and basal cells (*arrowhead*) with underlying lymphoid stroma and separated by cystic spaces.

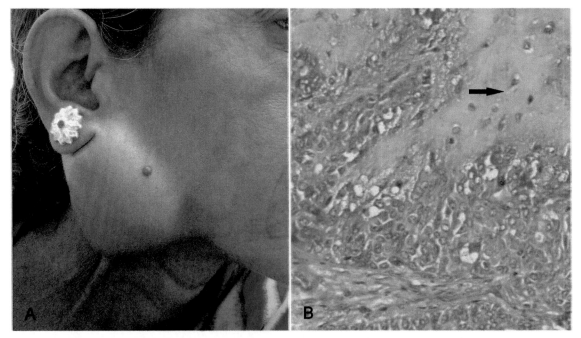

FIG. 3.6 Photograph showing pleomorphic adenoma (parotid gland). (a) Clinical presentation. (b) Histopathology showing highly cellular tumor with chondromyxoid matrix material (*arrow*). Background shows modified myoepithelial cells.

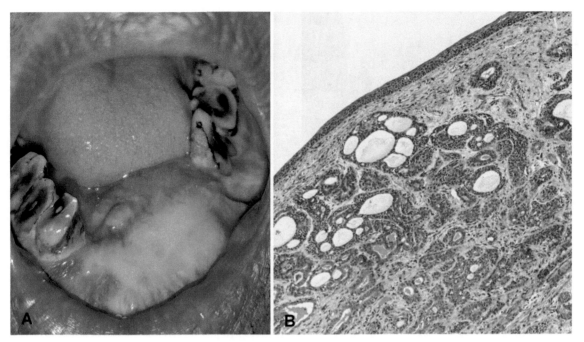

FIG. 3.7 Photograph showing adenoid cystic carcinoma (sublingual salivary gland). (a) Clinical presentation. (b) Histopathology showing cribriform and tubular patterns composed of inner ductal and outer myoepithelial cells. Myoepithelial cells show dark angulated nuclei and scanty cytoplasm.

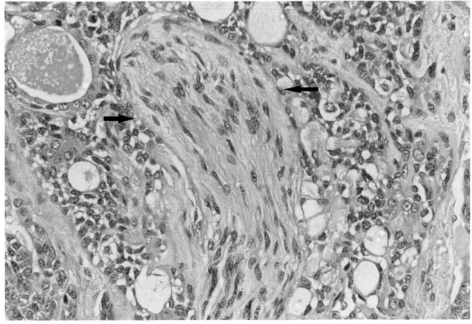

FIG. 3.8 Photograph of histopathology showing perineural invasion of tumor cells (*arrowheads*) in adenoid cystic carcinoma (salivary gland).

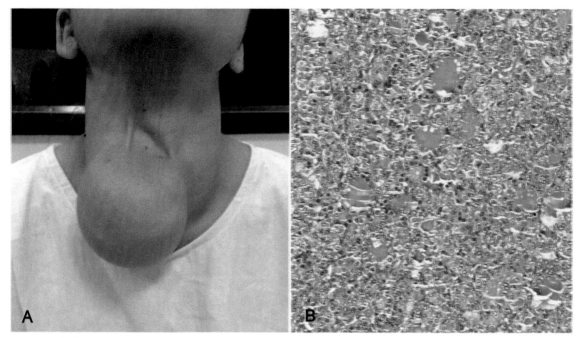

FIG. 3.9 Photograph showing follicular adenoma thyroid. (a) Clinical presentation. (b) Histopathology showing closely packed follicles lined with cuboidal to low columnar cells.

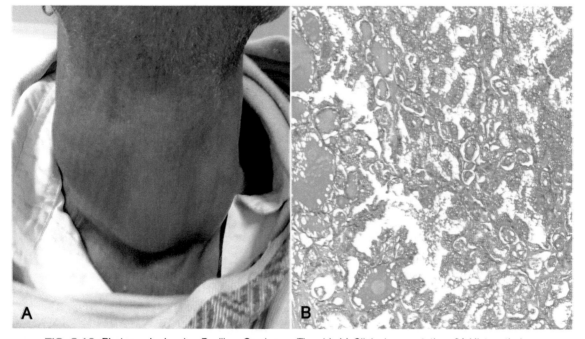

FIG. 3.10 Photograph showing Papillary Carcinoma Thyroid. (a) Clinical presentation. (b) Histopathology showing extensive branching papillae with fibrovascular cores and typical nuclear features i.e., nuclear enlargement, nuclear overlapping and nuclear clearing.

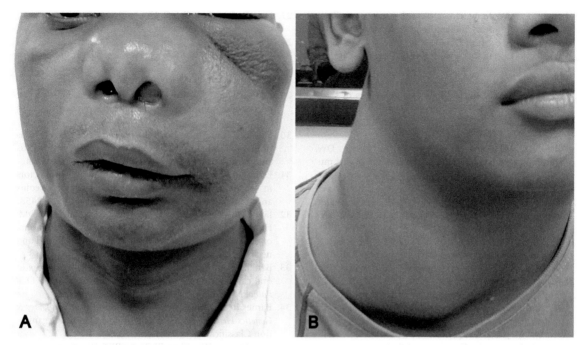

FIG. 3.11 Clinical photograph showing (a) rhabdomyosarcoma maxilla (b) Hodgkin's lymphoma (cervical swelling).

REFERENCES

1. Kumar B, Shukla A. Head and neck carcinoma and its association with environmental factors. *Int J Otorhinolaryngol Head Neck Surg.* 2019;5(6):1619−1623.
2. Ridge JA, Glisson BS, Lango MN, Feigenberg S. Head and neck tumors. *Cancer Network Home J Oncol;* 2011:1−82. https://www.cancernetwork.com/view/head-and-neck-tumors#.
3. Bussels B, Hermans R, Reijnders A, Dirix P, Nuyts S, Van den Bogaert W. Retropharyngeal nodes in squamous cell carcinoma of oropharynx: incidence, localization, and implications for target volume. *Int J Radiat Oncol Biol Phys.* 2006;65(3):733−738.
4. Geschickter CF. Tumors of the Nasal and Paranasal Cavities. 637−660.
5. Funk GF, Karnell LH, Robinson RA, Zhen WK, Trask DK, Hoffman HT. Presentation, treatment, and outcome of oral cavity cancer: a National Cancer Data Base report. *Head Neck.* 2002;24(2):165−180.
6. Ghoshal S, Mallick I, Panda N, Sharma SC. Carcinoma of the buccal mucosa: analysis of clinical presentation, outcome and prognostic factors. *Oral Oncol.* 2006;42(5): 533−539.
7. Chi AC, Day TA, Neville BW. Oral cavity and oropharyngeal squamous cell carcinoma—an update. *CA A Cancer J Clin.* 2015;65(5):401−421.
8. Blot WJ, Devesa SS, McLaughlin JK, Fraumeni JJ. Oral and pharyngeal cancers. *Cancer Surv.* 1994;19:23−42.
9. Gilyoma JM, Rambau PF, Masalu N, Kayange NM, Chalya PL. Head and neck cancers: a clinico-pathological profile and management challenges in a resource-limited setting. *BMC Res Notes.* 2015;8:772. https://doi.org/10.1186/s13104-015-1773-9.
10. Pai SI, Westra WH. Molecular pathology of head and neck cancer: implications for diagnosis, prognosis, and treatment. *Annu Rev Pathol.* 2009;4:49−70.
11. Helliwell TR, Giles TE. Pathological aspects of the assessment of head and neck cancers: United Kingdom National Multidisciplinary Guidelines. *J Laryngol Otol.* 2016; 130(Suppl. S2):S59−S65.
12. Wei WI, Ferlito A, Rinaldo A, et al. Management of the N0 neck—reference or preference. *Oral Oncol.* 2006;42(2): 115−122.
13. Huang SH, Hwang D, Lockwood G, Goldstein DP, O'Sullivan B. Predictive value of tumor thickness for cervical lymph-node involvement in squamous cell carcinoma of the oral cavity: a meta-analysis of reported studies. *Cancer Interdiscipl Int J Am Cancer Soc.* 2009;115(7): 1489−1497.
14. D'Cruz AK, Vaish R, Kapre N, et al. Elective versus therapeutic neck dissection in node-negative oral cancer. *N Engl J Med.* 2015;373(6):521−529.

15. Strome SE, To W, Strawderman M, et al. Squamous cell carcinoma of the buccal mucosa. *Otolaryngology-Head Neck Surg (Tokyo)*. 1999;120(3):375–379.

16. Shaw R, McGlashan G, Woolgar J, et al. Prognostic importance of site in squamous cell carcinoma of the buccal mucosa. *Br J Oral Maxillofac Surg*. 2009;47(5):356–359.

17. Jing J, Li L, He W, Sun G. Prognostic predictors of squamous cell carcinoma of the buccal mucosa with negative surgical margins. *J Oral Maxillofac Surg*. 2006;64(6):896–901.

18. Urist MM, O'Brien CJ, Soong S-J, Visscher DW, Maddox WA. Squamous cell carcinoma of the buccal mucosa: analysis of prognostic factors. *Am J Surg*. 1987;154(4):411–414.

19. Hao S-P, Cheng MH. Cancer of the buccal mucosa and retromolar trigone. *Operat Tech Otolaryngol Head Neck Surg*. 2004;15(4):239–251.

20. McMahon J, O'brien C, Pathak I, et al. Influence of condition of surgical margins on local recurrence and disease-specific survival in oral and oropharyngeal cancer. *Br J Oral Maxillofac Surg*. 2003;41(4):224–231.

21. Wong LS, McMahon J, Devine J, et al. Influence of close resection margins on local recurrence and disease-specific survival in oral and oropharyngeal carcinoma. *Br J Oral Maxillofac Surg*. 2012;50(2):102–108.

22. Bloom ND, Spiro RH. Carcinoma of the cheek mucosa: a retrospective analysis. *Am J Surg*. 1980;140(4):556–559.

23. Diaz Jr EM, Holsinger FC, Zuniga ER, Roberts DB, Sorensen DM. Squamous cell carcinoma of the buccal mucosa: one institution's experience with 119 previously untreated patients. *Head Neck*. 2003;25(4):267–273.

24. Hicks Jr WL, Loree TR, Garcia RI, et al. Squamous cell carcinoma of the floor of mouth: a 20-year review. *Head Neck*. 1997;19(5):400–405.

25. Sessions DG, Spector GJ, Lenox J, et al. Analysis of treatment results for floor-of-mouth cancer. *Laryngoscope*. 2000;110(10):1764–1772.

26. Woolgar JA, Triantafyllou A. A histopathological appraisal of surgical margins in oral and oropharyngeal cancer resection specimens. *Oral Oncol*. 2005;41(10):1034–1043.

27. Love R, Stewart I, Coy P. Upper alveolar carcinoma–a 30 year survey. *J Otolaryngol*. 1977;6(5):393–398.

28. Rao D, Shroff P, Chattopadhyay G, Dinshaw K. Survival analysis of 5595 head and neck cancers–results of conventional treatment in a high-risk population. *Br J Cancer*. 1998;77(9):1514–1518.

29. Li Q, Zhang X-R, Liu X-K, et al. Long-term treatment outcome of minor salivary gland carcinoma of the hard palate. *Oral Oncol*. 2012;48(5):456–462.

30. Simental Jr AA, Johnson JT, Myers EN. Cervical metastasis from squamous cell carcinoma of the maxillary alveolus and hard palate. *Laryngoscope*. 2006;116(9):1682–1684.

31. Eskander A, Givi B, Gullane PJ, et al. Outcome predictors in squamous cell carcinoma of the maxillary alveolus and hard palate. *Laryngoscope*. 2013;123(10):2453–2458.

32. Lindel K, Beer KT, Laissue J, Greiner RH, Aebersold DM. Human papillomavirus positive squamous cell carcinoma of the oropharynx: a radiosensitive subgroup of head and neck carcinoma. *Cancer*. 2001;92(4):805–813.

33. Bankfalvi A, Piffko J. Prognostic and predictive factors in oral cancer: the role of the invasive tumour front. *J Oral Pathol Med*. 2000;29(7):291–298.

34. Barnes L, Eveson JW, Reichart P, Sidransky D. *Pathology & Genetics Head and Neck Tumours*. World Health Organization Classification of Tumours; 2003.

35. Howe To VS, Wai Chan JY, Tsang RKY, Wei WI. Review of salivary gland neoplasms. *ISRN Otolaryngol*. 2012:6. https://doi.org/10.5402/2012/872982. Article ID 872982.

36. Bradley PJ. Frequency and histopathology by site, major pathologies, symptoms and signs of salivary gland neoplasms. *Adv Oto-Rhino-Laryngol*. 2016;78:9–16. https://doi.org/10.1159/000442120.

37. Nguyen QT, Lee EJ, Huang MG, Park YI, Khullar A, Plodkowski RA. Diagnosis and treatment of patients with thyroid cancer. *Am Health Drug Benef*. 2015;8(1):30–38.

38. Schiff BA. Overview of Head and Neck Tumors. MSD Manual Professional version.

CHAPTER 4

History of Plastic Surgery and General Concepts of Reconstruction

MOHAMMED FAHUD KHURRAM, MBBS, MS, MCH, DNB PLASTIC SURGERY

In the past few decades, the development of plastic surgery has taken place at a very high pace, but the origins of this specialty are very old. Often called "the father of plastic surgery," "Sushruta" in his compilation known as "Sushruta Samhita" has described the reconstruction of the nose with the help of a cheek flap. This technique was published in the "Gentleman's magazine" of Calcutta in October 1794,[1] and it was widely known as the "Indian method" of the nose job.

Perhaps the most significant improvements in plastic surgery techniques were introduced during the world wars. Archibald Mc Indoe and Harold Gilles[2] were the pioneers of this period. Military surgeons were required to treat extensive facial and head injuries caused by modern weapons. These grievous injuries necessitated newer innovations in reconstructive surgical procedures.

INTRODUCTION

Successful management of a head and neck cancer patient requires a team approach, which includes a medical oncologist, a surgical oncologist, a reconstructive surgeon, a prosthodontist, a psychologist, and a nutritionist. A careful preoperative assessment and development of a treatment plan are a must. The patient's age, tumor stage and prognosis, sex, body habitus, availability of donor sites, and psychological status of the patient are considered before formulating a plan. As far as reconstruction is considered, these are a few principles that should be followed:

1. Perform adequate excision/debridement prior to reconstruction, and this should include the removal of all barriers to tissue growth (infection, biofilm, dead cells).
2. Replace like with like—the tissue of same thickness, color match, and pliability.[3]
3. Preserve form and function. Recreate normal anatomy, obliterate dead spaces, and establish adequate blood supply to restore normal form and function.

4. Minimize donor site morbidity and protect the surgical site in postoperative period.[4]
5. Have a backup plan (plan A, plan B, plan C).[5]
6. Innovation—the plastic surgeon must strive to tailor every operation and make proper adjustments to standard procedures and techniques.[6]

The Reconstructive Ladder to a Reconstructive Elevator

A new paradigm, the reconstructive elevator is more appropriate than the reconstructive ladder as a guideline to reconstruct a complex defect. It emphasizes the selection of a technique that is safer and successfully reconstructs the defect to achieve appropriate form and function.

The reconstructive ladder describes a sequential approach to wound closure, and it starts with the simplest option and then proceeds upward in a stepwise manner. This concept dates back to ancient Egyptians. But with the advances in the understanding of wound healing and the development of advanced surgical techniques, the concept of the reconstruction ladder is now often replaced with the "reconstructive elevator."[5] It implies that the simplest may not be the best option. One can jump to the best suitable step/option to recreate and restore form and function. It should be a result of a creative and parallel thought process tailored for a particular patient and should not be generalized for all.

The reconstructive ladder is a conceptual tool used in plastic and reconstructive surgery to guide the selection of appropriate techniques for the reconstruction of defects or injuries. The ladder has five rungs, each representing a different level of complexity and invasiveness:

1. Primary closure: The simplest technique, in which the wound edges are brought together and sutured.
2. Skin grafts: The use of skin taken from a donor site and transferred to the wound.

Prosthetic Rehabilitation of Head and Neck Cancer Patients. https://doi.org/10.1016/B978-0-323-82394-4.00001-X

79

3. Local flaps: The use of nearby tissue that can be mobilized to cover the defect.
4. Regional flaps: The use of tissue from a more distant but related part of the body.
5. Free flaps: The most complex technique, in which tissue is taken from a remote part of the body and transplanted to the defect, along with its own blood supply.

The selection of the appropriate rung on the reconstructive ladder depends on various factors such as the size and location of the defect, the availability of donor tissue, the patient's overall health, and the desired cosmetic outcome. The ladder provides a framework for surgeons to choose the most appropriate technique for each individual case, balancing the complexity and invasiveness of the procedure against the potential benefits to the patient.

The reconstructive triangle concept (Fig. 4.1) primarily refers to a geometric principle used in plastic and reconstructive surgery to guide the reconstruction of facial defects. However, it is true that various techniques, including flaps, tissue expansion, and microsurgery, can be used in conjunction with the reconstructive triangle concept to achieve optimal outcomes in reconstructive surgery.

Flaps are a type of tissue transfer technique that involves moving tissue from one area of the body to another, often with an intact blood supply. Flaps can be used to reconstruct defects in various parts of the body, including the face, and are often guided by the principles of the reconstructive triangle.

Tissue expansion involves stretching the skin and soft tissue using a balloon-like device called an expander, which can create new tissue where there was a deficiency. Tissue expansion is often used in conjunction with other reconstructive techniques, including flaps, and can be guided by the principles of the reconstructive triangle.

Microsurgery is a technique used to transfer tissue from one part of the body to the other using anastomosis of very small blood vessels, often in the range of 1–3 mm in diameter. Microsurgery is particularly useful in the reconstruction of complex defects and can also be guided by the principles of the reconstructive triangle.

Overall, the reconstructive triangle concept provides a framework for the surgeon to plan and execute various reconstructive techniques, including flaps, tissue expansion, and microsurgery, in a way that optimizes both functional and esthetic outcomes.

PREOPERATIVE PLANNING
Introduction

A large population of patients with head and neck cancer is elderly with multiple comorbidities. Therefore, whenever planning a reconstruction, patient-related factors and tumor-related factors are considered. When selecting a reconstruction strategy, it is crucial to customize it not only to the defects but also to the individual patient.

Tumor-related factors

1. Site: It is the most significant factor that affects the decision-making while reconstructing a postoncologic resection defect. Broadly there are six subunits of the head and neck region:

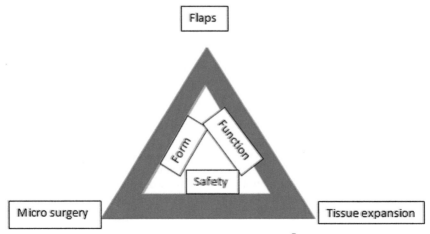

FIG. 4.1 Reconstructive triangle.[7]

i. *Intraoral region*: It includes defects of the tongue, the floor of the mouth, the inner cheek, and the lip. Pharyngeal (oropharynx, hypopharynx) and esophageal defects in the cervical region are too considered here. This region requires thin pliable flaps.

ii. *Mandibular*: It is further divided into central, lateral, and posterior defects. All these defects are usually reconstructed with free osteocutaneous flaps for the best results. These defects require maximum preoperative planning for best-fitting bone flaps.

Planning in such cases can be done with the help of computer-aided design and manufacturing (CAD/CAM). Mandible defects require dental implants for better esthetics and functional result. Small defects of the bony part may be recreated with free bone grafts or bridged with reconstruction plates. But the results are suboptimal as compared with free osteocutaneous flaps.

iii. *Midface/maxillary*: Reconstruction of the maxilla is usually aimed to separate the oral cavity from the nasal cavity and obliterate any dead space. Nose, orbit, and palate reconstruction is also considered in this region. Fasciocutaneous flaps are best suited, and if osseo-integrated implants are required, then free osteocutaneous flaps are considered.

iv. *Cranial*: Defects of anterior, middle, and cranial fossae are there in this region. The main aim of reconstruction is to separate cranial contents from the upper aerodigestive tract. Well-vascularized flaps are used here.

v. *Cutaneous and vi. Scalp*

Small skin flaps are reconstructed with local flaps (like Limberg, rotation, transposition, and advancement flaps), but large defects may require regional flaps or free flaps.

2. Tumor status and nodal status, metastases

The prognosis of the patient depends on the staging of the disease.

Patient-related factors

Systemic factors. ASA (American Society of Anesthesiologists) score is an important determinant of postoperative complications in long-duration surgery. Microvascular operation requires prolonged anesthesia time and is associated with an increased risk of complication.

Comorbidities such as diabetes, hypertension, ischemic heart disease, renal insufficiency, and pulmonary disease also increase the risk of complications and outcomes. History of alcohol intake and smoking should always be considered.

Local factors
- Irradiation
- Previously used local—regional free flaps/scars

Preoperative assessment and optimization. The patient needs to be assessed preoperatively for fitness regarding anesthesia and for feasibility of type of surgery that can be done.

Over the past few years, there has been a growing emphasis on predicting different risk factors in patients who are undergoing prolonged and intricate surgical procedures. Risk stratification should be done and discussed with all the team members. Identification of significant comorbidities and therapies requires specific preoperative management. Hypertension, history of ischemic heart disease, arrhythmias, cardiac and anticoagulant drug intake, history of heart failure, respiratory diseases, obstructive sleep apnea, diabetes, steroid therapy, history of stroke, rheumatoid arthritis—related neck instability, anemia, alcohol intake, smoking, and nutritional status are all considered, and appropriate measures are taken for preoperative optimization of the patient with all these conditions.

Defect analysis and choice of flap. Defects of the head and neck can be categorized into simple, complex, and composite. Depending on the tissue required, an appropriate reconstructive strategy can be selected.

Simple defects: These can be reconstructed with soft tissue flaps such as anterolateral thigh (ALT) flap and radial artery forearm flap (RAFF).

Complex defects: These required input of soft tissue as well as bone. Osteocutaneous free fibula, part of scapula based on dorsal scapular artery perforator, or iliac crest bone flap based on deep circumflex iliac artery can be utilized along with the skin paddle.

Multiple flaps requirement: If the defects require more flaps to reconstruct the different areas, then either multiple free flaps can be done, or one free flap and other regional or a local flap or a chimeric flap can be designed and used.

SCALP AND FOREHEAD RECONSTRUCTION

The scalp has one of the thickest skin in the body. This skin thickness of around 3—8 mm along with the galea aponeurotica limits the scalp pliability. Primary closure with adjacent hair-bearing tissue is always preferred in scalp reconstruction, but it can be done only with a defect of 3 cm or less. Galeal scoring can increase scalp pliability and reduces tension at closure lines, but it has its limitations. Broadly there are two techniques of scalp and forehead reconstruction: nonmicrosurgical procedures and microsurgical techniques.

Nonmicrosurgical Technique

1. Skin grafting: If the underlying calvarium is not exposed, then it can be covered with either a split-thickness graft or a full-thickness skin graft. If calvarium is exposed, another option is to do burring in the outer table up to diploe and then this area can be covered by STSG primarily or after the application of skin/dermal substitute as a secondary procedure.
2. Local flaps: They have the advantage of replacing like with like—the central tenet of reconstructive surgery. This also maintains the thickness of skin here, and more importantly, in the scalp, it will bear hair. This technique is also required where underlying bone is exposed. Most local flaps are pivotal-based flaps or based on advancement principles.
   a. Rotation flaps: Usually used for defects up to 6 cm. The defect is modified into an isosceles triangle. The flap size is usually 5–6 times the defect's base size. The secondary defect is closed primarily with or without the help of Burrow's triangle or back-cut. Multiple rotation flaps can be used especially for central defects.
   b. Transposition flaps: For defects larger than 6 cm, a transposition flap is used. The secondary defect here is covered with STSG. Standing skin deformity is usually seen. If based on named arteries, very large flaps can be raised.
   c. Other flaps:
      • Double opposing rotation flap
      • Pinwheel flap
      • O to Z, O to S, O to A flap
      • Orticochea flaps
      • Juri's temporoparietal occipital flap
   Unlike the scalp, special attention is given to brow position and anterior hairline, which reconstruct the forehead defects. The best cosmetic results are achieved by adhering to the principles of aesthetic subunit, aiming to minimize the visibility of scars.
3. Regional flaps
   There are few options available for the reconstruction of scalp and forehead defects with regional flaps.
   a. Temporalis flap—either temporoparietal fascial flap or temporalis muscle flaps can be used in adjacent areas.
   b. Trapezius myocutaneous or muscle flaps can be used for temporal, occipital, or mastoid defects.
   c. Pedicled latissimus dorsi flap can reach the defect in the occipital region.
4. Tissue expansion
   It has become a preferred technique in the secondary reconstruction of the scalp and forehead. The shape, size, and number of expanders required are based on the size and site of the defect. Expanders of various shapes and sizes are available, which are placed within subgaleal space.
   Tissue expansion is a valuable tool in scalp reconstruction, especially for the reconstruction of large scalp defects. The scalp is a common site of skin cancer and traumatic injuries, and reconstruction of scalp defects can be challenging due to the limited availability of local tissue and the importance of preserving the underlying bones, muscles, and nerves.
   Tissue expansion can be used to create new skin and soft tissue in areas where there is a deficiency, and can be particularly useful in scalp reconstruction because the scalp has a good blood supply and is able to accommodate the expansion of tissue without causing significant functional or aesthetic issues.
   The tissue expansion process typically involves placing a balloon-like device called an expander underneath the skin near the area to be reconstructed. Over time, the expander is gradually filled with sterile saline solution, which stretches the overlying skin and creates new tissue. Once the skin has been sufficiently stretched, the expander is removed, and the new tissue is used to reconstruct the defect.
   In scalp reconstruction, tissue expansion can be used to create large flaps of skin and soft tissue that can be rotated or transposed to cover the defect. The size and shape of the expander can be customized to match the specific requirements of the defect, and the placement of the expander can be carefully planned to optimize the final outcome.
   Tissue expansion is a safe and effective technique for scalp reconstruction that can reduce the need for more complex reconstructive techniques, such as free tissue transfer, while minimizing the risk of functional and aesthetic complications.
5. Microvascular flap technique
   - Free flaps are usually required in areas where locoregional options are not there. They are also used where local flaps have failed, which has led to excessive scarring in the surrounding areas. A

thorough preoperative planning is a must to select recipient vessels and choice of donor flaps.

- The choice of recipient vessel
  - Superficial temporal vessels (STVs)
  - Facial artery
  - Superior thyroid artery
  - Lingual artery
  - Except for STV, all others require a vein graft
- Choice of flaps
  - Latissimus dorsi myocutaneous or muscle-only flap
  - ALT flap
  - Rectus abdominis myocutaneous flap
  - Vastus lateralis muscle-only flap
  - Serratus anterior myocutaneous flap
  - Radial forearm flap (for relatively small defect)
  - Omentum flap for large defects

Forehead reconstruction can involve different techniques depending on the extent and type of deformity, including skin grafts, local tissue flaps, or microsurgical free flaps.

The primary goal of forehead reconstruction is to create a smooth and symmetrical appearance while maintaining proper facial proportions and avoiding functional impairments.

Techniques: Various surgical techniques can be used to reconstruct the forehead, including skin grafts, tissue expansion, local flaps, and free flaps (Figs. 4.2—4.5).

RECONSTRUCTION OF CALVARIUM[8–18]

The bony defect in this region can be the result of resection primary bone malignancies, bone metastasis, osteoradionecrosis, or soft tissue tumor of the scalp that invades the bone. The goals of reconstruction are to protect underlying brain parenchyma and to restore the normal contour of the skull.

Alloplastic materials are most commonly used to reconstruct calvarial defects. The abundant supply availability in all sizes and shapes and no donor site morbidity are the main advantages of this technique. Prevention of infection is a must to avoid extrusion.

The ideal implant is compatible with the surrounding bone and soft tissue, resistant to infection, easily shaped, and should remain stable over time. Examples of alloplastic materials are titanium mesh, polymethyl methacrylate, porous polyethylene, and calcium phosphate cement.

Autologous Technique

The reconstruction of calvarial bony defects can be a complex and challenging procedure that requires careful planning and execution to achieve optimal outcomes. Calvarial bony defects can be caused by a variety of factors, including trauma, tumor resection, and congenital anomalies, and can lead to significant functional and aesthetic issues if left untreated.

The reconstruction of calvarial bony defects typically involves the use of bone grafts or synthetic bone substitutes to replace the missing bone. The choice of graft material depends on the size and location of the defect, as well as the patient's medical history and preferences.

Autologous bone grafts, which are taken from the patient's own body, are often preferred because they have the best chance of integrating with the surrounding bone and providing long-term stability. Common sources of autologous bone grafts for calvarial reconstruction include the iliac crest, rib, and skull itself.

In some cases, synthetic bone substitutes, such as hydroxyapatite or calcium phosphate, may be used instead of or in combination with autologous bone grafts. These materials have the advantage of being readily available and avoiding the need for a second surgical site to harvest bone grafts.

Once the bone graft material has been selected, the reconstruction of the calvarial bony defect typically involves the use of plates, screws, or other fixation devices to stabilize the graft and promote healing. The plates and screws are typically made of titanium or other biocompatible materials and are placed in a way that maximizes the stability of the graft and minimizes the risk of complications, such as infection or displacement.

In some cases, tissue expansion may also be used to create new skin and soft tissue over the reconstructed area, particularly in cases where the defect is large or complex. This can help to improve the cosmetic outcome and reduce the risk of complications.

Overall, the reconstruction with the appropriate graft material and fixation devices, and using advanced techniques such as tissue expansion when necessary, plastic surgeons can help to restore both the form and function of the skull, improving the quality of life for patients who have suffered from calvarial bony defects. Reconstruction of calvarial bony defects is a complex and multistep procedure that requires careful planning and execution to achieve optimal outcomes.

RECONSTRUCTION OF EYELID[19–31]

Detailed understanding and knowledge of eyelid anatomy are required to select the appropriate reconstructive procedure along with a careful assessment of the patient's factors. The eyelids are thin, mobile folds of skin and muscle that cover and protect the eyes. They

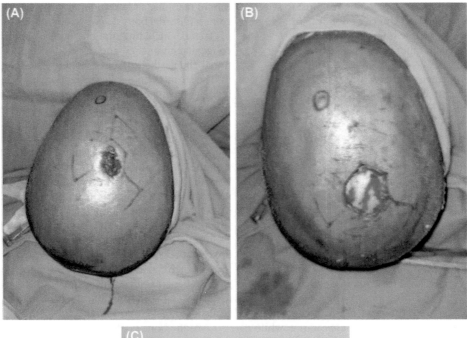

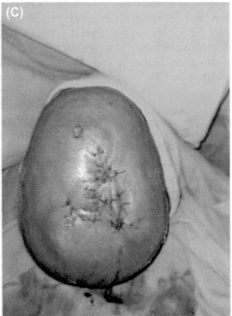

FIG. 4.2 (a) BCC scalp. (b) Hexagonal defect created after tumor excision and three Limberg's flap marked. (c) After closure.

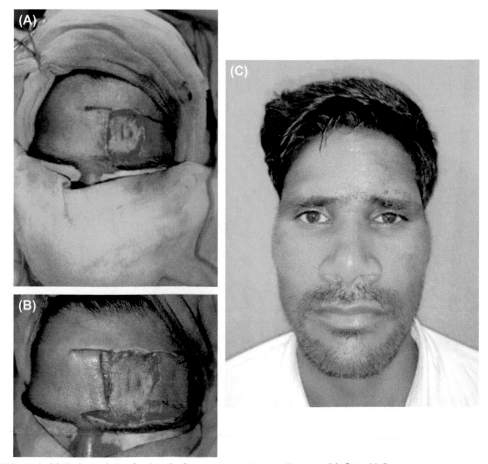

FIG. 4.3 (a) Defect of the forehead after excision of neurofibroma. (b) O to H flaps were planned and harvested. (c) After suture removal with good aesthetic outcome.

consist of several layers of tissue, including skin, muscle, connective tissue, and a thin inner lining called the conjunctiva.

The skin of the eyelids is the thinnest and most delicate on the body, and contains many tiny blood vessels and nerve endings. The skin is attached to a thin layer of muscle called the orbicularis oculi muscle, which encircles the eye and is responsible for closing the eyelids.

Underneath the muscle layer, there is a layer of connective tissue called the tarsus, which gives the eyelid its shape and rigidity. The tarsus is made up of dense fibrous tissue and contains many small glands that produce an oily substance that helps to lubricate the eye.

The inner lining of the eyelid is called the conjunctiva, which is a thin, transparent membrane that covers the white part of the eye (sclera) and the inner surface of the eyelids. The conjunctiva contains many small blood vessels and is responsible for producing mucus and tears, which help to keep the eye moist and protect it from irritation.

The eyelids are also equipped with several specialized structures that help to protect and maintain the health of the eye, including the eyelashes, which act as a barrier against debris and other irritants, and the meibomian glands, which produce oil that helps to prevent tear evaporation and maintain the stability of the tear film.

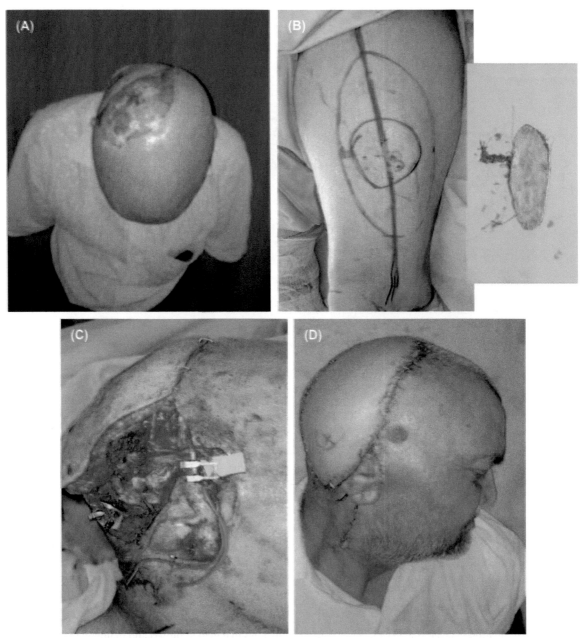

FIG. 4.4 (a) Recurrent squamous cell carcinoma of the scalp. (b) Free ALT flap was harvested to cover the defect; marking; free ALT flap harvested (on right side of the picture). (c) Arterial anastomosis with superficial temporal artery and vein graft was used to anastomosed the flap vein to the external jugular vein. (d) Day 14: Flap well taken up.

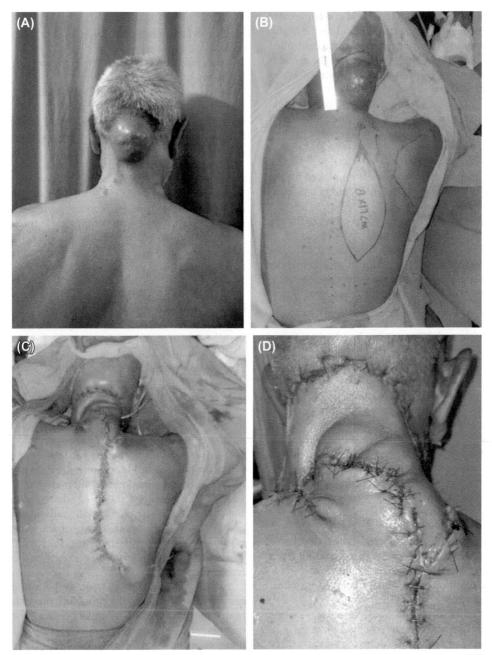

FIG. 4.5   (a) 80 years old patient presented to us as a case of spindle cell neoplasm malignant involving the occiput and upper back of neck. (b) Trapezius myocutaneous flap was planned. (c) Trapezius flap inserted and donor area closed primarily- intraoperative picture. (d) Trapezius flap after 7 days post-operative.

In general, the anatomy of the eyelid is complex and specialized, designed to protect and maintain the health of the eye while also allowing for precise and controlled movement. Understanding the anatomy of the eyelid is crucial for effective diagnosis and treatment of eyelid disorders and injuries.

The eyelid defects are divided into the partial thickness or full thickness defects, anterior or posterior lamellar defects.

Upper Eyelid Reconstruction

Mohs micrographic surgery is usually employed for the resection of tumors of eyelids. Small defects (<5 mm) can be left to heal secondarily.

Partial thickness defects: A defect of <50% of the upper eyelid can be closed primarily.

For defects >50%, full-thickness grafts are preferred. They can either be taken from other upper eyelids or postauricular repair to match the recipient area. Supraclavicular and upper trunk are other donor sites.

Full-thickness defects:
- Defects of around 25% may be closed primarily.
- A pentagonal defect may be created for better aesthetic correction. The lid margin is approximated separately. The tarsal plate and skin are closed to complete the layered reconstruction.
- 25%–75% defects of the upper eyelid can be closed with a modified Hugh's advancement flap/sliding transconjunctival flap with a skin graft or composite graft that is covered by myocutaneous advancement flap.
  - ➤ Key to successful closure of the upper eyelid is as follows:
    1. Reestablishment of the posterior mucosal layer
    2. A structural support layer
    3. Anteriorly a well-vascularized covering layer
  - ➤ Composite grafts can cover a larger area

Free tarsal graft or contralateral upper lid, conjunctival graft can also be used.

Nasal septal cartilage and hard palate are also the donor site for free grafts to replace tarsal plate.

The anterior covering is done by either using bipedicled skin—orbicularis oris muscle flap, paramedian forehead flaps, inverted or Tenzel flap, or Cutler Beard flap.

Defects of >75% area are difficult and challenging to reconstruct. The options include Cutler Beard flap, forehead flap, Fricke's flap (Lateral temporal flap), and glabellar flap.

Lower Eyelid Reconstruction

Smaller defects <30% can be closed primarily with or without cantholysis.

Moderate defects (30%–50%) are reconstructed in layers.

Hugh's tarso conjunctival flap is used for posterior lamella, and for anterior lamella, either cheek advancement flap, full-thickness graft, nasojugal flap, or Tripier flap is used. Tenzel semicircular flap is also used for moderate-sized defects.

Large defects are reconstructed with either a Mustarde cheek rotation flap in conjunction with a composite graft or Hughs flap. Mustarde flap should be anchored to the inferior orbital rim periosteum to prevent tension to cause ectropion or vertical shortening. Other options to reconstruct the lower eyelid include paramedian/median forehead flap, lateral temporal flap, and nasojugal flap (Fig. 4.6).

NOSE RECONSTRUCTION[11,32–57]

Reconstruction of the nose is a complex surgical procedure that is often required to restore the form and function of the nose following trauma or cancer surgery. The nose is a highly visible and important feature of the face, and any defects or deformities can have a significant impact on the patient's self-esteem and quality of life.

There are several techniques that can be used for nasal reconstruction, including local flaps, skin grafts, and tissue expansion. The specific technique used depends on the size and location of the defect, as well as the patient's individual needs and preferences.

Local flaps involve transferring adjacent skin and tissue to the defect site, while skin grafts involve transplanting skin from another area of the body. Tissue expansion involves stretching the skin over time to create additional tissue that can be used for reconstruction.

Nasal reconstruction is typically performed under general anesthesia, and the procedure may take several hours to complete. After the procedure, the patient may experience some discomfort and swelling, but these symptoms can usually be managed with pain medication and ice packs.

The overall goal of nasal reconstruction is to restore both the form and function of the nose, while minimizing scarring and achieving a natural-looking result. With careful planning and skilled execution, nasal reconstruction can be a highly successful procedure that can significantly improve the patient's quality of life.

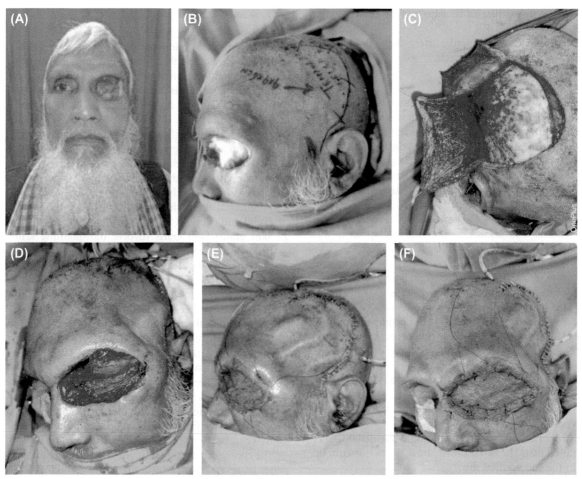

FIG. 4.6 (a) Patient of intra orbital tumor presented to us post excision with raw area in the left orbit. (b) Temporalis muscle with STSG was planned for lining of the orbit to fit orbital prosthesis at a later stage. (c) Temporalis muscle flap raised. (d) Flap insetted into the orbit. (e) Temporalis muscle flap covered with the STSG; donor area closed over the drain (lateral view). (f) Temporalis muscle flap covered with the STSG; donor area closed over drain (anterior view).

Because of its location, the nose is a common site for the development of basal cell carcinoma. The subunit concept is followed critically in nasal reconstruction.

While planning the reconstruction, three distinct anatomic layers are considered in the nose that is skin cover, cartilaginous/bony support, and nasal mucosal lining.

For composite, trilamellar defects, locoregional flaps are used.

Nasolabial flap or facial artery musculomucosal (FAMM) flaps can be used for the lining.

Workhorse flap is the forehead flap.

The small defect can be covered with full-thickness skin grafts from preauricular, postauricular, supraclavicular, or forehead region.

Upper defects of small size can be reconstructed with a dorsal nasal flap, glabellar flap, and Rieger flap and Miter flap.

A bilobed flap is used for lower third nose defects of small size.

Nasolabial flaps can be used to reconstruct the nasal lateral wall or ala. They can be either superior or inferiorly based.

Single-staged nasolabial flaps can be used for alar defects.

V–Y flap based on angular artery can be used for the lateral wall of the nose defects.

Forehead Flap

The use of the forehead flap for nasal reconstruction dates back to ancient India, where it was first described in the Sushruta Samhita, an ancient text on surgery and medicine. The technique was later reintroduced in the Western world by Italian surgeon Gaspare Tagliacozzi in the 16th century, and it has since been further refined and developed by numerous plastic surgeons over the centuries.

- This is the workhorse flap for nasal reconstruction.
- This is also known as the Indian flap as it was practiced in ancient India by Kumhar caste.
- This flap can be used for any nasal reconstruction from severe tip and alar loss to a lateral nasal defect.
- It can be raised in any desired shape.
- It is based on the supratrochlear vessels.

A vertical flap is designed if the height of the forehead is more than 3 inches, otherwise, it is planned obliquely. Planning in reverse is very critical before committing the incision.

If larger flaps are required, an incision delay is used.
Surgical steps:
- Handheld doppler helps in identifying and mark the vessels.
- After careful planning and marking, the distal flap is raised first. The flap is raised above the periosteum up to the supraorbital rim.
- Care should be taken to avoid injury to supratrochlear vessels.
- Dissection is continued till the flap reaches the desired area without tension.
- Donor area can be closed primarily or left as such for healing by secondary intention.
- In stage 2, the pedicle is divided after 3–4 weeks. The distal part is thinned, and the nasal defect is completely covered and closed with fine sutures. The proximal part is turned back toward the forehead to achieve a good brow match.

Other Options

Prefabricated and prelaminated free flaps are often the only option for nasal reconstruction where the foreheal flap is not available. The best option is the RAFF. Free fibula along with skin paddle can be used where the defects involved the maxilla.

CHEEK AND LIP DEFECTS[50,58–83]
Cheek Reconstruction

There are several surgical options available for reconstructing a cheek, and the choice of technique depends on the size and location of the defect, as well as the patient's individual needs and preferences. Some of the most common surgical options for cheek reconstruction include the following:
1. Local flaps: This technique involves transferring tissue from adjacent areas of the face to the defect site. The most commonly used flaps for cheek reconstruction include the nasolabial flap, which uses tissue from the cheek and upper lip, and the infraorbital flap, which uses tissue from the lower eyelid and cheek.
2. Skin grafts: Skin grafts involve transplanting skin from another area of the body, typically the thigh or abdomen, to the defect site. This technique is often used for larger defects that cannot be repaired with local flaps.
3. Microvascular free flaps: This technique involves transplanting tissue from another part of the body, such as the forearm or thigh, to the defect site using microsurgical techniques. This allows for a larger volume of tissue to be transferred, which can be useful for more extensive defects.
4. Tissue expansion: This involves stretching the skin over time using a silicone balloon or other device, which allows for the creation of additional tissue that can be used for reconstruction.

The choice of technique for cheek reconstruction depends on several factors, including the size and location of the defect, the patient's individual needs and preferences, and the experience and expertise of the surgeon. With careful planning and skilled execution, cheek reconstruction can be a highly successful procedure that can significantly improve the patient's quality of life.

Ideally, scars on the cheek should be carefully planned according to relaxed skin tension lines (RSTL).

Reconstruction options for reconstruction of cheek defects are as follows:
- Healing by secondary intention—for small and superficial defects.
- Primary closure depends on the location, size, and surrounding skin laxity. Even large defects in older patients can be closed primarily.
- Skin grafts: Full-thickness skin grafts are preferred.
- Local flaps
  - Pivotal-based, rotation, transposition flap
  - Advancement flap: V–Y advancement flaps

Transposition flaps such as bilobed flaps, banner flaps, and rhomboid flaps are all employed for various defects of the cheek.

Limberg flap: A classic rhomboid flap has two angles at 60 and 120°. The flap should be positioned in the direction of RSTL. Four options can be planned for a rhombus. Final work is done that is based on skin laxity and should be parallel to RSTL. A line is drawn that is an extension of the short diagonal of the rhombus. The length of this line is equal to the side of the rhombus. Another line is drawn, which is parallel to the adjacent side of the rhombus, and its length is similar to any side of the rhombus. The flap is raised in the subcutaneous region preserving the subdermal and papillary plexus. The donor area is closed primarily.

- Regional flaps
  - Cheek advancement and rotation flap
  - Cervicopectoral flap
  - Deltopectoral flap
  - Pectoralis major myocutaneous flap
  - Trapezius flap
  - Supraclavicular flap
  - Cervicothoracic flap
- Free flaps:
  - RAFF, ALT flap, gracilis myocutaneous flap, lateral arm flap
- Tissue expansion: For similar color and skin texture, it cannot be done simultaneously with tumor excision and it is a multistaged procedure (Figs. 4.7–4.12).

Lip reconstruction

Lips are among the principal aesthetic units of the face. Functionally, it is involved in verbal and nonverbal communication, deglutition, and oral competence. The goals of reconstruction are therefore to restore the aesthetic appearance and functional capabilities by aperture, mobility, sensation, and appearance. Various options to reconstruct the defects of the lip are as follows:

Superficial cutaneous defects of the lip can be closed either primarily or can be skin grafted.

Local flaps based on cheek advancement, nasolabial flap or lateral V–Y advancement can be used for deeper or complex defects.

Vermilion defects:
- Small defects are managed by musculomucosal advancement flaps.
- Lesions that are close to vermilion are excised vertically to facilitate white roll alignment.

- Undermining of buccal mucosa along with the advancement is used to resurface the mucocutaneous region.
- Other options are lip-sharing procedure, cross-lip mucosal flap, FAMM flap.

Small Full-thickness Defects

- Lower lip defects of <40% can be closed primarily.
- Upper lip defects of <25% are preferably closed primarily.
- Shield-shaped excision of small tumors/lesions is preferred for accurate alignment of all layers of the lip.
- W-plasty design may be incorporated during excision of lower lip lesion to avoid extension of scar inferiorly and labiomental crease may be preserved.

Intermediate/mid-sized full-thickness defects
Lower lip

1. Schuchardt procedure
2. Webster's technique
3. Bengt–Johansson staircase technique
4. Lip switch procedure—reverse abbe flap, Estlander flap (Fig. 4.13)
5. Gille's fan flap
6. Karapandzic flap
7. McGregor flap

Upper lip

1. Abbe's flap
2. Reverse Estlander
3. Reverse Karapandzic

The McGregor flap is a technique used for lip reconstruction, named after the plastic surgeon Ian McGregor who first described the technique in the 1970s. This flap is typically used for repairing defects on the lower lip, although it can also be used for upper lip reconstruction.

The McGregor flap is a type of local flap that involves transferring tissue from the adjacent area of the lip to the defect site. The flap is designed to include the orbicularis oris muscle, which is responsible for lip movement, as well as the underlying mucosa and submucosal tissue.

The flap is elevated and rotated into the defect site, and the donor site is closed primarily. The advantage of the McGregor flap is that it provides a reliable reconstruction that preserves the functional and aesthetic properties of the lip.

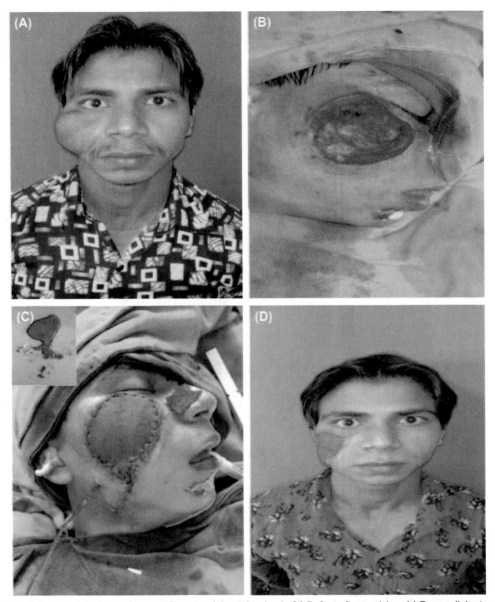

FIG. 4.7 (a) Young male with neurofibroma of the right cheek. (b) Defect after excision. (c) Free radial artery forearm fascio-cutaneous flap. (d) Follow-up photo after 3 months.

Another technique that can be used is the Abbe flap, which involves taking a segment of tissue from the inner cheek and rotating it into the defect area. This technique can be particularly useful if there is not enough tissue available in the lip for reconstruction.

There are several techniques that can be used for total lip reconstruction, but one of the most common is the Karapandzic flap. This involves taking a segment of tissue from the upper or lower lip and rotating it

into the defect area. The tissue is then sutured into place, and the blood supply is reestablished to ensure that the tissue remains alive and healthy.

Karapandzic flap is a surgical technique used for reconstructing defects in the lower lip. The technique was developed by Dr. Zoran Karapandzic, a Serbian plastic surgeon, in 1985.

The procedure involves taking a segment of tissue from the upper or lower lip and rotating it into the

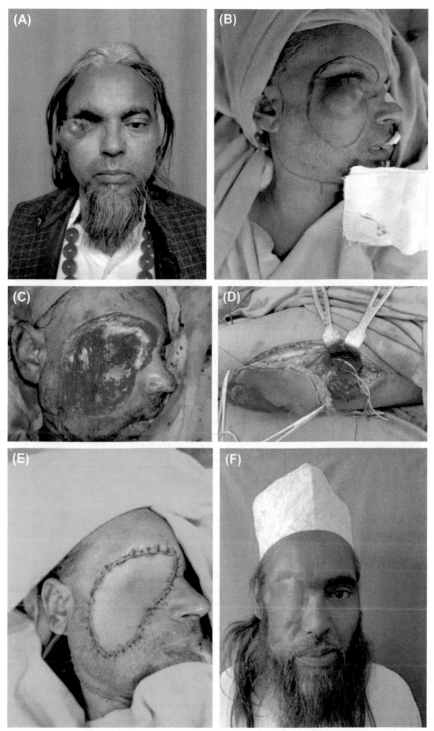

FIG. 4.8 (a) Recurrent squamous cell carcinoma (Rt) side cheek involving the infra orbital region. (b) Marking for wide local excision. (c) Defect after excision. (d) Free ALT flap harvesting. (e) Immediate postoperative photo. (f) Follow-up after 6 months.

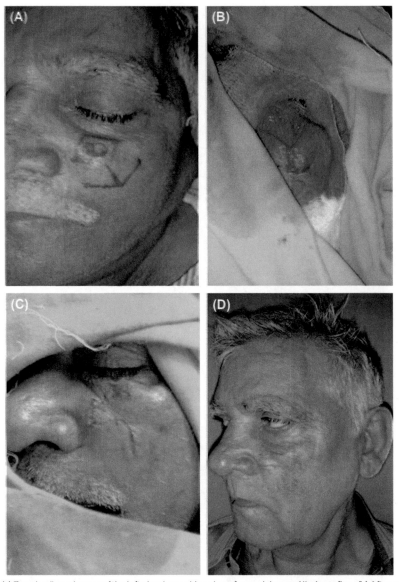

FIG. 4.9   (a) Basal cell carcinoma of the left cheek; marking done for excision and limberg flap. (b) After excision and flap harvesting. (c) Limberg's flap inplace sutured into the defect. (d) Post op photograph taken after 3 months.

defect area. The tissue is then sutured into place, and the blood supply is reestablished to ensure that the tissue remains alive and healthy. The flap can be used to repair a wide range of defects, including those caused by trauma or cancer excision.

One of the advantages of the Karapandzic flap is that it preserves the natural appearance and function of the lip, as the tissue used for the reconstruction is taken from the same area. The procedure also has a low rate of complications and can be performed under local anesthesia.

Overall, the Karapandzic flap is a valuable technique for reconstructing defects in the lower lip and has been widely adopted by plastic surgeons around the world (Figs. 4.14 and 4.15).

Gillies' fan flap is a surgical technique used for reconstructing defects on the cheek, particularly after the removal of skin cancer or other lesions. The technique was developed by Sir Harold Gillies, a pioneering plastic surgeon who is often referred to as the father of modern plastic surgery.

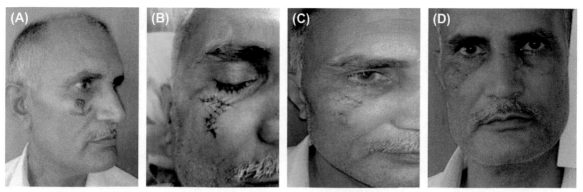

FIG. 4.10 (a) BCC right cheek. (b) Limberg's flap used to cover the defect. (c) After suture removal (post op day 8). (d) After 1 month showing well hidden scars.

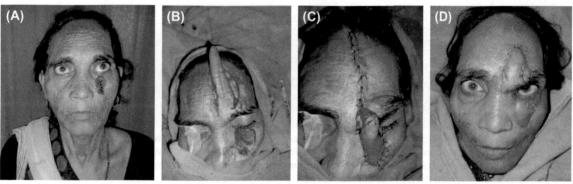

FIG. 4.11 (a) Basal cell carcinoma left cheek infra orbital region. (b) Paramedian forehead flap raised to cover the defect. (c) Forehead flap insetted into the defect. (d) After second stage of operation.

The procedure involves taking a triangular-shaped flap of skin and subcutaneous tissue from the cheek, which is then rotated into the defect area. The flap is designed to resemble a fan, with the apex of the triangle at the defect site and the base of the triangle at the donor site. The flap is then sutured into place and the blood supply is reestablished to ensure that the tissue remains alive and healthy.

One of the advantages of the Gillies' fan flap is that it provides a good match for the color and texture of the surrounding skin, as the tissue used for the reconstruction is taken from the same area. The procedure also has a low rate of complications and can be performed under local anesthesia.

In some cases, the surgeon may also use skin grafts or other tissue flaps to help rebuild the lip. The goal of total lip reconstruction is to restore the appearance and function of the lip, as well as to minimize scarring and other complications.

After the reconstruction surgery, the patient will typically need to stay in the hospital for a few days to monitor their progress and ensure that the tissue is healing properly. The patient will also need to follow a specific care plan, which may include taking medications, avoiding certain foods, and avoiding smoking or other activities that could interfere with the healing process.

Overall, total lip reconstruction is a complex and challenging procedure, but it can help patients regain their confidence and improve their quality of life after cancer or other lip-related issues. It is important to work with an experienced and qualified plastic surgeon who can provide personalized care and ensure the best possible outcome for each individual patient.

Total Lip Defects

Lip defects of more than 80% are difficult to reconstruct with lower locoregional flaps. Various options that can be considered are:

Bernard cheiloplasty.

Webster's modification of Bernard's procedure.

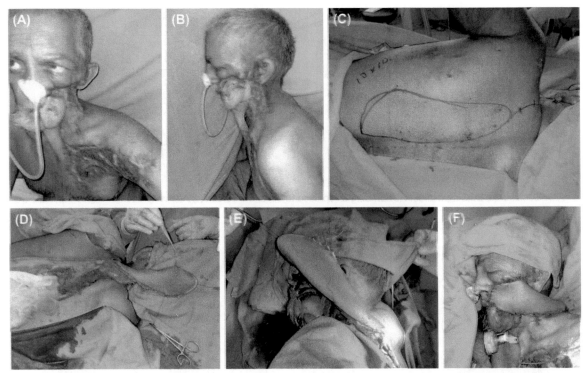

FIG. 4.12 (a) 85 years old patient presented to us as a case of failed deltopectoral flap with probable residual disease over the cheek. (b) Lateral view preoperative. (c) Trapezius myocutaneous flap was planned. Picture showing the markings of unusually large flap. (d) Flap raised based on the branch of transverse cervical artery. (e) Photograph showing the reach of this flap. (f) Flap insetted into the cheek defect.

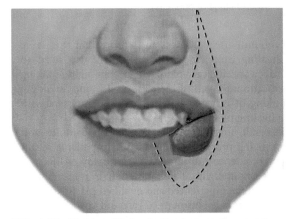

FIG. 4.13 Marking of Estlander flap for lower lip reconstruction; defect located on lateral aspect.

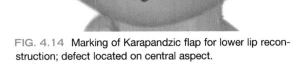

FIG. 4.14 Marking of Karapandzic flap for lower lip reconstruction; defect located on central aspect.

Nasolabial flaps—Fujimori's gate flap, Von Bran's flap.

Regional flaps—submental flap, deltopectoral flap (DP) flap.

Free flaps: RAFF, gracilis flap.

Vermilion is usually reconstructed at a later stage (Figs. 4.16—4.18).

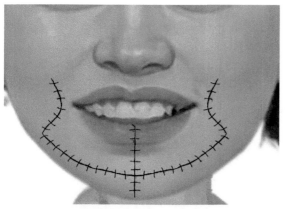

FIG. 4.15 Karapandzic flap for lower lip reconstruction; after closure of the defect.

MANDIBLE RECONSTRUCTION[84–96]

The primary objective of mandibular reconstruction is to achieve premorbid form and function. The newly reconstructed mandible should be able to support osteointegrated implants or dentures. The patient should be able to eat a normal diet and should have a normal appearance with the skin envelope. This is achieved by careful optimization of patient and recipient area and proper selection of donor site, appropriate surgical technique, and reconstructive schedule or timeline. There are two techniques of bony reconstruction:

Ist: Nonvascularized bone graft

IInd: Vascularized free tissue transfer

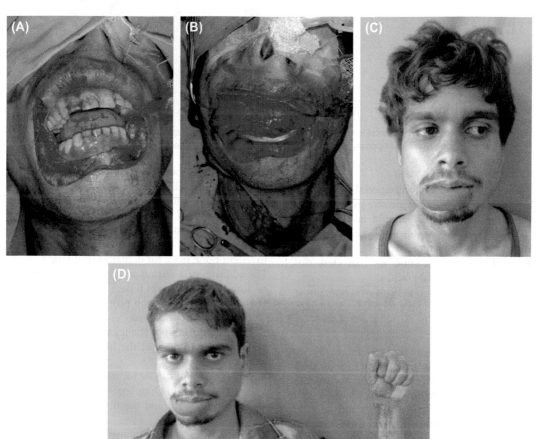

FIG. 4.16 (a) Defect of the lower lip after excision of SCC. Whole of the lower lip was removed for margin clearance. (b) Radial artery forearm flap along with palmaris longus tendon which was used as a sling to maintain the height of the neo-lower lip. (c) After 2 months of reconstruction. (d) After 3 months of reconstruction also showing the donor area of the forearm.

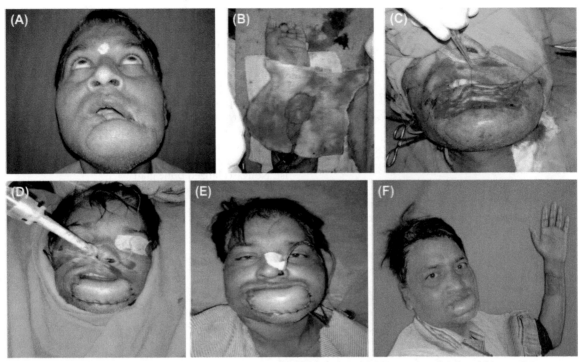

FIG. 4.17 (a) Post tumor excision lower lip defect. (b) RAFF elevated. (c) Flap cover of defect. (d) Immediate post operative photo. (e) Post operative photo after 1 week. (f) Follow-up photo after 2 months.

Nonvascularized Bone Grafts

Commonly used for small defects especially after a section of benign tumors or nonaggressive malignances.

Surrounding tissue usually should not have been disrupted; that is, it requires a healthy, well-vascularized bed and covering.

Potential donor sites are either the iliac crest, ribs, fibula, tibia, or split calvarial graft.

These should be avoided in patients who have undergone radiotherapy or might require adjuvant radiotherapy.

Vascularized Free Tissue Transfer

With improvement in microsurgical techniques, the use of vascular as bone flaps has increased in the past two - decades. It has several advantages over nonvascular bone graphs. Bony union time is less in cases with bone flaps, the risk of infection is less, and they can be used in compromised wound beds and where soft tissue deficiency is there.

Free fibula flap

First described in the late 1980s by Hidalgo, now it has become a standard procedure for mandible reconstruction.

The advantages of a free fibular flap are as follows:

The length of the bone can be up to 26 cm, length of the pedicle, and reliability.

Based on both endosteal blood supply and periosteal blood supply.

Multiple osteotomies can be made to shape it better.

A large skin pedal can also be raised with it.

Excellent bone stock for dental rehabilitation.

The addition of a second surgeon to harvest the fibula simultaneously saves time.

Use of CAD/CAM helps in proper planning.

Important surgical steps:

Patient positioning: The leg is bent at the knee joint and internally rotated at the hip joint and supported with a sand bag.

- Skin perforator can be located preoperatively with a hand-held audio Doppler.
- Proximally 6 cm and distally 8 cm of bone should be left intact.
- In the cases of osteocutaneous flap, the perforator should be identified first.
- During dissection in the flexor compartment, care should be taken to avoid injury to peroneal vessels.
- Distal and proximal osteotomies are done, and bone is retracted laterally and then the anterior interosseous membrane is divided.

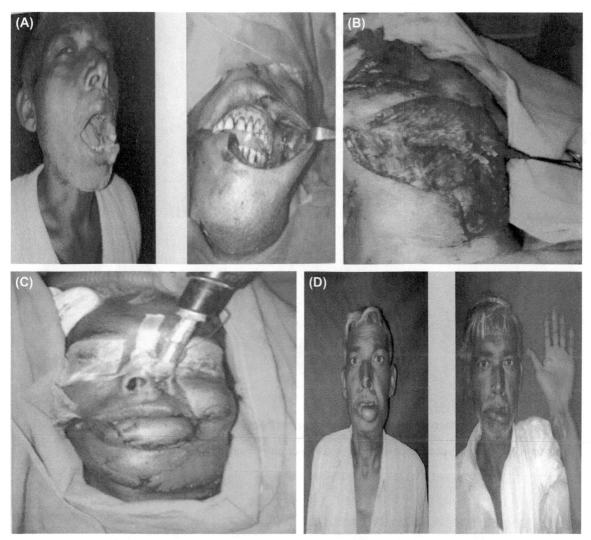

FIG. 4.18 (a) Carcinoma lower lip left side involving the commissure. (b) Flap raised and vascular anastomosis done with facial vessels. (c) Flap insetted. (d) Post op picture taken after 3 months.

- A cuff muscle is left over the fibula, and care should be taken to avoid striping of the periosteum from the fibula.
- Exposure of interosseous septum by bluntly separating the extensors over it. The septum is dived keeping a distance of 1 cm from the fibula.
- Careful dissection of all surrounding muscles.
- Distal pedicles may be ligated early or distal flow can be used during the reshaping of the fibula into the desired neomandible of the maxilla.
- A drain is inserted and if the skin paddle is small then the donor area can be closed primarily or else grafted (Figs. 4.19 and 4.20).

Iliac crest bone flap

- It is also used for extensive defects of the mandible and maxilla.
- It is an extensive source of bone in various shapes and sizes.
- CAD/CAM can be used for proper planning.
- Anatomy is well defined.
- There is less donor site morbidity.
  Disadvantages:
- It has a short pedicle.
- Unreliable venous drainage.
- Donor side morbidity if proper closure is not done.

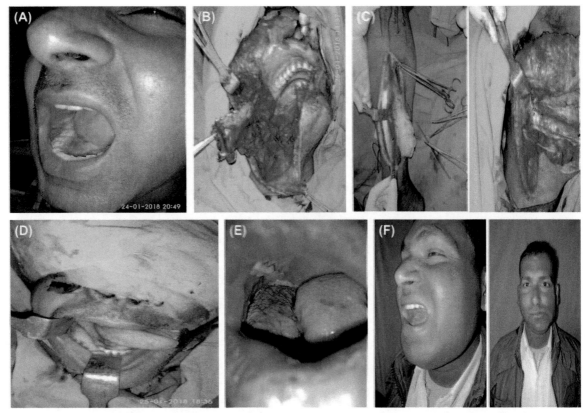

FIG. 4.19 (a) Right side carcinoma buccal mucosa involving the gingiva. (b) Intra operative photo with enbloc excision of tumor along with segmental mandibulectomy. (c) Free fibula fascio-cutaneous flap elevated and insetted. (d) Immediate post operative photo. (e) Follow-up after 1 month. (f) Follow-up after 6 months.

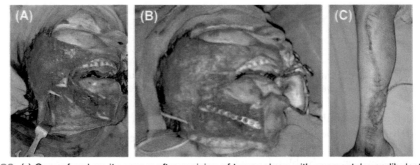

FIG. 4.20 (a) Case of oral cavity cancer after excision of tumor along with segmental mandibulectomy. (b) Free osteocutaneous fibular flap used for mandibular reconstruction. (c) Donor area of the fibula flap.

Scapular flap

- Based on the circumflex scapular artery, which itself is the branch of the axillary artery.
- A thin flap can be raised and a chimeric flap can be a plan for complex defects.
- Smaller mandible defects can be reconstructed with this flap.
- The skin component is good for intraoral reconstruction as it is hairless and less adipose tissue is there.
- The donor site can be closed primarily.
- It is also a good donor site for maxillary reconstruction.

MAXILLARY RECONSTRUCTION[97–106]

The reconstruction of the maxilla after tumor resection typically involves a multidisciplinary approach that may include the use of bone grafts, free tissue transfer, and dental implants. The specific technique used will depend on the extent of the defect and the individual needs of the patient.

In cases where the defect is small, a bone graft may be used to fill in the gap left by the tumor resection. This can be done using bone from the patient's own body, such as the iliac crest, or using bone from a donor.

For larger defects, a free tissue transfer may be necessary. This involves transferring a piece of tissue, often taken from the patient's thigh or abdomen, along with its blood supply, to the defect site. The transferred tissue may include bone, muscle, and skin, and it can be used to reconstruct the missing portion of the maxilla.

In cases where teeth have been lost due to the tumor resection, dental implants may be used to restore the patient's ability to eat and speak normally. Dental implants are artificial tooth roots that are implanted into the jawbone, and they can be used to support a prosthetic tooth or denture.

Reconstruction of the maxilla after tumor resection is a complex procedure that requires careful planning and coordination between the surgical team and other healthcare professionals, such as dentists and maxillofacial prosthodontists. Patients should work closely with their healthcare team to determine the best approach for their individual needs and goals.

Cordeiro's approach is a technique used for the reconstruction of large maxillary defects following tumor resection. The technique was developed by Dr. Peter G. Cordeiro, a plastic surgeon at Memorial Sloan-Kettering Cancer Center in New York.

The Cordeiro approach involves the use of a free tissue transfer, typically a fibula-free flap, which is a piece of tissue, including bone, muscle, and skin, taken from the patient's leg. The fibula is chosen because it is a long, straight bone that can be used to reconstruct the missing part of the maxilla.

During the procedure, the fibula is harvested along with its blood vessels and transferred to the defect site. The bone is then shaped to fit the contour of the maxilla, and the soft tissue is draped over the bone to provide coverage.

One of the advantages of the Cordeiro approach is that it allows for the reconstruction of large maxillary defects while preserving the patient's facial contour and symmetry. The technique also has a high success rate, with low rates of complications and donor site morbidity.

Like all surgical techniques, the Cordeiro approach requires careful planning and execution to achieve the best possible outcome. Patients considering this technique should discuss their options with a qualified plastic surgeon who can help determine whether the Cordeiro approach is the best choice for their individual needs and goals.

Reconstruction of the maxilla can be performed at the time of resection that is primaraxillary

reconstruction or it can be done at a later stage. It also depends on the disease process, patient preferences, preoperative and postoperative radiotherapy, and, more importantly on patients' general conditions.

The goals of midface reconstruction are first
- to provide oronasal separation,
- to support the eye.
- to form patent nasal airway,
- to restore facial esthetics,
- dental rehabilitation, and
- proper speech

Classification of Maxillary Defects

Brown at all described the defects of the maxilla into four classes based on vertical extent after the section and into three classes based on the horizontal extent of the resection.

Later on, they added classified as the orbit of the maxillary defect and class six as nasomaxillary defect.

The Cordeiro approach for the reconstruction of large maxillary defects is tailored to the specific type of defect being addressed. There are several types of maxillary defects, each of which may require a slightly different approach.

1. Midfacial defects: Midfacial defects refer to defects that involve the upper jawbone and the area surrounding the nose and eyes. These types of defects may require a fibula free flap or a scapula free flap, depending on the extent of the defect and the patient's individual needs.
2. Maxillary sinus defects: Maxillary sinus defects are defects that involve the sinus cavity located in the maxilla. These types of defects may require the use of a fibula free flap or a radial forearm free flap to reconstruct the bony structures surrounding the sinus cavity.
3. Orbital defects: Orbital defects refer to defects that involve the eye socket. These types of defects may require a scapula free flap or a latissimus dorsi flap, which can be used to reconstruct the soft tissue and bone around the eye.
4. Hemimaxillectomy defects: Hemimaxillectomy defects refer to defects that involve the removal of one half of the maxilla. These types of defects may require the use of a fibula free-flap, which can be used to reconstruct the missing bony structures of the maxilla.

Options for Maxillary Reconstruction
Locoregional tissue flaps

1. The temporalis flap is based on the deep temporal artery; it is a myofascial flap that reaches the oral cavity under the zygoma.
2. FAMM is based on the facial artery, consists of buccal mucosa and buccinator muscles, and it is suited for lateral palatal defects.

3. Palatal mucoperiosteal flap.
4. Buccal pad of fat.
5. Submental flap based on reverse flow from the facial artery.

Free flaps: For larger and more complex defects, free flaps are usually the first line of reconstruction.

i. Radial artery forearm fasiocutaneous flap (RAFF): RAFF flap provided thin and supple tissue for intraoral and external defects. Small portion of radius bone can also be harvested to reconstruct maxillary bone defects.
ii. Fibular flaps: It can be used for orbital and alveolar reconstruction. Osteocutaneous flap can be used to cover the soft tissue defects.
iii. Illac crest flap.
iv. Scapular flap.
v. Rectus abdominis flap.
vi. ALT flap: It is used to reconstruct large defects and obliterate the large cavity.

Summary of maxillary reconstruction according to different defects (Cordeiro's)

Type I: Limited maxillectomy
Reconstructed with bone graft and cavity is filled with RAFF.

Type II: Subtotal maxillectomy
RAFF with part of the radial bone to reconstruct anterior wall of the maxilla for good aesthetic outcome.

Type III (A): Total maxillectomy with orbital contents intact
Rectus abdominis free flap or pedicled temporalis flap is used to obliterate the space and bone graft is used to reconstruct the orbital floor.

Type III (B): Total maxillectomy with orbital exenteration
Reconstruction with rectus abdominis free flap.

Type IV: Orbitomaxillectomy with intact palate
Rectus abdominis free flap with or without skin paddle.

In general, the Cordeiro approach for the reconstruction of large maxillary defects involves the use of a free tissue transfer, typically a fibula free flap, to reconstruct the missing bony structures and soft tissue of the maxilla. The specific approach used will depend on the type and extent of the defect, as well as the patient's individual needs and goals.

RECONSTRUCTION OF THE ORAL CAVITY[107–115]

The oral cavity consists of the upper lip, lower lip, alveolar ridges of the mandible and maxilla, buccal mucosa, hard palate, floor of the mouth, retromolar trigone, and anterior two-thirds of the tongue. Defects of various sizes and composition are created after the resection of involved buccal mucosa, retromolar trigone, floor of the mouth, and tongue cancer. These defects often require aesthetic and functional reconstruction or correction.

Reconstructive Goals and Choices of the Flap

Buccal mucosa and retromolar trigone

Buccal mucosa acts as a barrier between facial muscles and the oral cavity. This also contributes for the symmetry of the face, smile creation, and vocalization.

Flap choices include grafts for the small defects and local flaps such as FAMM, submental, tongue flap, and thin supraclavicular flap. Large defects can be reconstructed with free radial forearm flap, MSAP, lateral arm flap, and thin ALT flap. Pedicled flaps such as DP flap and PMMC flap may also be used.

Floor of the mouth

Defects usually are found in association with resection of tongue and the mandible. It is reconstructed to separate the oral cavity from the contents of the neck.

Free flaps (composite and chimeric)
Pedicled PMMC
Local flaps are not available due to the ligation of facial artery

Glossectomy defects

One of the most common intraoral defects.
Reconstruction is required for speech and swallowing functions.
The remnant tongue will play a role in future tongue function.
Donor flaps need to be supple, thin, and pliable.
Sensate flaps are a good option to reconstruct the defect, as the lingual nerve stump can be used for coaptation with the donor sensory nerve.

Flap choices. Defect may be closed primarily if the resected tongue is less than one-third of the total or it can be grafted.

If floor of the mouth is also involved, then small flap is required to separate the oral cavity from the neck.

For hemiglossectomy defects, free RAFF or thin ALT are good options as they are pliable and can easily be folded to create lingual sulcus.

For subtotal and total glossectomy defects, thick flaps are required to provide the bulk to obliterate the large space created after resection of the tongue, floor of the mouth, and sometimes mandible. ALT flap, thick radial artery flap (if present), rectus abdominis flap and muscle-only free flap with STSG (Figs. 4.21–4.25).

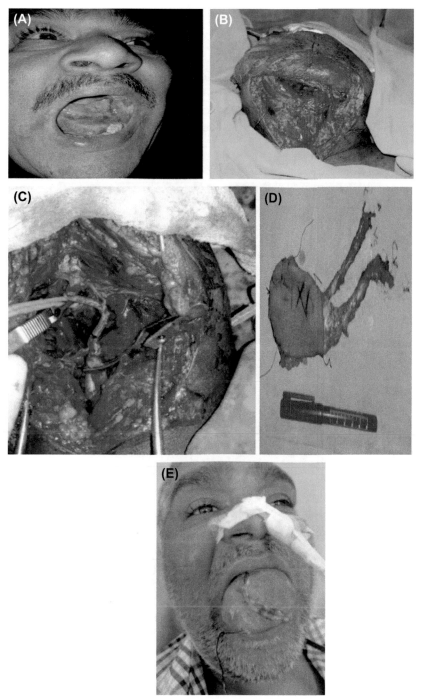

FIG. 4.21   (a) Case of carcinoma tongue involving the left lateral border. (b) Post-wide local excision defect. (c) Free radial forearm flap harvested; flap vessels anastomosed to the facial vessels. (d) Two weeks post-op picture. The bulk of the flap usually reduces after the radiation therapy.

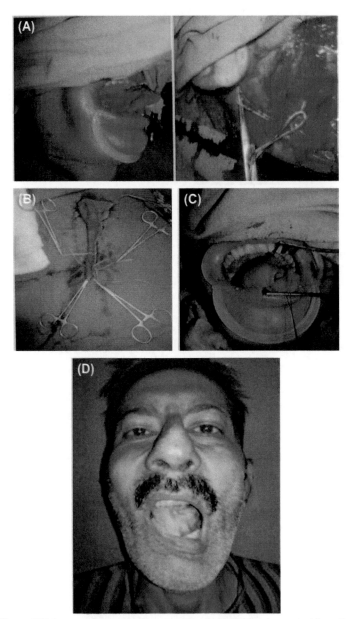

FIG. 4.22 (a) Case of CA tongue of the right lateral border. (b) RAFF flap harvested from the left forearm. (c) Flap insetted to reconstruct the tongue. (d) Follow-up after 3 months.

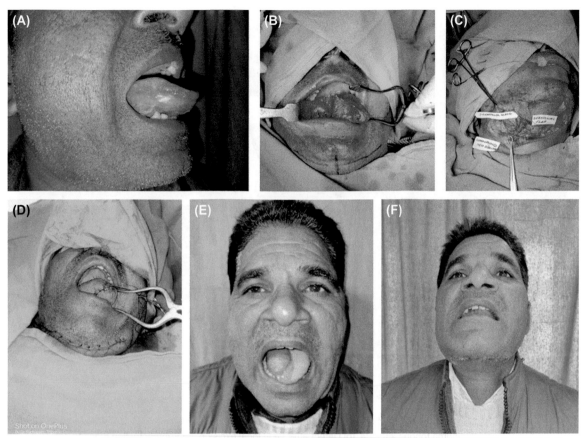

FIG. 4.23 (a) Carcinoma tongue left side. (b) Defect after wide local excision. (c) Submental flap raised. (d) Immediate post operative. (e) One month follow-up. (f) Two months follow-up showing the minimal neck scar.

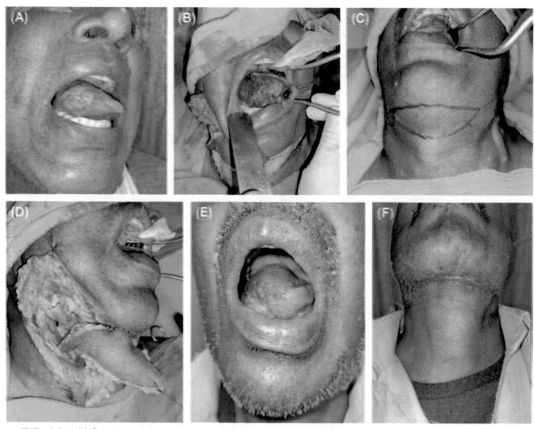

FIG. 4.24 (a) Carcinoma tongue left side. (b) Defect after wide local excision. (c) Submental flap marking. (d) Submental flap raised. (e) Three months follow-up. (f) Three months follow-up showing the minimal neck scar.

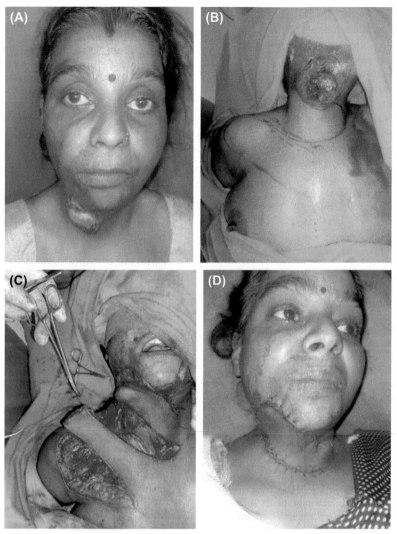

FIG. 4.25 (a) Case of MArjolin's ulcer (SCC) over the neck. (b) Local flaps were planned in such a way that whole of the area is closed primarily using two flaps. (c) Flaps raised; superior flap was raised to cover the defect after excision of the tumor and the second flap which is a deltopectoral flap raised to cover the secondary defect. (d) After flap insetting. This has the advantage over the two staged procedure that the patient can receive early adjuvant radiotherapy.

SUMMARY

Head and neck reconstruction is a complex surgical procedure aimed at restoring structures in the head and neck area that have been affected by trauma or cancer surgery. Various techniques can be used, including local flaps, skin grafts, microvascular free tissue transfer, and bone grafts, depending on the extent and location of the defect and the patient's overall health. Local flaps are used for small- to medium-sized defects and preferred in facial defects. Microvascular-free tissue transfer is a more complex technique that involves transplanting tissue from another part of the body, and small vessels are anastomosed at the recipient site. Bone grafts or vascularized bones are used to reconstruct bone defects. To attain the best outcomes, a competent multispecialty surgical team is needed, and patients may require physical and emotional recovery assistance from other healthcare professionals.

ABBREVIATIONS

ALT	Anterolateral thigh flap
ASA	American Society of Anesthesiologists
CAD/CAM	Computer-aided design and manufacturing
DP	Deltopectoral
FAMM	Facial artery musculomucosal
MSAP	Medial sural artery perforator
PMMC	Pectoral muscle myocutaneous
RAFF	Radial artery forearm flap
RSTL	Relaxed skin tension lines
STSG	Split-thickness skin graft
STV	Superficial temporal vessel

REFERENCES

1. Aylward JD. The gentleman's magazine. *Not Quer.* 1974; 8(20):891–892.
2. Chambers JA, Ray PD. Achieving growth and excellence in medicine: the case history of armed conflict and modern reconstructive surgery. *Ann Plast Surg.* 2009;63: 473–478.
3. &NA The principles and art of plastic surgery. *South Med J.* June 1958;51(6):805–806.
4. Harrison B, Khansa I, Janis JE. Evidence-based strategies to reduce postoperative complications in plastic surgery. *Plast Reconstr Surg.* 2016;137(1):351–360.
5. Gottlieb LJ, Krieger LM. From the reconstructive ladder to the reconstructive elevator. *Plast Reconstr Surg.* 1994;93: 1503–1504.
6. Kung TA, Bueno RA, Alkhalefah GK, Langhals NB, Urbanchek MG, Cederna PS. Innovations in prosthetic interfaces for the upper extremity. *Plast Reconstr Surg.* 2013;132(6):1515–1523.
7. Mathes S. *Reconstructive Surgery: Principles, Anatomy & Technique.* New York: Churchill Livingstone; 1997.
8. Orticochea M. Four flap scalp reconstruction technique. *Br J Plast Surg.* 1967;20(C):159–171.
9. Muresan C, Hui-Chou HG, Dorafshar AH, Manson PN, Rodriguez ED. Forehead reconstruction with microvascular flaps: utility of aesthetic subunits. *J Reconstr Microsurg.* 2012;28(5):319–326.
10. Kumar AR, Bradley JP, Harshbarger R, et al. Warfare-related craniectomy defect reconstruction: early success using custom alloplast implants. *Plast Reconstr Surg.* 2011;127(3):1279–1287.
11. Menick FJ, Burget GC. A 10-year experience in nasal reconstruction with the three-stage forehead flap. *Plast Reconstr Surg.* 2002;109(6):1856–1861.
12. Kane W, Mccaffrey TV, Wang TD, Koval TM, Shimotakahara SG, Larrabee WF. The effect of tissue expansion on previously irradiated skin. *Arch Otolaryngol Neck Surg.* 1992;118(5):534–535.
13. Sosin M, Schultz BD, De La Cruz C, et al. Microsurgical scalp reconstruction in the elderly. *Plast Reconstr Surg.* March 2015;135(3):856–866. http://journals.lww.com/00006534-201503000-00040.
14. Simunovic F, Eisenhardt SU, Penna V, Thiele JR, Stark GB, Bannasch H. Microsurgical reconstruction of oncological scalp defects in the elderly. *J Plast Reconstr Aesthetic Surg.* July 2016;69(7):912–919. https://linkinghub.elsevier.com/retrieve/pii/S1748681516300110.
15. Chao AH, Yu P, Skoracki RJ, Demonte F, Hanasono MM. Microsurgical reconstruction of composite scalp and calvarial defects in patients with cancer: a 10-year experience. *Head Neck.* December 2012;34(12): 1759–1764.
16. Lee EI, Chao AH, Skoracki RJ, Yu P, Demonte F, Hanasono MM. Outcomes of calvarial reconstruction in cancer patients. *Plast Reconstr Surg.* March 2014;133(3): 675–682.
17. Rubin JP, Yaremchuk MJ. Complications and toxicities of implantable biomaterials used in facial reconstructive and aesthetic surgery: a comprehensive review of the literature. *Plast Reconstr Surg.* 1997;100(5): 1336–1353.
18. Hanasono MM, Goel N, DeMonte F. Calvarial reconstruction with polyetheretherketone implants. *Ann Plast Surg.* 2009;62(6):653–655.
19. Lowry JC, Bartley GB, Garrity JA. The role of second-intention healing in periocular reconstruction. *Ophthalmic Plast Reconstr Surg.* 1997;13(3):174–188.
20. Morley AMS, deSousa JL, Selva D, Malhotra R. Techniques of upper eyelid reconstruction. *Surv Ophthalmol.* 2010;55(3):256–271.
21. Fogagnolo P, Colletti G, Valassina D, Allevi F, Rossetti L. Partial and total lower lid reconstruction: our experience with 41 cases. *Ophthalmologica.* October 2012;228(4): 239–243.
22. Meadows AER, Manners RM. A simple modification of the glabellar flap in medial canthal reconstruction. *Ophthalmic Plast Reconstr Surg.* 2003;19(4):313–315.
23. Spinelli HM, Jelks GW. Periocular reconstruction: a systematic approach. *Plast Reconstr Surg.* 1993;91(6): 1017–1024.
24. Rathore DS, Chickadasarahilli S, Crossman R, Mehta P, Ahluwalia HS. Full thickness skin grafts in periocular reconstructions: long-term outcomes. *Ophthalmic Plast Reconstr Surg.* 2014;30(6):517–520. http://www.embase.com/search/results?subaction=viewrecord&from=export&id=L53274697%0Ahttps://doi.org/10.1097/IOP.0000000000000237.
25. Alghoul M, Pacella SJ, McClellan WT, Codner MA. Eyelid reconstruction. *Plast Reconstr Surg.* August 2013;132(2): 288e–302e. https://linkinghub.elsevier.com/retrieve/pii/S0030666505000241.
26. Paarlberg JC, van den Bosch WA, Paridaens D. Reconstruction following subtotal full-thickness upper eyelid resection with preservation of the lid margin. *Orbit.* 2007;26(4):319–321. http://www.embase.com/search/results?subaction=viewrecord&from=export&id=L35101376.
27. Patrinely JR, O'Neal KD, Kersten RC, Soparkar CNS. Total upper eyelid reconstruction with mucosalized tarsal graft and overlying bipedicle flap. *Arch Ophthalmol.* 1999; 117(12):1655–1661.

28. Poh EWT, O'Donnell BA, McNab AA, et al. Outcomes of upper eyelid reconstruction. *Ophthalmology*. 2014;121(2):612–613.e1. http://www.embase.com/search/results?subaction=viewrecord&from=export&id=L601063603%0Ahttps://doi.org/10.1016/j.ophtha.2013.10.010.

29. Elliot D, Britto JA. Tripier's innervated myocutaneous flap 1889. *Br J Plast Surg*. September 2004;57(6):543–549.

30. Santos G, Goulão J. One-stage reconstruction of full-thickness lower eyelid using a Tripier flap lining by a septal mucochondral graft. *J Dermatol Treat*. 2014;25(5):446–447.

31. Hawes MJ, Grove AS, Hink EM. Comparison of free tarso-conjunctival grafts and hughes tarsoconjunctival grafts for lower eyelid reconstruction [cited 2022 Dec 26] *Ophthalmic Plast Reconstr Surg*. May 2011;27(3):219–223. https://journals.lww.com/op-rs/Fulltext/2011/05000/Comparison_of_Free_Tarsoconjunctival_Grafts_and.18.aspx.

32. Parrett BM, Pribaz JJ. An algorithm for treatment of nasal defects [cited 2022 Dec 26] *Clin Plast Surg*. July 2009;36(3):407–420. https://pubmed.ncbi.nlm.nih.gov/19505611/.

33. Pribaz J, Stephens W, Crespo L, Gifford G. A new intraoral flap: facial artery musculomucosal (famm) flap. *Plast Reconstr Surg*. 1992;90(3):421–429.

34. Walton RL, Burget GC, Beahm EK. Microsurgical reconstruction of the nasal lining. *Plast Reconstr Surg*. 2005;115(7):1813–1829.

35. Guo L, Pribaz JR, Pribaz JJ. Nasal reconstruction with local flaps: a simple algorithm for management of small defects. *Plast Reconstr Surg*. 2008;122(5).

36. Menick FJ. Nasal reconstruction: forehead flap. *Plast Reconstr Surg*. 2004;113(6):100e–111e.

37. Menick FJ. Nasal reconstruction. *Plast Reconstr Surg*. April 2010;125(4):138e–150e. http://journals.lww.com/00006534-201004000-00031.

38. Marchac D, Toth B. The axial frontonasal flap revisited. *Plast Reconstr Surg*. 1985;76(5):686–694.

39. Rohrich RJ, Muzaffar AR, Adams WP, Hollier LH. The aesthetic unit dorsal nasal flap: rationale for avoiding a glabellar incision. *Plast Reconstr Surg*. 1999;104(5):1289–1294.

40. Zimany A. The bi-lobed flap. *Plast Reconstr Surg*. 1953;11(6):424–434.

41. McGregor JC, Soutar DS. A critical assessment of the bilobed flap. *Br J Plast Surg*. 1981;34(2):197–205.

42. Zitelli JA. The bilobed flap for nasal reconstruction. *Arch Dermatol*. 1989;125(7):957–959.

43. Burget GC, Menick FJ. The subunit principle in nasal reconstruction. *Plast Reconstr Surg*. August 1985;76(2):239–247. http://journals.lww.com/00006534-198508000-00010.

44. Zook EG, Van Beek AL, Russell RC, Moore JB. V–Y advancement flap for facial defects. *Plast Reconstr Surg*. 1980;65(6):786–797.

45. Pribaz JJ, Chester CH, Barrall DT. The extended V-Y flap. *Plast Reconstr Surg*. 1992;90(2):275–280.

46. Herbert DC, DeGeus J. Nasolabial subcutaneous pedicle flaps. *Br J Plast Surg*. 1975;28(2):90–96.

47. Herbert DC. A subcutaneous pedicled cheek flap for reconstruction of alar defects. *Br J Plast Surg*. 1978;31(2):79–92.

48. Hofer SOP, Posch NA, Smit X. The facial artery perforator flap for reconstruction of perioral defects. *Plast Reconstr Surg*. April 2005;115(4):996–1003. http://journals.lww.com/00006534-200504010-00002.

49. Malard O, Lanhouet J, Michel G, Dreno B, Espitalier F, Rio E. Full-thickness nasal defect: place of prosthetic reconstruction. *Ann Fr d'Oto-Rhino-Laryngologie Pathol Cervico-Faciale*. 2015;132(2):83–87.

50. Menick FJ. Defects of the nose, lip, and cheek: rebuilding the composite defect. *Plast Reconstr Surg*. 2007;120(4):887–898.

51. Singh DJ, Bartlett SP. Aesthetic considerations in nasal reconstruction and the role of modified nasal subunits. *Plast Reconstr Surg*. 2003;111(2):639–648.

52. Rohrich RJ, Griffin JR, Ansari M, Beran SJ, Potter JK. Nasal reconstruction - beyond aesthetic subunits: a 15-year review of 1334 cases. *Plast Reconstr Surg*. November 2004;114(6):1405–1416. http://journals.lww.com/00006534-200411000-00006.

53. Taghina A, Pribaz J. Complex nasal reconstruction. *Plast Reconstr Surg*. 2008:15–27.

54. Burget GC, Menick FJ. Nasal support and lining: the marriage of beauty and blood supply. *Plast Reconstr Surg*. 1989;84(2):189–203.

55. Menick FJ. Anatomic reconstruction of the nasal tip cartilages in secondary and reconstructive rhinoplasty. *Plast Reconstr Surg*. 1999;104(7):2187–2198.

56. Burget GC, Menick FJ. Nasal reconstruction: seeking a fourth dimension. *Plast Reconstr Surg*. 1986;78(2):145–157.

57. Menick FJ. The use of skin grafts for nasal lining. *Otolaryngol Clin*. 2001;34(4):791–804.

58. MB FIFF Neligan PC. Strategies in lip reconstruction. *Clin Plast Surg*. 2009;36(3):477–485. 10.1016/j.cps.2009.02.013.

59. Webster JP. Crescentic peri-alar cheek excision for upper lip flap advancement with a short history of upper lip repair. *Plast Reconstr Surg*. 1955;16(6):434–464.

60. Blomgren I, Blomqvist G, Lauritzen C, Lilja J, Peterson L-E, Holmström H. The step technique for the reconstruction of lower lip defects after cancer resection:A follow-up study of 165 cases. *Scand J Plast Reconstr Surg*. January 8, 1988;22(1):103–111. http://www.tandfonline.com/doi/full/10.3109/02844318809097942.

61. Abbè R. A new plastic operation for the relief of deformity due to double harelip. *Plast Reconstr Surg*. 1968;42:481–483.

62. Estlander JA. Eine Methode aus der einen Lippe Substanzverluste der anderen zu ersetzen. *Nord Med Ark*. 2009;4(17):1–12. http://doi.wiley.com/10.1111/j.0954-6820.1872.tb00981.x.

63. Jabaley ME, Clement RL, Orcutt TW. Myocutaneous flaps in lip reconstruction. Applications of the Karapandzic principle. *Plast Reconstr Surg*. 1977;59(5):680–688.

64. Webster RC, Coffey RJ, Kelleher RE. Total and partial reconstruction of the lower lip with innervated muscle-bearing flaps. *Plast Reconstr Surg.* 1960;25(3):360–371.

65. Iii EFW, Setzen G, Michael J. Modified bernard-burow cheek advancement and cross-lip flap for total lip reconstruction. *Arch Otolaryngol head neck.* 2015;122(11):1155–1277.

66. Chang KP, Lai CS, Tsai CC, Lin TM, Lin SD. Total upper lip reconstruction with a free temporal scalp flap: long-term follow-up. *Head Neck.* 2003;25(7):602–605.

67. Sadove RC, Luce EA, McGrath PC. Reconstruction of the lower lip and chin with the composite radial forearm-palmaris longus free flap. *Plast Reconstr Surg.* 1991;88(2):209–214.

68. Jeng SF, Kuo YR, Wei FC, Su CY, Chien CY. Total lower lip reconstruction with a composite radial forearm-palmaris longus tendon flap: a clinical series. *Plast Reconstr Surg.* 2004;113(1):19–23.

69. Carroll CM, Pathak I, Irish J, Neligan PC, Gullane PJ. Reconstruction of total lower lip and chin defects using the composite radial forearm–palmaris longus tendon free flap. *Arch facial Plast Surg Off Publ Am Acad Facial Plast Reconstr Surgery, Inc Int Fed Facial Plast Surg Soc.* 2000;2(1):53–56.

70. Lengelé BG, Testelin S, Bayet B, Devauchelle B. Total lower lip functional reconstruction with a fabricated gracilis muscle free flap. *Int J Oral Maxillofac Surg.* 2004;33(4):396–401.

71. Jeng SF, Kuo YR, Wei FC, Su CY, Chien CY. Reconstruction of extensive composite mandibular defects with large lip involvement by using double free flaps and fascia lata grafts for oral sphincters. *Plast Reconstr Surg.* 2005;115(7):1830–1836.

72. Ninkovic M, Di Spilimbergo SS, Ninkovic M. Lower lip reconstruction: introduction of a new procedure using a functioning gracilis muscle free flap. *Plast Reconstr Surg.* 2007;119(5):1472–1480.

73. Roth DA, Longaker MT, Zide BM. Cheek surface reconstruction: best choices according to zones. *Operat Tech Plast Reconstr Surg.* 1998;5(1):26–36.

74. Furnas DW. The retaining ligaments of the cheek. *Plast Reconstr Surg.* 1989;83(1):11–16.

75. Pontes L, Ribeiro M, Vrancks JJ, Guimarães J. The new bilaterally pedicled V-Y advancement flap for face reconstruction. *Plast Reconstr Surg.* 2002;109(6):1870–1874.

76. Schulte DL, Sherris DA, Kasperbauer JL. The anatomical basis of the Abbé flap. *Laryngoscope.* March 2001;111(3):382–386. http://doi.wiley.com/10.1097/0000 5537-200103000-00004.

77. Chandawarkar RY, Cervino AL. Subunits of the cheek: an algorithm for the reconstruction of partial thickness defects [cited 2022 Dec 26] *Br J Plast Surg.* March 1, 2003;56(2):135–139. http://www.jprasurg.com/article/S0007 122603000262/fulltext.

78. Sugg KB, Cederna PS, Brown DL. The V-Y advancement flap is equivalent to the Mustardé flap for ectropion prevention in the reconstruction of moderate-size lid-cheek junction defects. *Plast Reconstr Surg.* 2013;131(1).

79. Dyer PV, Irvine GH. Cervicopectoral rotation flap. *Br J Plast Surg.* 1994;47(1):68.

80. Becker DW. A cervicopectoral rotation flap for cheek coverage. *Plast Reconstr Surg.* 1978;61(6):868–870.

81. Anand AG, Amedee RG, Butcher RB. Reconstruction of large lateral facial defects utilizing variations of the cervicopectoral rotation flap. *Ochsner J.* 2008;8(4):186–190.

82. McIvor NP, Fong MW, Berger KJ, Freeman JL. Use of tissue expansion in head and neck reconstruction. *J Otolaryngol.* 1994;23(1):46–49.

83. Argenta LC, Watanabe MJ, Grabb WC. The use of tissue expansion in head and neck reconstruction. *Ann Plast Surg.* 1983;11(1):31–37.

84. Akinbami B. Reconstruction of continuity defects of the mandible with non-vascularized bone grafts. Systematic literature review. *Craniomaxillofacial Trauma Reconstr.* 2016;9(3):195–205.

85. Foster RD, Anthony JP, Sharma A, Pogrel MA. Vascularized bone flaps versus nonvascularized bone grafts for mandibular reconstruction: an outcome analysis of primary bony union and endosseous implant success. *Head Neck.* 1999;21(1):66–71.

86. Cordeiro PG, Disa JJ, Hidalgo DA, Hu QY. Reconstruction of the mandible with osseous free flaps: a 10-year experience with 150 consecutive patients. *Plast Reconstr Surg.* 1999;104(5):1314–1320.

87. Metzler P, Geiger EJ, Alcon A, Ma X, Steinbacher DM. Three-dimensional virtual surgery accuracy for free fibula mandibular reconstruction: planned versus actual results. *J Oral Maxillofac Surg.* 2014;72(12):2601–2612.

88. Craig ES, Yuhasz M, Shah A, et al. Simulated surgery and cutting guides enhance spatial positioning in free fibular mandibular reconstruction. *Microsurgery.* 2015;35(1):29–33.

89. Moura LB, Carvalho PHdA, Xavier CB, et al. Autogenous non-vascularized bone graft in segmental mandibular reconstruction: a systematic review. *Int J Oral Maxillofac Surg.* 2016;45(11):1388–1394.

90. van Gemert JTM, van Es RJJ, Vc EM, Nonvascularized RK. Bone grafts for segmental reconstruction of the mandible-A reappraisal. *J Oral Maxillofac Surg.* 2009;67(7):1446–1452. http://ovidsp.ovid.com/ovidweb.cgi? T=JS&PAGE=reference&D=emed9&NEWS=N&AN=2009 287277.

91. Hidalgo DA, Rekow A. A review of 60 consecutive fibula free flap mandible reconstructions. *Plast Reconstr Surg.* 1995;96(3):585–596.

92. Ferretti C, Muthray E, Rikhotso E, Reyneke J, Ripamonti U. Reconstruction of 56 mandibular defects with autologous compressed particulate corticocancellous bone grafts. *Br J Oral Maxillofac Surg.* 2016;54(3):322–326.

93. Gadre PK, Ramanojam S, Patankar A, Gadre KS. Nonvascularized bone grafting for mandibular reconstruction: myth or reality? *J Craniofac Surg.* 2011;22(5):1727–1735.

94. ShihHeng C, HungChi C, ShyueYih H, et al. Reconstruction for osteoradionecrosis of the mandible: superiority of free iliac bone flap to fibula flap in postoperative infection and healing. *Ann Plast Surg.* 2014;73(Suppl. 1): S18–S26. http://journals.lww.com/annalsplasticsurgery/Abstract/2014/09001/Reconstruction_for_Osteoradionecrosis_of_the.5.aspx.

95. Shpitzer T, Neligan PC, Gullane PJ, et al. The free iliac crest and fibula flaps in vascularized oromandibular reconstruction: comparison and long-term evaluation. *Head Neck.* 1999;21(7):639–647.

96. Fujiki M, Miyamoto S, Sakuraba M, Nagamatsu S, Hayashi R. A comparison of perioperative complications following transfer of fibular and scapular flaps for immediate mandibular reconstruction. *J Plast Reconstr Aesthetic Surg.* 2013;66(3):372–375.

97. Brown JS, Shaw RJ. Reconstruction of the maxilla and midface: introducing a new classification. *Lancet Oncol.* 2010;11(10):1001–1008.

98. Hanasono MM, Silva AK, Yu P, Skoracki RJ. A comprehensive algorithm for oncologic maxillary reconstruction. *Plast Reconstr Surg.* 2013;131(1):47–60.

99. Cordeiro PG, Santamaria E. A classification system and algorithm for reconstruction of maxillectomy and midfacial defects. *Plast Reconstr Surg.* 2000;105(7):2331–2346.

100. Spiro RH, Strong EW, Shah JP. Maxillectomy and its classification. *Head Neck.* 1997;19(4):309–314.

101. Moreno MA, Skoracki RJ, Hanna EY, Hanasono MM. Microvascular free flap reconstruction versus palatal obturation for maxillectomy defects. *Head Neck.* 2010; 32(7):860–868.

102. Okay DJ, Genden E, Buchbinder D, Urken M. Prosthodontic guidelines for surgical reconstruction of the maxilla: a classification system of defects. *J Prosthet Dent.* 2001;86(4):352–363.

103. Ahmad FI, Means C, Labby AB, et al. Osteocutaneous radial forearm free flap in nonmandible head and neck reconstruction. *Head Neck.* 2017;39(9):1888–1893.

104. Chang EI, Hanasono MM. State-of-the-art reconstruction of midface and facial deformities. *J Surg Oncol.* 2016; 113(8):962–970.

105. Kirby EJ, Turner JB, Davenport DL, Vasconez HC. Orbital floor fractures: outcomes of reconstruction. *Ann Plast Surg.* 2011;66(5):508–512.

106. Mericli AF, Gampper TJ. Treatment of postsurgical temporal hollowing with high-density porous polyethylene. *J Craniofac Surg.* 2014;25(2):563–567.

107. Patel UA, Hartig GK, Hanasono MM, Lin DT, Richmon JD. Locoregional flaps for oral cavity reconstruction: a review of modern options. *Otolaryngol Head Neck Surg.* 2017;157(2):201–209.

108. Chang EI, Ibrahim A, Papazian N, et al. Perforator mapping and optimizing design of the lateral arm flap: anatomy revisited and clinical experience. *Plast Reconstr Surg.* 2016;138(2):300e–306e.

109. Wu JCW, Huang JJ, Tsao CK, Abdelrahman M, Kolios G, Cheng MH. Comparison of posteromedial thigh profunda artery perforator flap and anterolateral thigh perforator flap for head and neck reconstruction. *Plast Reconstr Surg.* 2016;137(1):257–266.

110. Tarsitano A, Battaglia S, Cipriani R, Marchetti C. Microvascular reconstruction of the tongue using a free anterolateral thigh flap: three-dimensional evaluation of volume loss after radiotherapy. *J Cranio-Maxillofacial Surg.* 2016;44(9):1287–1291.

111. Yu P, Chang EI, Selber JC, Hanasono MM. Perforator patterns of the ulnar artery perforator flap. *Plast Reconstr Surg.* 2012;129(1):213–220.

112. Manrique OJ, Leland HA, Langevin CJ, et al. Optimizing outcomes following total and subtotal tongue reconstruction: a systematic review of the contemporary literature. *J Reconstr Microsurg.* 2017;33(2): 103–111.

113. Fernández–Riera R, Hung SY, Wu JCW, Tsao CK. Free profunda femoris artery perforator flap as a first-line choice of reconstruction for partial glossectomy defects. *Head Neck.* 2017;39(4):737–743.

114. Ito R, Huang JJ, Wu JCW, Lin MCY, Cheng MH. The versatility of profunda femoral artery perforator flap for oncological reconstruction after cancer resection—clinical cases and review of literature. *J Surg Oncol.* 2016; 114(2):193–201.

115. Yang XD, Zhao SF, Wang YX, et al. Use of extended lateral upper arm free flap for tongue reconstruction after radical glossectomy for tongue cancer. *Aesthetic Plast Surg.* 2015; 39(4):562–569.

FURTHER READING

1. Antonyshyn O, Gruss JS, Zuker R, Mackinnon SE. Tissue expansion in head and neck reconstruction. *Plast Reconstr Surg.* 1988;82(1):58–68.

CHAPTER 5

Radiotherapy Treatment: Planning and Posttreatment Care

SHAHID A. SIDDIQUI, MD • MOHSIN KHAN, MD

The management of patients with head and neck cancers (HNCs) is complex and warrants a multidisciplinary approach. Patients need access to all the specialists including head and neck surgeons, radiation/medical oncologists, dentistry/prosthodontics, plastic and reconstructive surgery, physical medicine and rehabilitation, speech and swallowing therapy, radiology, clinical social work, nutrition, and various other adjunctive disciplines. Outcomes are improved when patients are given full range of support services ranging from general medical care, pain management, nutritional support, dental care, smoking and alcohol cessation, and psychiatric and social support.[1]

According to the GLOBOCAN report 2018, there are 834,860 cases per year of HNCs, with 431,131 deaths per year around the world. HNCs account for 30%–40% of all cancer sites in India,[2] with the highest incidence (60.7%) reported for the lip and oral cavity sites. Tobacco consumption, whether smokeless, smoked, or chewable along with alcohol is one of the major risk factors for HNCs. Majority of these epithelial malignancies will have squamous cell histology. Surgery and radiotherapy are the most commonly applied treatment strategies either alone or in combination depending upon the site/stage of the disease, histopathological characteristics, and some patient-related factors (e.g., performance status, consent, etc.). Radiotherapy, often with concurrent chemotherapy, has a significant role in the "curative" management of HNC. Primary chemoradiation allows the preservation of organs, and in turn functions of the site involved. It is the treatment of choice for tumors arising in the oropharynx, nasopharynx, hypopharynx, and larynx. In oral cavity cancers, the best cure rates are obtained using surgical techniques with adjuvant or postoperative radiotherapy (with or without chemotherapy). Radiotherapy also plays an important role in the palliation of symptoms in patients with advanced/incurable HNC[3,4] (Fig. 5.1).

PHYSICAL AND BIOLOGICAL BASIS OF RADIOTHERAPY

Radiotherapy is a clinical modality dealing with the use of ionizing radiation in the treatment of patients with malignant and occasionally benign diseases.[5] The characteristic feature of this **ionizing radiation** is the localized release of large amounts of energy, which when transferred to the orbital electrons can eject them from the atoms or molecules in the process known as ionization. If any form of radiation—be it X-rays or γ-rays (the designation of x-or γ-rays reflects the ways they are produced), charged particles or uncharged particles—is absorbed in biological material, there is a possibility that it will interact with the critical targets in the cells (e.g., DNA). The atoms of these critical targets may be directly ionized by the radiation in what is known as direct action of radiation, or the radiation may first interact with some other molecule (especially water because of its abundance), producing free radicals, which then can damage the critical targets—the indirect action of radiation (Fig. 5.2).

Ionizing radiation (IR) deposits its energy randomly. This can lead to damage of all the molecules in the cell. However, molecules such as water, proteins, and RNA have multiple copies in the cellular system and undergo continuous rapid turnover, limiting the consequences of damaging to just a few molecules of one type. In contrast, DNA, which is central to all biological functions, has limited turnover, with only two copies, thereby providing the biggest target for ionizing radiation to act. Thus, if DNA gets damaged by the ionizing radiation, the results can be permanent and lethal.[6]

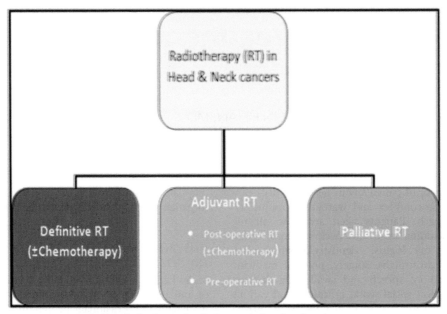

FIG. 5.1 Indications of radiotherapy in head and neck cancers.

A spectrum of lesions ranging from base damage, single-strand breaks (SSBs), double-strand breaks (DSBs), intrastand cross-links, etc., can result from lesions produced by IR in DNA. Out of these, DSBs are considered the most lethal, as they constitute breaks that will disrupt the chromosome segregation during mitosis (Fig. 5.3). To give a better perspective of relative damage, 1 Gray (Gy), usual dose of X-ray used clinically, can induce around 1000 base damages and SSBs and around 40 DSBs per cell. On the contrary, cells have intricately evolved a series of sensor and repair pathways to respond to each type of radiation-induced damage.

The *dose* of radiation, the SI unit of which is Gy, is the amount of radiation/energy deposited per unit mass as a result of an exposure to ionizing radiation. Thus, 1 Gy = 1 J/kg. Delivering a single large dose of 60 Gy to a malignant lesion, for example, on tongue, can sterilize the lesion site from cancer cells, but at the same time will result in unacceptable and at times permanent normal surrounding tissue damage. Fractionation of this large dose into daily small fractions over a period of weeks can, thus, relatively spare the normal tissues. This occurs due to repair of the sublethal damage between dose fractions and repopulation of cells if overall treatment time is sufficiently long. In parallel to this, dividing a dose into a number of fractions increases damage to the tumor because of reoxygenation and redistribution of the cells into the more

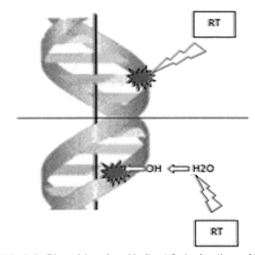

FIG. 5.2 Direct (above) and indirect (below) actions of RT.

radiosensitive phases of cell cycle. Prolongation of treatment thereby spares early normal tissue reactions. However, excessive prolongation can negate the aforementioned advantages by allowing surviving tumor cells to proliferate.

A variety of autocrine, paracrine, and endocrine sequences of events in combination with cell killing are responsible for the *effects* of irradiation on normal tissues. After irradiation, a variety of growth and

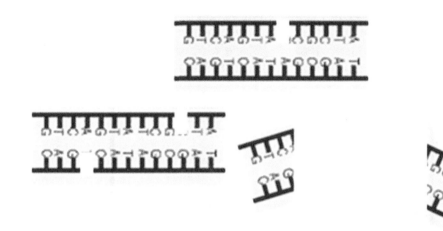

FIG. 5.3 (Above) RT-induced single-strand break. (Below) RT-induced double-strand breaks. If these breaks lie opposite to each other or are separated by only few base pairs, the chromatin tears apart.

simultaneously inhibitory factors are released; also there occurs modulation of cell receptors, and this dysregulation of the tissue microenvironment is translated into postreceptor cytoplasmic, nuclear, and interstitial events.[7] Therefore, cell killing, alterations in gene expression, and release of proinflammatory and profibrotic cytokines determine the fate of normal tissues/structures (Fig. 5.4).

The response of normal tissues to radiation depends on both the treatment-related factors and patient (tissue)-related factors. The treatment-related factors include (1) the total radiation dose and the fraction size—the effects of increasing severity become apparent if the doses or doses per fraction rise above a threshold level; (2) the total duration of radiation; (3) the time interval between radiation fractions; and (4) the dose rate. Patient-related factors include (1) the volume of irradiation—killing a small number of cells in a tissue matters very little; however, the visible damage becomes evident if a large proportion of cells are killed; (2) the kinetics of the tissue being irradiated—radiation mainly effects cells when they attempt to divide, damage becomes quickly evident in tissues with rapid turnover, e.g., bone marrow, skin, whereas tissues that rarely divide, radiation damage can remain latent for quiet a long period of time; (3) the structural organization of tissue—the tolerance of normal tissues depends on the ability of clonogenic cells to maintain a sufficient number of mature cells so as to sustain the organ function; and (4) the inherent or intrinsic radio sensitivity of the cells.

The majority of the radiation effects can be broadly classified as (1) early effects and (2) late effects.[8] Early effects occur within days to weeks of radiation initiation and occur mainly in tissues with rapid turnover. Examples include skin, hematopoietic system, and gastrointestinal epithelium, where the mature functional cells, having short life span, are rapidly replenished by the underlying stem cells in a hierarchal cell lineage organization. In contrast, late effects appear after a delay of months and years and occur in slowly proliferating tissues, for example, the heart, liver, lungs, etc. Loss of parenchymal cells in combination with the vascular damage forms the main pathogenesis for occurrence of late effects (Fig. 5.4).

In practice, it is the tolerance of the normal tissues that are necessarily irradiated with the tumor tissue, which limits the amount of radiation to be given. Risk versus benefit approach, also known as *therapeutic ratio*, determines the conceptual framework for an optimal radiation treatment plan. As such, a balance must be obtained between what is deemed as an acceptable probability of radiation-induced normal tissue complication and the probability of adequate tumor control (Fig. 5.5.). An ideal situation is the one in which the radiation plan is able to maintain the graphs of tumor control and normal tissue complications, on a dose response curve as far separated as possible. This is the basic premise on which the latest technological advancements in the field of radiotherapy have taken place. These technological improvements have allowed delivery of large doses to tumor or lower doses to normal tissues.

The combination of chemotherapy with the radiation has perhaps made the strongest impacts on current cancer radiation therapy practice. Concurrent

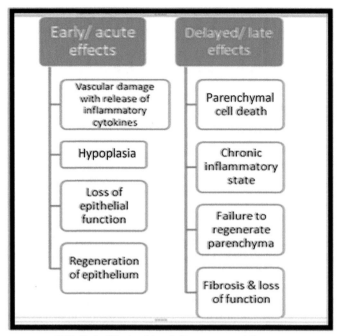

FIG. 5.4 Effects of irradiation on normal tissues.

chemoradiotherapy in many recent trials has not only shown better results in terms of locoregional control (LRC) of disease but has also shown improvement in patient survival. This stands true even for the HNCs, where concurrent chemoradiotherapy improved the progression-free survival and/or the overall survival (OS) at different sites/subsites and stages.[9,10] Combining chemotherapeutic drugs with radiation has strong biological rationale. These drugs are cytotoxic to the tumor cells, and they even sensitize these cells to the effects of radiation. However, the extended benefits are not without additional side effects. Damage to the normal tissue is often accentuated when these two cytotoxic agents are combined especially when they affect the same tissue.

Oral Cavity Cancers

The oral cavity consists of the upper and lower lips, gingivobuccal sulcus, buccal mucosa, upper and lower gingival (including alveolar ridge), retromolar trigone, hard palate, floor of mouth, and anterior two-thirds of the tongue. According to the GLOBO-CAN 2018 report,[11] out of the total reported HNC cases, lip and oral cavity sites are the most common reported with 60.7% incidence. Majority (around 90%) of these cases are squamous cell carcinomas. These are moderately radiosensitive. Staging and treatment recommendations for lip cancers vary slightly from rest of the subsites. However, in general, primary surgery followed by adjuvant therapy as indicated is the standard of care in operable/resectable disease.[12] In unresectable lesions, concurrent chemo-RT is the preferred regimen.

Postoperative radiation (RT) has shown superior results as compared with preoperative RT. Tupchong et al.[13] in a randomized controlled trial reported that postoperative RT significantly improved the LRC as compared with preoperative RT (58%—70%). Indications for postoperative RT alone include pathological T3/4 disease, close margins, nodal N2/3 status, neck nodal level IV-V, perineural invasion or lymphovascular space invasion.[14,15] Postoperative concurrent chemoradiotherapy is usually indicated for positive margins, gross residual disease, and/or extracapsular extension.[16,17]

EORTC 22931 trial[16] randomized 334 patients with operable HNCs to post-op RT versus post-op chemo-RT. Chemo-RT improved 5-year disease-free survival (DFS) from 36% to 47%, OS from 40% to 53%, and LRC from 69% to 82%. Similarly, RTOG 95-01 trial[17] in 459 operable HNCs demonstrated that concurrent chemo-RT improved DFS, LRC, at 10 years follow-up. Combined analysis of these two trials by Bernier et al.[18] showed that post-op chemo-RT improved OS, DFS, and LRC

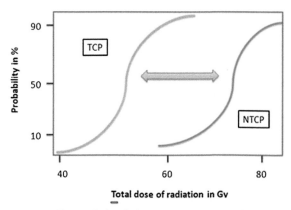

FIG. 5.5 The goal of radiation plan is to separate the above two curves as far as possible by shifting that of tumor control probability (TCP) to left and simultaneously the curve of normal tissue complications probability (NTCP) to extreme right.

versus RT alone in subset of patients with positive margins and/or extracapsular extension.

RADIATION PLANNING AND TECHNIQUES

Once the indication for RT is met, it is important to decide on three basic aspects of radiation planning—volume, dose, and technique. The volume of tissue to be treated is mainly governed by the stage, subsite, histopathological correlates, the locoregional spread and the possible microscopic spread of the disease, the lymphatic drainage of a particular site, and the other possible pathways or routes of spread. Next in line is the dose, radiation dose selection is a complex issue. The treating physician must determine the correct dose to achieve the intended goal. One must carefully select the total dose, dose per fraction, numbers of fraction, striking a balance between sufficient tumoricidal dose, and acceptable risk of side effects. Decisions concerning these factors will be driven in part, by the fundamentals of radiation physics and biology.

The next question that the treating physician faces is what appropriate technique is required? Radiation is generally delivered by two techniques. The first is *teletherapy*, where the source of radiation is placed at a distance from the patient and usually delivered by external beam sources of cobalt-60 machine or a linear accelerator. External beam teletherapy plans must be appropriately selected so as to achieve the intended goals. Improvements in diagnostic radiology and computer software technology have revolutionized the RT planning and delivery with external beam sources. Highly conformal treatment plans can be realized and delivered with these techniques. Another technique of radiation is *brachytherapy*. It refers to placement of radioactive sources at or near the target tissue. Early work in oral cavity tumors demonstrated acceptable control rates with brachytherapy alone or in combination with external beam therapy. Pernot et al.[19] reported local control rates of 96% for T1, 85% for T2, and 64% for T3 lesions of oral cavity treated with brachytherapy and neck dissection. Melzner et al.[20] found an OS of 83% and LC of 93% in patients treated with post-op or definitively with brachytherapy.

Simulation and Planning

Either a two-dimensional or three-dimensional computed tomography (CT)–based planning technique is utilized. Before planning, patients are simulated in treatment position using thermoplastic masks in supine position with extended neck. CT planning with fusion to MRI (magnetic resonance imaging), contrast-enhanced, and/or PET scans (positron emission tomography scans) is usually recommended. Generally, the target tissue includes the clinical or radiographic gross disease including primary and nodes, the entire post-op bed (if operated), areas of close/positive margins, entire flap, and areas of extranodular extension with margin. Elective irradiation of the neck including ipsilateral with or without contralateral is recommended based on the high-risk factors and more or less in conjunction with principles of extent of surgical neck dissection (Fig. 5.6).

In recent years, there has been increasing use of intensity-modulated radiation therapy (IMRT) for the treatment of head and neck regions. In particular for oral cavity lesions, IMRT offers the opportunity to limit the normal tissue complications, including damage to major salivary glands and to the mandible.

Dose and Fractionation

When definitive external beam radiation therapy is used as the treatment modality, doses around 66–70 Gy are usually required to obtain reliable local controls. For earlier lesions, boosting the primary with brachytherapy as a part of treatment has reliably shown improved local control rates.[21,22] When post-op RT is used, 2Gy per fraction is utilized. Operative bed should ideally receive up to 60 Gy. However, for close or positive microscopic margins or ENE, a sequential 6.0 Gy localized boost should be considered. If there is gross residual disease, either further surgical resection or focal boosting up to 70 Gy may be necessary. Regions of somewhat lesser

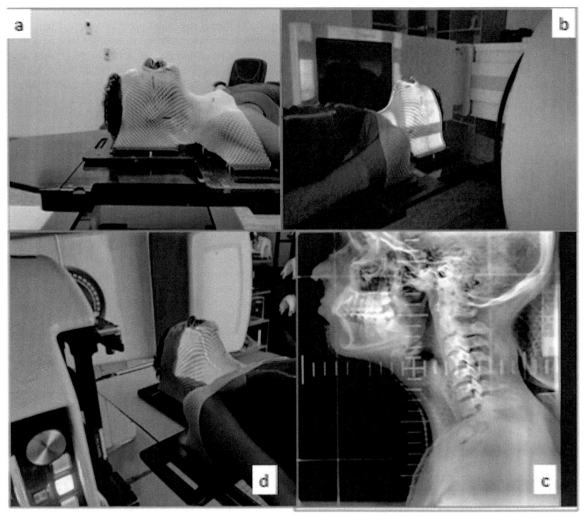

FIG. 5.6 (a,b) Patient undergoing simulation for RT with thermoplastic mask in place. (c) Simulation film of the same patient, depicting the region of interest, (d) patient receiving treatment in same position.

risk (i.e., clinically or pathologically uninvolved necks) should receive dose on the order of 54–56 Gy.

Brachytherapy

Brachytherapy has played an important role, historically, in the treatment of HNCs, especially for oral cavity sites. In carefully selected early lesions, it can be used as sole modality.[23] It is also used to boost the primary site before or after external beam RT. When used alone, doses of 65–75 Gy are commonly prescribed over 6–7 days using low dose rate or can be converted to equivalent high dose rate dosages in accordance with the radiobiological principles. Rigid cesium needles or iridium-192 sources after-loaded into angiocaths are commonly used and inserted with free hand or custom templates for source and dose optimization.

Intraoral Cone

Another tool to boost radiation doses especially, for anterior oral cavity lesions, is the use of intraoral cone. Accessible lesions up to 3 cm can be boosted with this technique. It employs either low-energy X-rays of 100–250 kV or electron beam therapy. The advantage with intraoral cone over brachytherapy is it being noninvasive avoids the needle trauma to the patient.

DENTAL EVALUATION

A thorough oral and dental, clinicoradiological evaluation is vital before initiating radiation therapy. Preventive dental care and extractions are warranted to minimize subsequent risk of osteoradionecrosis. Teeth with advanced caries and significant periodontal disease should be removed in addition to impacted teeth, unopposed teeth especially, when they lie in regions of high dose of radiation. Extraction of marginal teeth should also be considered in patients who will not be able to maintain adequate oral hygiene. Pre-RT dental care should also include patient education regarding meticulous oral hygiene and diet counseling (Fig. 5.7).

Radiation can impair bone healing and diminish the capacity to repair following trauma. Therefore, elective oral surgical procedures must be carefully planned before RT. It is usually recommended to complete dental extractions/procedures at least 10–14 days prior to start of RT. Radiation can induce several chronic effects in the oral cavity including xerostomia, which can alter the normal physiology of oral cavity and hence warrants routine surveillance. Long-term prognosis of teeth and patient motivation should be considered.

Frequent dental follow-up examinations and cleaning, flossing, brushing, and eliminating potential sources of infection should be integral to post- RT care.

PRERADIATION PROSTHODONTIC CARE

Definitive prosthodontic care is tremendously indispensable prior to radiation of head and neck region. It is extremely essential to evaluate the acceptable prosthodontic standards of existing prosthesis in patient's mouth. Progressive mucositis developed during and after the radiotherapy can affect patient's ability to bear the prosthesis due to compromised condition of oral mucosa. Relining of ill-fitting prosthesis with temporary relining material such as silicone should be avoided as it will not only affect the oral hygiene maintenance but also acts as a source for active fungal growth, leading to unwarranted mucosal discomfort. Those patients who have fixed prosthesis in their mouth can suffer from backscatter of radiation, leading to redundant irradiation to adjacent normal tissues. Suitable use of prosthetic stent can be implemented to curtail the radiation exposure to surrounding normal tissues.

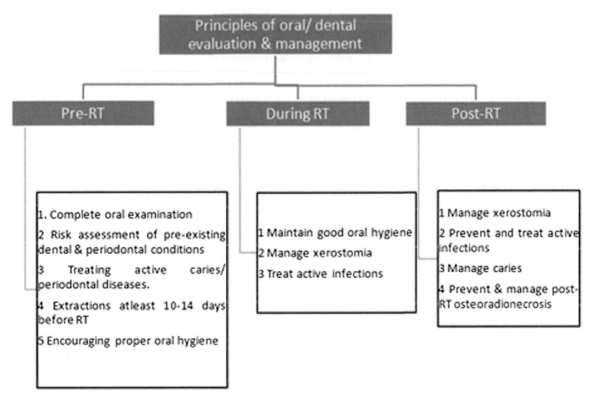

FIG. 5.7 Principles of oral/dental evaluation and management.

Fluoride application trays can also be used to relocate the normal soft tissue in buccal and lingual directions. If any patient has implants in the region of head and neck to be irradiated, then it should be precisely examined clinically as well as radiographically as it will aid to decide whether removal of any implant is necessary. Radiation carrier prosthesis can be fabricated with acrylic to position the radioactive source near the tumor site during brachytherapy. Tubing is incorporated within this device to carry the radiation over short distance utilizing radioisotopes positioned in close proximity to the tumor with the assistance of radiation carrier.

PATIENT CARE DURING AND AFTER RT

Radiation therapy is one of the established modality for cancer treatment. The effects get potentiated when it is combined with chemotherapeutic agents. This is true even for the normal tissues, which develop complications during the course of treatment. Almost every course of treatment has some risk of acute and late ill effects. When these occur, they must be properly documented. Thus, every patient should be clinically examined for any untoward side effects at least once a week during the course of treatment and thereafter as per the follow-up schedule, in addition to the response evaluation. There are various techniques/scales available for documenting adverse effects of the treatment. However, two of the most commonly used criteria in clinical practice are Radiation Therapy Oncology Group (RTOG)/European Organisation for Research and Treatment of Cancer (EORTC) Radiation Toxicity Grading[24] (Tables 5.1 and 5.2), or the NCI-CTCAE criteria (National Cancer Institute—Common Terminology Criteria for Adverse Events)[25] (Table 5.3).

A variety of normal tissue changes are induced by ionizing radiation. Some of the clinically relevant effects are discussed in the following along with their relevant pathophysiology and preventive and management strategies.

Skin and Soft Tissue

Clinical features: Acute radiation injury can occur within days to weeks after radiation exposure, and the pattern of skin manifestation is mainly related to the

---

TABLE 5.1
Acute Toxicity Criteria of the Radiation Therapy Oncology Group (RTOG) and the European Organisation for Research and Treatment of Cancer (EORTC)[24]

RTOG ACUTE RADIATION MORBIDITY				
Tissue	**Grade 1**	**2**	**3**	**4**
Skin	Follicular, faint or dull erythema/epilation/dry desquamation/ decreased sweating	Tender or bright erythema, patchy moist desquamation/ moderate edema	Confluent, moist desquamation other than skin folds, pitting edema	Ulceration, hemorrhage, necrosis
Mucous membrane	Irritation/may experience mild pain not requiring analgesic	Patchy mucositis that may produce an inflammatory serosanguinous discharge/may experience moderate pain requiring analgesia	Confluent fibrinous mucositis/may include severe pain requiring narcotic	Ulceration, hemorrhage or necrosis
Salivary gland	Mild mouth dryness/ slightly thickened saliva/ may have slightly altered taste such as metallic taste/these changes not reflected in alteration in baseline feeding behavior, such as increased use of liquids with meals	Moderate to complete dryness/thick, sticky saliva/markedly altered taste	(None)	Acute salivary gland necrosis

For all: 0—no symptoms, 5—death directly related to radiation effects.

TABLE 5.2
Late Toxicity Criteria of the Radiation Therapy Oncology Group (RTOG) and the European Organisation for Research and Treatment of Cancer (EORTC)[24]

RTOG LATE RADIATION MORBIDITY				
Tissue	Grade 1	2	3	4
Skin	Slight atrophy; pigmentation change; some hair loss	Patch atrophy; moderate telangiectasia; total hair loss	Marked atrophy; gross telangiectasia	Ulceration
Subcutaneous tissue	Slight induration (fibrosis) and loss of subcutaneous fat	Moderate fibrosis but asymptomatic; slight field contracture; <10% linear reduction	Severe induration and loss of subcutaneous tissue; field contracture >10% linear measurement	Necrosis
Mucous membrane	Slight atrophy and dryness	Moderate atrophy and telangiectasia; little mucous	Marked atrophy with complete dryness	Ulceration
Salivary glands	Slight dryness of mouth; good response on stimulation	Moderate dryness of mouth; poor response on stimulation	Complete dryness of mouth; no response on stimulation	Fibrosis

For all: 0—no symptoms, 5—death directly related to radiation effects.

radiation dose. Acute skin reaction may appear as erythema, inflammation, dry/moist desquamation, dermal necrosis, and ulceration (Fig. 5.8). First noticeable sign (erythema) usually appears around second to third week of standard fractionation schedule. Sterile sites will begin to epithelize within 10–14 days after exposure. Late skin changes evolve during months to years and manifests as telangiectasia, dense dermal fibrosis, loss of hair follicles, altered melanin deposition, and ulceration/dermal necrosis.[26]

Pathophysiology: Reactive oxygen species (ROS), proinflammatory cytokines, and the activated growth factors, all work in tandem to initiate and propagate the radiation induced skin injury. Acute radiation reactions appear as a diminution and degeneration of basal epithelial cells, accompanied with edema, inflammation, and vascular dilatation. Later destruction of microvasculature, atrophy, dense dermal fibrosis, and progressive arterial and venous lesions ensue.[27]

Prevention: Carefully selecting the total dose and fractionation, using conformal radiation delivery techniques such as IMRT, can physically decrease the total dose delivered to normal tissues. Avoiding friction/rubbing, sunlight can decrease adverse events. However, the evidence is not so strong. Some products such as Wobe-Mugos E, topical steroids, and oral zinc may play role in injury prevention.[28]

Treatment: Use of HBOT (hyperbaric oxygen therapy) has shown improvements in soft tissue necrosis in patients undergoing radiation.[29] Short wave infrared light (red light phototherapy) improves hemangiectasis and tissue circulation increasing wound healing and ulcer recovery.[30] Dye laser treatment is sometimes beneficial in relieving late-onset radiodermatitis.[31] Hydrogel membranes containing hyaluronic acid and synthetic hydrophilic macromolecules enhance reepithelialization, and soft silicone dressings promote granulation tissue, dissolve fibrotic/necrotic tissue, and aid in wound healing.[32] Many other bioactivators such as vitamin E, plasma, and interleukin-12 have been utilized for radiation-induced skin damage but with mixed results. Finally, surgical reconstruction using free flap–based grafts may be required in progressive ulcers.

Mucositis
Clinical features: Oral mucositis starts as erythema of the oral mucosa in the first 2–3 weeks of RT and progresses to ulceration as the dose of radiation increases (Fig. 5.8). Nonkeratinized oral tissues are more susceptible.[33] Use of concurrent chemotherapy may accelerate the process and can increase the duration too. Pain associated with mucositis negatively impacts the nutrition, compromising the function significantly. Quality

TABLE 5.3
The NCI Common Terminology Criteria for Adverse Events (CTCAE) v5.0[25]

CTCAE-COMMON TERMINOLOGY CRITERIA FOR ADVERSE EVENTS				
Tissue/term	**Grade1**	**2**	**3**	**4**	**5**
Dermatitis radiation	Faint erythema or dry desquamation	Moderate to brisk erythema; patchy moist desquamation, mostly confined to skin folds and creases; moderate edema	Moist desquamation in areas other than skin folds and creases; bleeding induced by minor trauma or abrasion	Life-threatening consequences; skin necrosis or ulceration of full-thickness dermis; spontaneous bleeding from involved site; skin graft indicated	Death
Mucositis oral	Asymptomatic or mild symptoms; intervention not indicated	Moderate pain or ulcer that does not interfere with oral intake; modified diet indicated	Severe pain; interfering with oral intake	Life-threatening consequences; urgent intervention indicated	Death
Trismus	Decreased ROM (range of motion) without impaired eating	Decreased ROM requiring small bites, soft foods or purees	Decreased ROM with inability to adequately aliment or hydrate orally	-	-
Osteonecrosis	Asymptomatic; clinical or diagnostic observations only; intervention not indicated	Symptomatic; medical intervention indicated (e.g., analgesics or bisphosphonates); limiting instrumental ADL	Severe symptoms; limiting self-care ADL; elective operative intervention indicated	Life-threatening consequences; urgent intervention indicated	Death

of life can be affected, requiring breaks in treatment and hospitalization.[34]

Pathophysiology: RT with or without chemotherapy induces cellular damage with ROS formation within the basal epithelial and submucosal cells. This activates p53 and nuclear factor-κB, which propagates the damage response. This results in the production of inflammatory cytokines, which induces damage and cell death. Lesions at this stage become apparent in the mucosa and, if bacterial colonization occurs, can further complicate ulcer formation.

Prevention: Good oral hygiene and nutrition are prudent preventive strategies. Early professional dental assessment and prophylactic care is mandated. Brushing with soft tooth brush twice a day, rinsing with bland solutions such as normal saline, and sodium bicarbonate at least four times per day are recommended.[35]

Treatment: For established mucositis, MASCC/ISOO (Multinational Association of Supportive Care

in Cancer/International society of Oral Oncology) has provided treatment guidelines.[33] Benzydamine mouthwash can be used in patients undergoing RT. For pain relief, 0.2% morphine and 0.5% doxepin mouthwashes can be used. No recommendation was given for combination mouthwashes (magic mouthwash) containing lidocaine and other ingredients. Use of sucralfate mouthwash, topical antimicrobials, chlorhexidine, and misoprostol mouthwashes is not recommended. Systemic oral zinc may benefit patients receiving RT.[36,37] Low-level laser therapy can also be utilized for its antiinflammatory and analgesic effects in addition to healing ulcer.

Salivary Glands

Clinical features: Xerostomia, the subjective experience of dry mouth, is one of the most common and distressing adverse effect of RT. It is caused by salivary gland dysfunction. It causes difficulties in mastication and

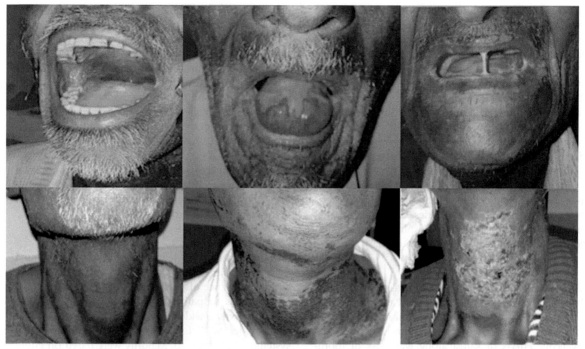

FIG. 5.8 (Above) Acute mucosal reactions RTOG Grade1 to 3, (below) acute skin reactions RTOG Grade 1 to 3.

swallowing and enhances dental problems affecting the quality of life, especially in long-term survivors after RT.

Pathophysiology: Radiation doses to the salivary glands (parotid and submandibular in particular) cause the loss and atrophy of acinar cells and granules.[38] Inflammatory changes and fibrosis are observed in periductal and intralobular areas. Late damage, on the other hand, results from depletion of stem cells.

Prevention: Total treatment volume, RT dose, and the initial volume and function of salivary gland influence the extent of salivary dysfunction. Methods such as limiting the mean dose to the parotids and use of IMRT can decrease the long-term risk of xerostomia. Surgically transplanting submandibular glands in the submental space prior to RT can prevent xerostomia.[39] Intravenous amifostine, a thiol-containing radioprotectant, administered before RT reduced acute and chronic xerostomia.[40]

Treatment: Timely and effective assessments of the xerostomia during and after RT are important for optimal patient care. Morphology and salivary flow rate can be measured in addition to subjective assessment in to assess the salivary gland changes and xerostomia condition. Dietary modifications such as avoiding

hard, spicy foods, consuming cold, tepid, and soft food and beverages are preferred. Saliva substitutes such as water, artificial saliva containing carboxymethylcellulose, xanthum gum mucin, etc. can be used. With residual salivary function, vitamin c lozenges, sugarless candies, and chewing gums can stimulate natural saliva. Systemic salivary gland stimulants such as pilocarpine, bethanechol, cevimeline, and other sialogogues have been used but with mixed results.[41] Acupuncture has also shown benefit even in pilocarpine-resistant xerostomia and improve quality of life.[42,43]

Dental Caries

Clinical features: NCI-CTCAE 5.0 defines treatment-induced dental caries as a disorder characterized by the decay of a tooth, in which it becomes softened, discolored, and/or porous[25] Hyposalivation induced by RT hastens the process of caries infection and increases its severity. Untreated caries can further progress to pulpitis and periapical abscess with subsequent loss of tooth. It also increases the risk for osteonecrosis of the mandible.

Pathophysiology: Radiation caries develop and progress rapidly, involving usually nonclassical surfaces of teeth such as cusp tips and gum line cavities.[44] Increased demineralization of the teeth, increased mineral loss, poor oral hygiene, and shift to more cariogenic flora accentuate the process.

Prevention: Comprehensive oral examination with early identification of carious lesions, fluoride, and calcium applications can prevent the progression of demineralization. The application of fluoride can be done using fluoride trays, high fluoride toothpastes, fluoride varnishes, or complex fluoride slow-release devices.[45] Grossly carried teeth should be extracted at least 2 weeks before the start of RT.

Treatment: Proper oral hygiene, managing xerostomia, and frequent oral hydration are initial key steps in the management of dental caries. Use of remineralizing products such as calcium and phosphate, in addition to topical fluoride, can be considered.[46]

Periodontal Disease

Clinical features: Periodontal disease is a disorder of the gingival tissue around the teeth. Patients receiving RT are at an increased risk for periodontal disease as compared with general population. Loss of the protective effects of saliva along with loss of tooth-supporting tissue predisposes RT patients to periodontitis. It can culminate in pain, with infection around the

dental roots and tooth loss. It can trigger osteoradionecrosis.[47]

Pathophysiology: The risk of periodontal disease in patients undergoing RT is dose dependent. Chronic inflammation with superadded microbial infection especially in a preexisting periodontitis can cause increased tooth and supporting tissue loss. This results in progressive gingival recession, bone loss, bleeding culminating in tooth loss, and finally giving predisposing patient to osteoradionecrosis of the maxilla or mandible.

Prevention and treatment: Thorough examination by dentist before, during and following RT, with extractions of teeth with severely compromised periodontium before treatment is recommended.[48]

Osteoradionecrosis

Osteoradionecrosis is defined as the exposed irradiated bone that fails to heal over a period of 3 months without evidence of persisting or recurrent tumor.[49] It can progress to pathological fracture (Fig. 5.9). The prevalence varies widely from 0.4% to 56% and usually affects elderly.[50,51] In the past, several scoring/staging systems were proposed. Majority were based on either response of the lesion to HBOT, degree of damage to bone, clinicoradiological characteristics of lesion,

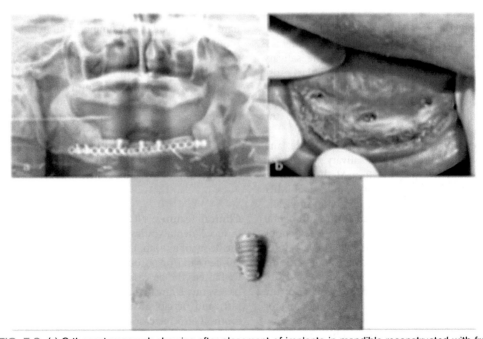

FIG. 5.9 (a) Orthopantomograph showing after placement of implants in mandible reconstructed with free fibula flap. (b) Placement of titanium implants in irradiated mandible reconstructed with free fibula flap. (c) Failure of implant osseointegration due to osteoradionecrosis.

TABLE 5.4
Clinical Staging Classification for Osteoradionecrosis (ORN)[57]

RECENT CLASSIFICATION FOR OSTEORADIONECROSIS (ORN)		
Stage I	ORN confined to alveolar bone	Based on clinical findings
Stage II	ORN limited to the alveolar bone and/or mandible above the level of inferior alveolar canal	
Stage III	ORN involving the mandible below the level of the inferior alveolar canal and/or skin fistula and/or pathological fracture	

etc.[52–54] The most recent staging systems are those proposed by Shwartz et al.[55] and Notani et al.[56] (Table 5.4).

Clinical features: Pain, trismus, and infection at the site of exposed bone and mucosa are initially appreciable. Impacted food particles, halitosis and altered taste sensation along with pain, dysesthesia, or anesthesia are usually present. Progressive lesions can culminate in pathological fracture of the bone with difficulty in mastication and speech. Superadded microbial infection can further lead to intra- or extraoral fistulae, cellulitis, and severe pain. Biopsy, to rule out residual or progressive lesion, is mandatory to diagnose osteoradionecrosis.

Pathophysiology: Ischemic necrosis is the hallmark of the lesion. Chronic inflammation with increased endothelial cell activity at the site of lesion, i.e., the prefibrotic phase, is followed by increased abnormal fibroblastic activity and finally fibroatrophic remodeling of the bone, which ends in loss of osteocytes. Thus, hyperemia, endarteritis, and thrombosis can be seen initially followed by fibrosis, hypovascularity, and progressive cell loss.[58,59] Radiologically, initial lesions are characterized by increased radiodensity, which progresses over time to radiolucent areas representing bone destruction.[49] On CT scans, cortical interruptions with focal lytic areas with associated soft tissue thickening can be appreciated.[60] CT scans, at times, cannot reliably differentiate between recurrent tumors and osteoradionecrotic lesions. Therefore, MRI (magnetic resonance imaging) scans with contrast, having better soft tissue delineation and high spatial resolution characteristics,

aid in the differential diagnosis.[61] Bone scintigraphy using 99mTc-marked diphosphonates (99mTc-MDP) shows high sensitivity (up to 100%) but low specificity (about 60%) for diagnosis of osteoradionecrosis.[61] PET (positron emission tomography) can reliably differentiate between tumor recurrence and osteoradionecrotic lesion.[57]

Prevention: Maintaining good oral hygiene, treating any existing oral disease before treatment, and stabilizing oral health during RT can decrease the incidence of osteoradionecrosis. The main goal of comprehensive dental care should be to minimize the need of invasive interventions (like extraction) and dental inflammatory disease/infection during and after RT for the life of the patient.[44] Utilizing modern RT techniques such as IMRT can further decrease the incidence of osteoradionecrosis.[62]

Treatment: Management varies widely from the use of antifibrotic medications such as pentoxifylline, tocopherol, clodronate, and antioxidants initially on completion of RT to using HBOT, surgical resection, and reconstruction for advanced, nonresponding lesions. Low-level laser therapy can promote bone and soft tissue repair.[63] Bone marrow–derived stem cells and bone morphogenetic protein-2 can facilitate healing, but these are still experimental.[64] Initial treatment should always be conservative. Resection with reconstruction may become necessary in advanced, severe cases especially those with pathological fracture or threatening fracture despite nonsurgical measures.

Trismus
RT-induced trismus varies widely, ranging from 5% to as high as 45%.[65] A cutoff point of <35 mm for mouth opening is used to define trismus in clinical studies.[44] Fibrosis of the muscles of mastication including masseter, temporalis, and medial and lateral pterygoids and/or the temporomandibular joint can cause RT-induced trismus. It significantly affects the oral articulation of the patient including speech and swallowing and limits the effective dental care and delivery (Fig. 5.10).

Patho-physiology: Plethora of normal tissue complications including vessels, muscles, nerves, and lymphatics, ensuing in post-RT fibrosis is the main cause for trismus.

Prevention and treatment: The shift of RT from two-dimensional to three-dimensional to intensity-modulated radiotherapy (IMRT) has gradually shifted the weighted prevalence of RT-induced trismus.[66] Pentoxifylline and vitamin E can reduce fibrosis, but level of evidence is not sufficient.[66] Tongue blades/dynamic

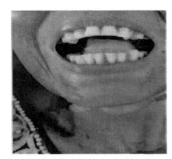

FIG. 5.10 Treatment-related trismus.

bite opening devices can be used to gradually increase mouth opening. Photobiomodulation or low light laser therapy can both prevent and treat RT-induced trismus.[67]

Postradiation Prosthodontic Care

The main goal of postradiation prosthodontic care is to adequately maintain the oral function and health of the patient including rehabilitation of RT-induced normal tissue complications. Patients often require partial or complete new dentures. However, oral tissues should be adequately healed before initiation of any prosthodontic plan. Ideally, it requires a minimum of 6 months for the oral soft tissues to repair the damage. Thus, a window period of 6–12 months should be provided post-RT to initiate any prosthodontic procedure.[68]

CONCLUSION

Radiotherapy plays a vital role in the treatment of head and neck malignancies either exclusively or as adjuvant to surgery. Dose sculpting to the target/treatment volume especially using IMRT not only improves the disease control probability, but it also allows protection of healthy organs, thereby avoiding a variety of normal tissue complications. Comprehensive follow-up strategies including dental care for RT effects are imperative to the prevention and management of treatment-related sequelae.

REFERENCES

1. *NCCN Clinical Practice Guidelines in Oncology;* 2020. https://www.nccn.org/professionals/physician_gls/pdf/head-and-neck.pdf/. Accessed December 3, 2020.
2. Prabhash K, Babu G, Chaturvedi P, et al. Indian clinical practice consensus guidelines for the management of squamous cell carcinoma of head and neck. *Indian J Cancer.* 2020;57(Suppl S1):1–5.
3. Lefebvre JL. Laryngeal preservation in head and neck cancer: multidisciplinary approach. *Lancet Oncol.* September 2006;7(9):747–755.
4. Ordoñez R, Otero A, Jerez I, et al. Role of radiotherapy in the treatment of metastatic head and neck cancer. *OncoTargets Ther.* 2019;12:677–683.
5. Halperin EC, Perez CA, Brady LW, eds. *Perez and Brady's Principles and Practice of Radiation Oncology.* 5th ed. Philadelphia: Lippincott Williams & Wilkins; 2008.
6. Joiner MC, vanderKogel AJ, eds. *Basic Clinical Radiobiology.* 5th ed. United Kingdom: CRC Press; 2018.
7. Rubin P, Finkelstein JN, Williams JP. In: Tobias J, Thomas P, eds. *Paradigm Shifts in the Radiation Pathophysiology of Late Effects in Normal Tissues: Molecular vs. Classic Concepts.* London: Arnold; 1998.
8. Hall EJ, Giaccia AJ, eds. *Radiobiology for the Radiologist.* 7th ed. Philadelphia: Lippincott Williams & Wilkins; 2012.
9. Al-Sarraf M, LeBlanc M, Giri PG, et al. Chemoradiotherapy versus radiotherapy in patients with advanced nasopharyngeal cancer: phase III randomized Intergroup study 0099. *J Clin Oncol.* 1998;16(4):1310–1317.
10. Denis F, Garaud P, Bardet E, et al. Final results of the 94-01 French Head and Neck Oncology and Radiotherapy Group randomized trial comparing radiotherapy alone with concomitant radiochemotherapy in advanced-stage oropharynx carcinoma. *J Clin Oncol.* 2004;22(1):69–76.
11. Bray F, Ferlay J, Soerjomataram I, et al. Global cancer statistics 2018: GLOBOCAN estimates of incidence and mortality worldwide for 36 cancers in 185 countries. *CA Cancer J Clin.* 2018;68:394–424.
12. Iyer NG, Tan DSW, Tan VK, et al. Randomized trial comparing surgery and adjuvant radiotherapy versus concurrent chemoradiotherapy in patients with advanced, non-metastatic squamous cell carcinoma of the head and neck: 10-year update and subsetanalysis. *Cancer.* 2015;121(10):1599–1607.
13. Tupchong L, Scott CB, Blitzer PH, et al. Randomized study of preoperative versus postoperative radiation therapy in advanced head and neck carcinoma: long-term follow-up of RTOG study 73-03. *Int J Radiat Oncol Biol Phys.* 1991;20:21–28.
14. Peters LJ, Goepfert H, Ang KK, et al. Evaluation of the dose for postoperative radiation therapy of head and neck cancer: first report of a prospective randomized trial. *Int J Radiat Oncol Biol Phys.* 1993;26(1):3–11.
15. Ang KK, Trotti A, Brown BW, et al. Randomized trial addressing risk features and time factors of surgery plus radiotherapy in advanced head-and-neck cancer. *Int J Radiat Oncol Biol Phys.* 2001;51:571–578.
16. Bernier J, Domenge C, Ozsahin M, et al. Postoperative irradiation with or without concomitant chemotherapy for locally advanced head and neck cancer. *N Engl J Med.* 2004;350:1945–1952.
17. Cooper JS, Zhang Q, Pajak TF, et al. Long-term follow-up of the RTOG 9501/intergroup phase III trial: postoperative concurrent radiation therapy and chemotherapy in high-risk squamous cell carcinoma of the head and neck. *Int J Radiat Oncol Biol Phys.* 2012;84(5):1198–1205.

18. Bernier J, Cooper JS, Pajak TF, et al. Defining risk levels in locally advanced head and neck cancers: a comparative analysis of concurrent postoperative radiation plus chemotherapy trials of the EORTC (#22931) and RTOG (# 9501). *Head Neck.* 2005;27(10):843–850.

19. Pernot M, Verhaeghe JL, Guillemin F, et al. Evaluation of the importance of a systematic neck dissection in carcinomas of the oral cavity treated by brachytherapy only for the primary lesion (about a serie of 346 patients). *Bull Cancer Radiother.* 1995;82:311–317.

20. Melzner WJ, Lotter M, Sauer R, et al. Quality of interstitial PDR brachytherapy-implants of head-and-neck-cancers: predictive factors for local control and late toxicity. *Radiother Oncol.* 2007;82:167–173.

21. Wendt CD, Peters LJ, Delclos L, et al. Primary radiotherapy in the treatment of stage I and II oral tongue cancers: importance of the proportion of therapy delivered with interstitial therapy. *Int J Radiat Oncol Biol Phys.* 1990; 18(6):1287–1292.

22. Grabenbauer GG, Rodel C, Brunner T, et al. Interstitial brachytherapy with Ir-192 lowdose- rate in the treatment of primary and recurrent cancer of the oral cavity and oropharynx.Review of 318 patients treated between 1985 and 1997. *Strahlenther Onkol.* 2001;177:338–344.

23. Lefebvre JL, Coche-Dequeant B, Buisset E, et al. Management of early oral cavity cancer. Experience of Centre Oscar Lambret. *Eur J Cancer B Oral Oncol.* 1994;30B(3): 216–220.

24. Cox JD, Stetz J, Pajak TF. Toxicity criteria of the radiation therapy oncology Group (RTOG) and the European organization for Research and treatment of cancer (EORTC). *Int J Radiat Oncol Biol Phys.* March 30, 1995;31(5): 1341–1346.

25. Common Terminology Criteria for Adverse Events (CTCAE). https://ctep.cancer.gov/protocoldevelopment/ electronic_applications/docs/ctcae_v5_quick_reference_ 5x7.pdf; 2020. Accessed December 3, 2020.

26. Ryan JL. Ionizing radiation: the good, the bad, and the ugly. *J Invest Dermatol.* 2012;132:985–993.

27. Gottlober P, Krahn G, Peter RU. Cutaneous radiation syndrome: clinical features, diagnosis and therapy. *Hautarzt.* 2000;51:567–574.

28. Chan RJ, Webster J, Chung B, et al. Prevention and treatment of acute radiation-induced skin reactions: a systematic review and meta-analysis of randomizedcontrolled trials. *BMC Cancer.* 2014;14:53.

29. Tahir AR, Westhuyzen J, Dass J, et al. Hyperbaric oxygen therapy for chronicradiation-induced tissue injuries: Australasia's largest study. *Asia Pac J Clin Oncol.* 2015;11: 68–77.

30. Zhang X, Li H, Li Q, et al. Application of red light phototherapy in the treatment ofradioactive dermatitis in patients with head and neck cancer. *World J Surg Oncol.* 2018;16:222.

31. Seite S, Bensadoun RJ, Mazer JM. Prevention and treatment of acute and chronicradio-dermatitis. *Breast Cancer.* 2017; 9:551–557.

32. Diggelmann KV, Zytkovicz AE, Tuaine JM, et al. Mepilex-Lite dressings for themanagement of radiation-induced erythema: a systematic inpatient controlledclinical trial. *Br J Radiol.* 2010;83:971–978.

33. Lalla RV, Saunders DP, Peterson DE. Chemotherapy or radiation induced oral mucositis. *Dent Clin.* 2014;58: 341–349.

34. Elting LS, Cooksley CD, Chambers MS, et al. Risk, outcomes, and costs of radiation induced oral mucositis among patients with headandneck malignancies. *Int J Radiat Oncol Biol Phys.* 2007;68:1110–1120.

35. Bensinger W, Schubert M, Ang KK, et al. NCCN Task Force Report. Prevention and management of mucositis in cancer care. *J Natl ComprCancNetw.* 2008;6:S1–S21. quiz S22-S24.

36. Khan M, Siddiqui SA, Akram M, et al. Can zinc supplementation widen the gap between control and complications in head and neck cancer patients treated with concurrent chemo-radiotherapy. *J Med Sci.* 2019;39:267–271.

37. Yarom N, Ariyawardana A, Hovan A, et al. Systematic review of natural agents for the management of oral mucositis in cancer patients. *Support Care Cancer.* 2013;21: 3223–3232.

38. Wang X, Eisbruch A. IMRT for head and neck cancer: reducing xerostomia and dysphagia. *J Radiat Res.* 2016; 57(Suppl. 1):i69–i75.

39. Zhang Y, Guo CB, Zhang L, et al. Prevention of radiation-induced xerostomia by submandibular gland transfer. *Head Neck.* 2012;34(7):937–942.

40. Brizel DM, Wasserman TH, Henke M, et al. Phase III randomized trial ofamifostine as a radioprotector in head and neck cancer. *J Clin Oncol.* 2000;18(19):3339–3345.

41. Jensen SB, Pedersen AM, Vissink A, et al. A systematic review of salivarygland hypofunction and xerostomia induced by cancer therapies:management strategies and economic impact. *Support Care Cancer.* 2010;18(8): 1061–1079.

42. Johnstone PA, Peng YP, May BC, et al. Acupuncture for pilocarpine resistant xerostomia following radiotherapy for head and neck malignancies. *Int J Radiat Oncol Biol Phys.* 2001;50(2):353–357.

43. Meng Z, Garcia MK, Hu C, et al. Randomized controlled trial of acupuncture for prevention of radiation-induced xerostomia among patients with nasopharyngeal carcinoma. *Cancer.* 2012;118(13):3337–3344.

44. Sroussi HY, Epstein JB, Bensadoun RJ, et al. Common oral complications of head and neck cancer radiation therapy: mucositis, infections, saliva change, fibrosis, sensory dysfunctions, dental caries, periodontal disease, and osteoradionecrosis. *Cancer Med.* 2017;6(12):2918–2931.

45. Chambers MS, Mellberg JR, Keene HJ, et al. Clinical evaluation of the intraoral fluoride releasing system in radiation-induced xerostomic subjects. Part 1: fluorides. *Oral Oncol.* 2006;42:934–945.

46. Deng J, Jackson L, Epstein JB, et al. Dental demineralization and caries in patients with head and neck cancer. *Oral Oncol.* 2015;51:824–831.

47. Katsura K, Sasai K, Sato K, et al. Relationship between oral health status and development of osteoradionecrosis of the mandible: a retrospective longitudinal study. *Oral Surg Oral Med Oral Pathol Oral Radiol Endod.* 2008;105:731–738.

48. Hong CH, Napeñas JJ, Hodgson BD, et al. A systematic review of dental disease in patients undergoing cancer therapy. *Support Care Cancer.* 2010;18:1007–1021.

49. Chronopoulos A, Zarra T, Ehrenfeld M, et al. Osteoradionecrosis of the jaws: definition, epidemiology, staging and clinical and radiological findings. A concise review. *Int Dent J.* 2018;68:22–30.

50. Reuther T, Schuster T, Mende U, et al. Osteoradionecrosis of the jaws as a side effect of radiotherapy of head and neck tumour patients—a report of a thirty year retrospective review. *Int J Oral Maxillofac Surg.* 2003;32:289–295.

51. Grötz KA, Riesenbeck D, Brahm R, et al. Chronic radiation effects on dental hard tissue (radiation caries). Classification and therapeutic strategies. *Strahlenther Onkol.* 2001;177:96–104.

52. Marx RE. Osteoradionecrosis; a new concept of its pathophysiology. *J Oral Maxillofac Surg.* 1983;41:283–288.

53. Morton ME, Simpson W. The management of osteoradionecrosis of the jaws. *Br J Oral Maxillofac Surg.* 1986;24:332–341.

54. Store G, Boysen M. Mandibular osteoradionecrosis: clinical behavior and diagnostic aspects. *ClinOtolaryngol.* 2000;25:378–384.

55. Schwartz HC, Kagan AR. Osteoradionecrosis of the mandible: scientific basis for clinical staging. *Am J ClinOncol.* 2002;25:168–171.

56. Notani K, Yamazaki Y, Kitada H, et al. Management of mandibular osteoradionecrosis corresponding to the severity of osteoradionecrosis and the method of radiotherapy. *Head Neck.* 2003;25:181–186.

57. Minn H, Aitasalo K, Happonen RP. Detection of cancer recurrence in irradiated mandible using positron emission tomography. *Eur Arch Oto-Rhino-Laryngol.* 1993;250:312–315.

58. Zheng WK, Inokuchi A, Yamamoto T, et al. Taste dysfunction in irradiated patients with head and neck cancer. *Fukuoka Igaku Zasshi.* 2002;93:64–76.

59. Panayiotou H, Small SC, Hunter JH, et al. Sweet taste (dysgeusia). The first symptom of hyponatremia in small cell carcinoma of the lung. *Arch Intern Med.* 1995;155:1325–1328.

60. Tobias JS, Thomas PRM. *Current Radiation Oncology.* Vol. 2. London: Arnold; 1996.

61. Bachmann G, Rossler R, Klett R, et al. The role of magnetic resonance imaging and scintigraphy in the diagnosis of pathologic changes of the mandible after radiation therapy. *Int J Oral Maxillofac Surg.* 1996;25:189–195.

62. Widmark G, Sagne S, Heikel P. Osteoradionecrosis of the jaws. *Int J Oral Maxillofac Surg.* 1989;18:302–306.

63. Gomez DR, Estilo CL, Wolden SL, et al. Correlation of osteoradionecrosis and dental events with dosimetric parameters in intensity modulated radiation therapy for head and neck cancer. *Int J Radiat Oncol Biol Phys.* 2011;81:e207–e213.

64. Hey J, Seidel J, Schweyen R, et al. The influence of parotid gland sparing on radiation damages of dental hard tissues. *Clin Oral Invest.* 2013;17:1619–1625.

65. Dijkstra PU, Kalk WW, Roodenburg JL. Trismus in head and neck oncology: a systematic review. *Oral Oncol.* 2004;40:879–889.

66. Bensadoun RJ, Riesenbeck D, Lockhart PB, et al. A systematic review of trismus induced by cancer therapies in head and neck cancer patients. *Support Care Cancer.* 2010;18:1033–1038.

67. Zecha JA, Raber-Durlacher JE, Nair RG, et al. Low level laser therapy/photobiomodulation in the management of side effects of chemoradiation therapy in head and neck cancer: part 2: proposed applications and treatment protocols. *Support Care Cancer.* 2016;24:2793–2805.

68. Devi S, Singh N. Dental care during and after radiotherapy in head and neck cancer. *Natl J Maxillofac Surg.* 2014;5:117–125.

CHAPTER 6

Prosthetic Rehabilitation of Mandibular Defects

PANKAJ PRAKASH KHARADE, MDS, FJPS.

Prosthetic rehabilitation of mandibular defects due to surgical resection or trauma is usually very complex procedure. Rehabilitation is the process of getting back to a healthy or better lifestyle, or the procedure of assisting the patients to do this. Mandibular defects induce paradigm shift in the lifestyle of patient due to functional, biological, esthetic, and social consequences of the treatment. Augmentation of the understanding and advancement of new technology has fostered the rehabilitation of these defects. Interdisciplinary approach is essential for a successful rehabilitation, which includes surgical intervention, radiation therapy, and/or chemotherapy followed by prosthetic restoration. Patients with postsurgical defects can return to as close to normal if all possible and constant customized modifications are made precisely. Apart from that, it may also necessitate additional surgical procedures to improve the treatment outcome. Surgical reconstruction of defect with free bone grafts, pedicle bone grafts, particulate bone cancellous marrow grafts, reconstruction plates, and microvascular free flaps is possible where these procedures involve harvesting of bone and soft tissues from donor sites. Among all these procedures, surgical reconstruction with microvascular free flaps is considered most recent. There are chances of significant morbidity, which can affect the acceptance of the treatment by the patient. Diagnosis and treatment planning should be executed in a precise manner to improve the prognostic factor. Curtis and Cantor in 1974 mentioned regarding the problems-associated treatment planning of mandibular defects. Recent advances in the field of surgical reconstruction and prosthetic rehabilitation have improved the treatment outcome as compared with clinical procedures in the past. It is essential to assess various clinical situations associated with mandibular defects and treat appropriately to improve the quality of life for these patients. Prosthetic rehabilitation for restoration of normal function as well as esthetics is a principal challenge in the rehabilitation of patients who have lost their teeth and part of mandible after surgical resection of cyst or tumor.[1] Whenever the extent of edentulous span and length of defect increases, rehabilitation with fixed or removable prosthesis becomes further complicated. Anatomic deformities in addition to adverse biomechanics in the proximity of resection area add to incongruence. Disabilities resulting due to resection often lead to loss of mandibular continuity, which further leads to facial disfigurement, uncoordinated movement, difficulty in chewing, impaired speech, and frontal plane rotation of teeth[2] (Fig. 6.1).

TYPES OF MANDIBULAR DEFECTS

a. Marginal mandibulectomy (continuity defect) (Fig. 6.2)

Segmental mandibulectomy (discontinuity defect): These defects affect function as well as esthetics extensively after resection of mandible due to lack of continuity due to resection of mandibular segment (Fig. 6.3).

b. Hemimandibulectomy (discontinuity defect):

Such cases need rigid reconstruction after hemimandibulectomy.

Hemimandibulectomy with discontinuity defects affects the muscular balance of facial muscles, leading to disfigurement of face if reconstruction is not done.

Such cases are usually reconstructed with reconstruction plates (Fig. 6.5).

The most extensively documented classification system is the HCL classification by Jewer and colleagues.[3] This HCL classification was amended by JB Boyd and colleagues with addition of three lower case letters o (neither skin nor mucosa, m (mucosa) and s (skin)), which represents epithelial involvement.[4]

Prosthetic Rehabilitation of Head and Neck Cancer Patients. https://doi.org/10.1016/B978-0-323-82394-4.00004-5

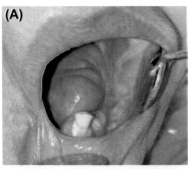

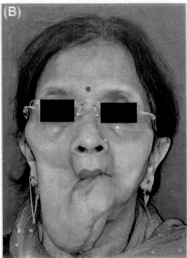

FIG. 6.1 (a) Deviation of mandible due to muscle pull. (b) Disfigured face after surgical resection of mandible.

There has been mention of several mandibular defect classifications in various documents. Pavlov has classified mandibular defects into three classes grounded on number of residual bone fragments.[5] David and colleagues have given the classification of six types of defects, which is based on the segments of resected mandible.[6] In1991, Urken et al. proposed a widespread classification of mandibular defects based on anatomical, functional as well as esthetic considerations. The classification consists of mandibular defects (S-symphysis, SH, R-ramus, C-condyle, B-body) and soft tissue defects in addition to neurological defects.[7] Iizuka and colleagues classified the resection of mandible into four classes centered on osteotomies for mandibular fibula free flap reconstruction with the help of endosseous implants.[8]

Hashikawa and colleagues suggested the CAT classification in the year 2008, which was illustrative of loss of condylar head (C), angle as well (A) as mental tubercle (T). The hemimandibulectomy was symbolized as CAT.[9] In 2011, Baumann DP et al. proposed the classification of the mandibular bone defects resulting to osteoradionecrosis into four types, viz., type I a, type I b, type II a, and type II b in reference to loss of condyle, mucosa, and overlying skin.[10]

In 2015, Schultz and colleagues proposed the classification of the mandibular defects based on their complex nature into four types with two subsections depending on the availability or insufficiency of ipsilateral vasculature for reconstruction.[11]

In recent times, Brown and colleagues suggested a classification, which showed upsurge in size as well as complexity and proliferation in morbidity in terms of esthetics and functional outcome as the classes proceed from class I to class IV. This classification has been claimed to be one of the most simple as well as logical while considering clinical applicability.[3]

Despite continuous attempts in classifying mandibular defects, an unanimously recognized classification, mandibular defect, is still arguable. It is very indispensable to recognize the characteristics of the surgical treatment and prosthodontic restrictions for accurate clinical management of patients with mandibular defects.[12]

SEQUELAE OF MANDIBULAR RESECTION

Loss of esthetic as well as function is obvious consequence of mandibular resection. Apart from that, what remains overlooked is the psychological, social, and financial influence of these defects after resection of mandible. Total or partial loss of a portion of mandible leads to compromised masticatory, deglutition, and speech function. In conjunction with these issues, the patient has to deal with the major social as well as mental aftereffects of mandibular resections. The following clinical features are seen after resection of mandible (Fig. 6.4):

a. Mandibular deviation toward the surgical side.
b. Destroyed balance.
c. Altered mandibular movements.
d. Facial asymmetry and malocclusion.
e. Frontal plane rotation

If the mandibular discontinuity is not restored, the additional impairment of tongue function in most of the patients may lead to severely compromised masticatory function. Frontal plane rotation is most commonly associated with lateral discontinuity defect of the mandible. Such type of deviation takes place regardless

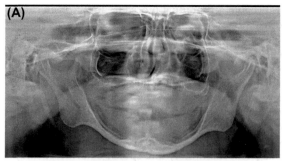

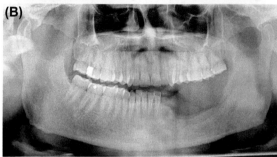

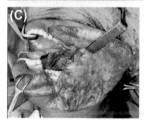
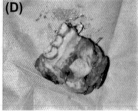

FIG. 6.2 (a) Mandibular resection has not affected continuity of mandible. (b) Mandibular continuity defect. (c) Marginal resection of mandible. (d) Section of mandible after marginal resection.

of whether the surgical site after resection has been closed primarily or by incorporating free or myocutaneous flaps. Lack of restoration of mandibular discontinuity after surgical resection may lead to variable degree of severe as well as permanent deviation of mandible. Several complex factors are responsible for such type of deviation of mandible, which includes method of closure, amount of hard and soft tissue resection, and so on. Incorporation of free or myocutaneous during closure of surgical site will help to achieve acceptable occlusal relationship in patients even in the absence of adjunctive therapy, whereas primary closure

of surgical site causes unstable and inappropriate interocclusal relationship in patients (Chart 6.1).

MANAGEMENT FOR THE DEVIATION OF MANDIBLE

1. **Guide flange prosthesis**
   Guide flange prosthesis is used to correct the deviated mandible due to unilateral muscle pull after resection of tumor.
2. **Physiotherapy to diminish fibrosis**
   Prosthetic management and exercise program should be started 2 weeks after the surgery. This exercise program helps to release scar contracture and reduce the severity of trismus and also helps to improve maxillomandibular relationships (Fig. 6.6).
3. **Reconstruction with reconstruction plates**
   Reconstruction plates can serve as provisional means of reconstruction after resection of mandible (Fig. 6.8a). Probability of fracture or loosening of these plates is high if they are used as the only means of reconstruction and left over for longer duration. Apart from that, chances of failure increase due to greater length of missing segment, i.e., more than 5 cm and postresection radiotherapy treatment.[13,14] Exposure of the reconstruction plate can be seen either due to lack of bony flap in combination with reconstruction plate or in patients who have undergone radiotherapy treatment (Figs. 6.7 and 6.8b).
4. **Intermaxillary fixation**
   This method is used less frequently nowadays as it may cause dental ailments and excessive discomfort to the patient. It is considered an effective method during initial healing period after surgical resection to maintain the sense of proprioception to restore the interocclusal relationship. Intermaxillary fixation is maintained 5–7 weeks after resection of tumor. Intermaxillary fixation is effective when there is minimal loss of tissue after resection of tumor as fibrosis due to scarring is less. Apart from that, abundant tissue is available for primary closure without scar formation, and imbalance related to muscles is less severe. It has been used in the past as one of the effective methods to minimize the deviation after resection of tumor. Maxillomandibular fixation is not indicated in patients undergoing radiotherapy after composite resection with radicle neck dissection and in situations where oral surgical

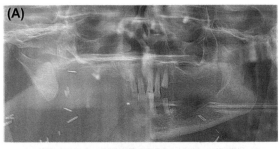

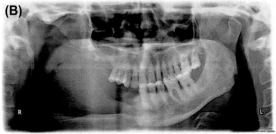

FIG. 6.3 (a) Marginal resection of mandible- Radiograph showing segmental resection. (b) Radiograph showing segmental resection without reconstruction.

site is closed primarily. Scar contracture formed due to primary closure of big defects contributes more toward deviation of mandible as compared with muscular imbalance and loss of proprioception to maintain occlusal relationship (Fig. 6.8).

5. **Reconstruction with soft tissue free flaps** (Fig. 6.9)
6. **Reconstruction with free vascularized bone flap** (Fig. 6.10)

SURGICAL RECONSTRUCTION OF MANDIBLE

Resection of a segment of the mandible, which is leading to mandibular discontinuity, is very destructing in nature.[15] An ameloblastoma is an extremely common and exceptionally aggressive odontogenic tumor of epithelial origin. Ameloblastoma is commonly found in posterior region of mandible and most frequently treated with surgical excision of the tumor.[16] Mandibular reconstruction is essential to restore facial symmetry, arch alignment in addition to stable occlusion, but masticatory function frequently remains compromised.[17,18] There is paucity of literature related to reconstruction of mandible with fibula graft as well as restoration of esthetics, speech intelligibility, swallowing, and masticatory performance.[19–25] The fibula graft was made popular by Hidalgo in the 1990s and

has become very routine procedure for reconstruction nowadays.[26] Soft tissue dehiscence is one of the significant concerns, which needs to be paid attention for patients who wear entirely soft tissue borne prosthesis over the area reconstructed with free fibula graft. Implant-retained prosthesis in free fibula flap helps to prevent tissue dehiscence due to appropriate distribution of masticatory load. Even though denture bearing area was not favorable to achieve satisfactory retention as well as stability, implant-retained prosthesis helps to augment masticatory and speech outcome. A study conducted at Tata Memorial Hospital to assess the quality of life (EORTC QlQ-C30) after implant-retained prosthetic rehabilitation in reconstructed jaws post cancer treatments has achieved favorable outcomes after reconstruction with free fibula graft. In this study, speech was assessed objectively and swallowing was assessed by using a questionnaire. It was seen that the patient's voice resonance was enhanced, and they could endure phonation for longer duration without difficulty after prosthetic rehabilitation in grafted mandible. Eating ability was found to be better; consumption of solid, semisolid, and overcooked food was considerably improved with the prosthesis.[27]

Whenever anterior part of mandible is resected, it should be reconstructed simultaneously as discontinuity in the anterior region of mandible leads to severe form of disability. Anterior resection leaves unsupported fragments of posterior mandible, which are pulled in medial direction by mylohyoid muscle and superiorly by muscles of mastication. Additionally, retrusion of tongue in posterior direction due to loss of anterior attachments creates occlusion of airway and difficulty in fabrication of prosthesis. Primary closure should be avoided in such situations as it can impair mobility of tongue and loss of vestibule will be seen in the anterior region. Primary closure makes mastication impossible. Also there is continuous drooling of saliva, and speech is impaired. Cosmetic appearance is extensively affected, creating illusion of loss of lower third of the face accentuating facial disfigurement (Fig. 6.11).

Restoration of occlusion and prosthetic rehabilitation is very much complicated for patients with anterior mandibular defect without surgical reconstruction. Such defects can be reconstructed using free fibula graft. Advances in the field of prosthesis have made use of recently introduced materials such as polyetherketone-ketone (PEKK) possible for fabrication of prosthetic framework using dental implants to rehabilitate such defects and achieve favorable esthetics and functional results.[28–35] Use of vascular flaps for surgical

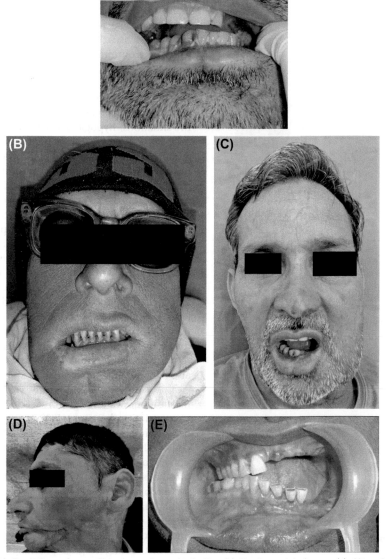

FIG. 6.4 (a) Deviation of mandible toward surgical site. (b) Destroyed balance. (c) Altered mandibular movements. (d) Facial asymmetry and malocclusion. (e) Frontal plane rotation.

reconstruction allows tension-free closure and osseointegration of dental implants for prosthetic rehabilitation.[36,37] Various studies have shown that reconstruction of mandibular segmental defects with dental implants and vascularized autogenous grafts is a successful treatment to restore oral function.[38–42]

In certain situations, even though continuity of mandible is restored with surgical reconstructions without causing tongue morbidity, compromised posture as well as function of lower lip is seen due to affected sensory and motor supply of tongue. It is very essential to maintain bulk of the anterior tongue during surgical resection as it can affect the function even if the continuity of mandible is maintained. During surgical reconstruction, precautions should be taken not to alter the pattern of closure as it can affect functions such as

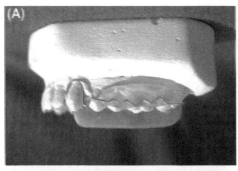

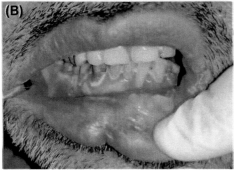

FIG. 6.5 (a) Guide flange prosthesis. (b) Correction of deviation with guide flange prosthesis.

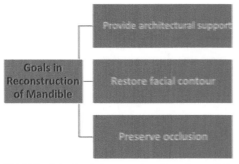

CHART 6.1 Goals in reconstruction of mandible.

mastication, deglutition, and speech to certain extent. In short, it is very vital to maintain the tongue mobility as it can lead to functional deficiencies. In most of these situations, sensory and motor innovations of tongue are not compromised, whereas reverse is true for sensory and motor innovations of lower lip, which makes them incompetent and unable to control salivary secretions. When extent of tumor is limited to the alveolar ridge, resultant disability due to resection of tumor is minimal as continuity of mandible is maintained in

marginal mandibulectomy. These defects can be rehabilitated using conventional removable prosthesis. Usually, there is obliteration of buccal or lingual sulci. These resections cause less morbidity and damage to inferior alveolar nerve. If the tumor in the alveolar region is extensive, then resection of such tumors will lead to discontinuity of the mandible causing deviation of mandible due to muscular imbalance. In these situations, tongue can be used for normal functioning as chances of resection excessive bulk of tongue are very less causing minimal injury to hypoglossal. In most of the situations, hypoglossal nerve remains intact. If the bulk of the tongue remains intact and motor functions are not affected, tongue can perform most of the visual functions without any significant dysfunction.

Whenever mandibular deviation is associated with muscular imbalance as the primary reasons along with compromised proprioception, it can be corrected with the help of mandibular guidance prosthesis. Proportion of correction of mandibular deviation is associated with the timing of prosthetic rehabilitation. Minimum amount of initial deviation leads to better the correction.[43] The extent of scarring depends on use of free flaps and dose of radiotherapy incorporated for particular patient. Well-designed free vascularized flaps in consultation with the prosthodontist can appropriately resolve the problem of mandibular discontinuity and make prosthetic rehabilitation possible. In certain situations, flaps also help in restoration of lost buck of tongue due to surgical resection, and subsequently, vital functions such as mastication, swallowing, and speech can be restored in a very operational manner. In this way, vascularized flap helps to improve the quality of life of head–neck cancer patients. Novel techniques such as transport disc, distraction osteogenesis, tissue engineering, and modular endoprosthesis are being developed and verified to minimize the morbidity of the donor site.[44] It is very unfortunate that usually all mandibulectomy interventions are executed without considering the prognosis of a subsequent prosthetic rehabilitation. Hence, it is very significant that during surgical planning, the clinical team should figure out some surgical procedures to enhance prosthetic prognosis. The inclusion of free fibula bone graft, osseointegrated implants, and digital technologies may aid to improve the prognosis of such prosthetic rehabilitation. The treatment planning should be aimed at evaluating the surgical modifications to augment the prosthetic prognosis as well as functional outcome in patients with mandibular defects after mandibular resection. Alterations in surgical interventions will definitely help to improve the prosthetic prognosis in patients suffering with mandibular defects.[45] The prognosis of

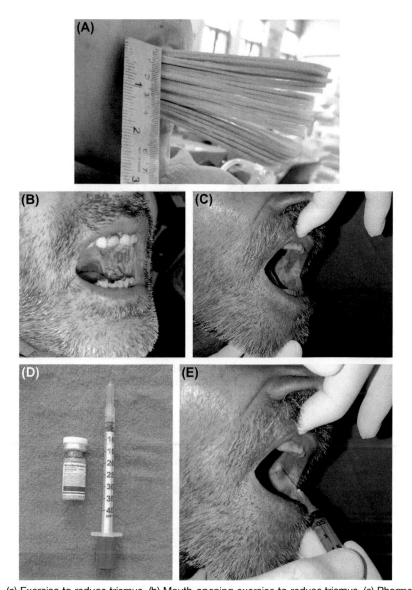

FIG. 6.6 (a) Exercise to reduce trismus. (b) Mouth-opening exercise to reduce trismus. (c) Pharmacological management of trismus. (d) Hyaluronidase injection to manage trismus. (e) Intralesional hyaluronidase injection to manage trismus.

removable prosthesis for patients who have undergone resection of mandible and tongue is variable. For certain patients, only esthetics can be enhanced due to lack of retention and support for the prosthesis. Patients who undergo reconstruction with free vascularized fibula flaps and improved mastication can be judiciously achieved.[46–49]

The obliteration of the mandibular sulcus often necessitates a skin graft and an immediate stent prosthesis

to stabilize and maintain the graft during the healing period.[50]

PROSTHETIC REHABILITATION OF MANDIBULAR DEFECTS

Obturator Prosthesis for Mandibular Defect

Sometimes, resection of mandibular tumors leads to smaller defects in body region if mandible. Such defects

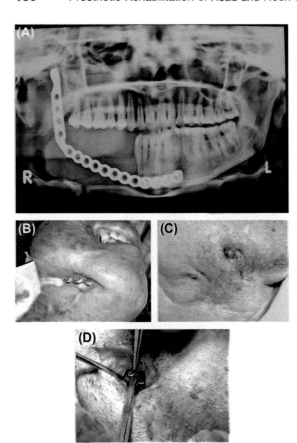

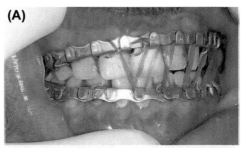

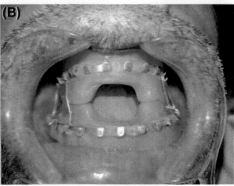

FIG. 6.8 (a) Intermaxillary fixation to prevent deviation of the mandible. (b) Gunning splint improves deviation in edentulous patient with discontinuity defect.

FIG. 6.7 (a) Radiograph after reconstruction with plate. (b) Exposure of reconstruction plate. (c) Skin lesion due to infection related to reconstruction plate. (d) Removal of screw is necessary before implant placement in the fibula.

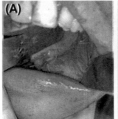

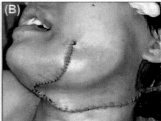

FIG. 6.9 (a) Reconstruction with soft tissue flap avoids contracture. (b) Extra oral suturing after reconstruction with free flap.

if not reconstructed properly remain permanent in the oral cavity. For such defects, hygiene maintenance is the major issue, which is worsened by food accumulation. It also leads to delayed healing during initial healing period. Fabrication of a prosthesis, which will obturate the mandibular defect, leads to satisfactory outcome as inconvenience of the patient is rectified.

After complete cleaning of the defect, impression of the defect is made with suitable elastic impression material. Mold is prepared by pouring that impression, and this mold is used for fabrication of obturator prosthesis. It is made hollow by using the hollowing technique. A loop can be attached to hold the prosthesis. Such kind of prosthesis can be prescribed for the patients who are not mentally prepared for surgical closure of the defect with bone grafting or if surgery is contraindicated due to any general or local ailment of the patient (Fig. 6.12).

In patients with impaired tongue tissue and movement, centric occlusion should be established at a decreased vertical dimension of occlusion to enable the tongue to interact more effectively with palatal structures.[51] For a patient who has undergone segmental mandibulectomy, appropriate fabrication of removable partial denture will provide a comfortable as well as economical treatment option. It is mandatory for the patient to attend regular follow-up visits for postinsertion assessment. Proper coordination between

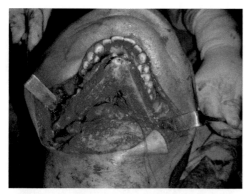

FIG. 6.10 Reconstruction with free fibula graft.

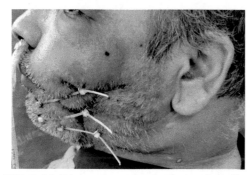

FIG. 6.11 Primary closure leading to scar formation.

the surgeon and prosthodontist will simplify the rehabilitation procedure.[52]

IMPLANT-SUPPORTED FIXED PROSTHESIS AFTER MARGINAL MANDIBULECTOMY

Interdisciplinary approach by oncosurgeon and prosthodontist can restore patient's dentition to perform various functions. If prosthodontic planning is missing during surgical reconstruction of mandibular defect to treat discontinuity, restoration of occlusion becomes impossible, which in turn affects overall esthetics of patient. Benign tumors usually have favorable prognosis as in most of the situations as they are limited to bone structure only and soft tissue loss is very less making restoration of esthetics possible after surgical reconstruction with free graft or free vascularized flaps. The extent of disability increases with the amount of mandibular resection. Mandibular guidance therapy with prosthesis and free flaps can be used effectively as a primary treatment depending on the situation and other health parameters related to patients. Drooling of saliva is difficult to control as in most of the

situations it is associated with compromised motor and sensory innovations of lower lip on the side of resection (Fig. 6.13).

Presurgical planning for prosthetic rehabilitation is extremely important to achieve minimum resection of mandible, which in turn reduces facial disfigurement, defective speech as well as mastication. Resection line of the mandible should be planned as posterior as possible as it will enhance the prognosis of prosthetic rehabilitation due to more amount of residual mandible especially in edentulous patients. Also bony cuts in the dentulous portion should be planned at intraseptal region rather than interproximal so that tooth next to the resection line can act as a sound abutment for prosthetic rehabilitation. Interdisciplinary approach by plastic surgeon and prosthodontist can accomplish effective reconstruction of mandibular defects. Prosthetic stents can be fabricated with the help of maxilla–mandibular relationship so that implants can be placed in fibula before actual reconstruction and same stent can be used to perform precise osteotomy of fibula to reconstruct the resected mandible. Such approach is essential for precise rehabilitation of speech, deglutition, and mastication. Resultant morbidity is less if mandibular continuity is restored especially in case of lateral mandibular body defects. Patient's occlusion, masticatory performance, and esthetics can be restored successfully by prosthetic rehabilitation if maxilla–mandibular relationship is maintained close to its original state (Fig. 6.14).

PROSTHETIC REHABILITATION AFTER RECONSTRUCTION WITH FIBULA GRAFT

Even though immediate mandibular reconstruction helps to reinstate facial symmetry, masticatory function remains compromised in several situations. In the middle of 1980s, free flaps (free tissue transfers) were introduced basically for the restoration of large soft and hard tissue defects created after resection of tongue and mandible. These flaps will replace the tissue lost due to resection of tumor. Improved blood supply was the most noteworthy advantage of this flap as compared with other flaps. This high vascularity of the flap is beneficial not only for the tissue being transferred but also to the recipient site, which in turn safeguards improved mobility of the reconstructed portion of the tongue or mandible without scarring. Inadequate tissue in the absence of free flap will lead to formation of contracture and inadequate closure of the defect (Fig. 6.15).

It results in better movement and shaping of the flap portion related to remaining musculature. Speech

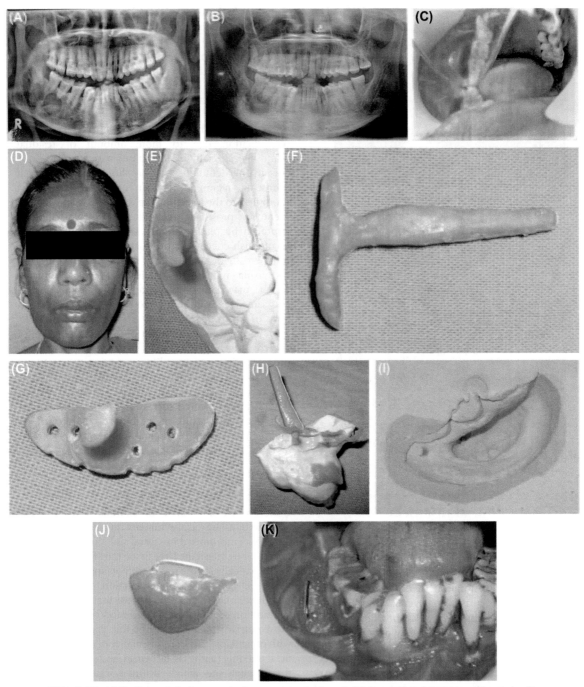

FIG. 6.12 (a) Radiograph before surgical management of cyst. (b) 5 months' follow-up radiograph after surgical management of cyst. (c) Intraoral defect. (d) Extraoral view. (e) Diagnostic impression was used to fabricate custom tray. (f) Custom tray to make impression of the defect. (g) Holes prepared in custom tray for retention. (h) Final impression with elastomer. (i) Final cast. (j) Final obturator prosthesis. (k) Final obturator prosthesis in the defect.

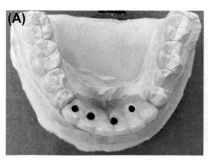 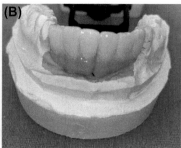 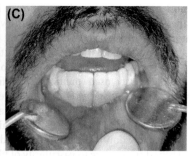

FIG. 6.13 (a) Implant-supported screw retained prosthesis for mandibular continuity defect after marginal mandibular resection. (b) Labial view of implant-supported screw retained prosthesis. (c) Mandibular continuity defect after marginal mandibular resection rehabilitated with implant-supported fixed prosthesis.

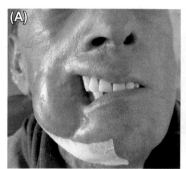 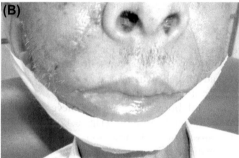

FIG. 6.14 (a) Well-maintained occlusion after reconstruction with free fibula graft. (b) Optimum esthetics after reconstruction with free fibula graft.

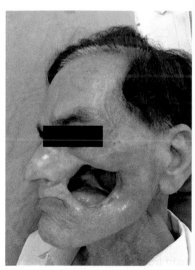

FIG. 6.15 Inadequate tissue in the absence of free flap leads to formation of contracture and inadequate closure of the defect.

restoration is close to normal in several cases after reconstruction with free flaps. Apart from that, better wound healing and survival in irradiated patients is seen due to improved blood supply after reconstruction with free flaps. Defects involving tongue and combination of tongue as well as mandible can be effectively restored with free flaps. Numerous free vascularized flaps, for example, fibula, scapula, radial forearm, thigh, and rectus abdominis, have been used for reconstruction of mandible subsequent to surgical resection. In the 1960s, the development of thoracoacromial (delto-pectoral) flaps and forehead flaps took place due to search for other means of wound closure.[53,54] Incorporation of these flaps in the surgical reconstruction helps the oncosurgeons to get more liberty in resection of affected tissue, resulting in better survival rates of the patients. As everyone is aware regarding the scarcity of studies related to resection of mandible followed by reconstruction with various graft materials, it is necessary to follow such patients meticulously. Apart from that, whatever studies have been done, they fail to report precise data regarding improvement in terms of esthetics, speech intelligibility, swallowing, and masticatory performance. With collective understanding regarding mandibular reconstruction, the vascularized bone flaps have been proved to be better compared with previously used methods. The fibula graft was made very popular by Hidalgo in the 1990s due to the benefits of free fibula graft. Fibula flap has countless advantages such as adequate length available for reconstruction, low donor site morbidity, and profuse periosteal blood supply due to vascularity of fibula that allows multiple osteotomies; addition of a skin island permits for absolute tension-free intraoral closure, which helps to improve tongue mobility and allows monitoring of the otherwise buried flap with extra precision. Combination with radiographic studies done using axial computed tomographic images of the mandible can be used to prepare 3D printed models of mandible and planned resection of mandible to guide the intraoperative procedure, precise contouring of the free flap, and also the postoperative procedures. But soft tissue reconstruction may lead to unesthetic appearance due to lack of adequate support (Fig. 6.16).

Rigid reconstruction with bony flap helps to achieve good esthetics due to adequate support (Fig. 6.17). Apart from that, prosthetic rehabilitation with implant-supported prosthesis is also possible as they can be shaped in the form of jaw (Figs. 6.18–6.24).

Centric Relation Record

The occlusal vertical dimension is maintained closed:

Closed or reduced vertical dimension will facilitate the interaction of the tongue with the palatal structures during speech and swallowing. Apart from that, it will make it easier for the tongue to position the bolus onto the occlusal table, leading to improved masticatory performance.

Occlusal Scheme

Monoplane scheme of occlusion was incorporated. Reduced vertical overlap of the anterior teeth was maintained to prevent interference during mandibular movements (Fig. 6.25).

PROSTHETIC REHABILITATION AFTER RECONSTRUCTION WITH RECONSTRUCTION PLATE WITHOUT BONE FLAP

However, the drawback of the fibula bone is the inadequate height; it can offer for reconstruction procedure of

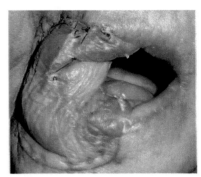

FIG. 6.16 Compromised appearance due to soft tissue reconstruction.

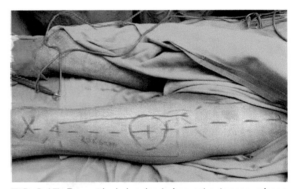

FIG. 6.17 Presurgical planning to harvest autogenous bone flap for reconstruction.

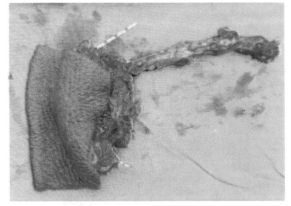

FIG. 6.18 Osteotomy of fibula into desirable contour with the help of prosthetic guide.

mandible. Apart from that, excess bulk of free fibula flap can affect the esthetics as well as prosthetic treatment outcome (Figs. 6.26 and 6.27a).

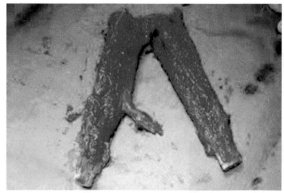

FIG. 6.19 Adequate length is available with free fibula graft.

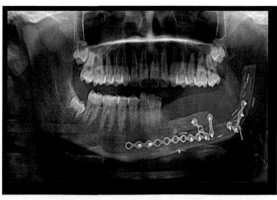

FIG. 6.22 Radiograph showing mandible reconstructed with fibula graft using double barrel technique.

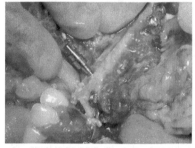

FIG. 6.20 Implant placement in grafted fibula for reconstruction of mandible.

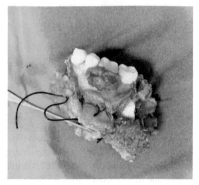

FIG. 6.23 Resected segment of mandible leading to discontinuity defect.

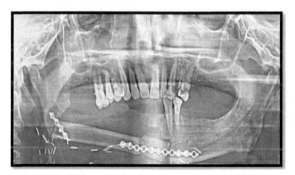

FIG. 6.21 Radiograph showing mandible reconstructed with fibula graft.

Prosthetic options for rehabilitation of patients with segmental resection of partially edentulous mandible reconstructed with free fibula graft include removable partial denture, fixed dental prosthesis, and an implant-retained prosthesis. However, fixed partial denture and implant-retained prosthesis are not reasonable in several cases, predominantly for patients with excessive bulk of grafted tissue, patients undergoing radiation treatment, and also due to financial constraints. For such state of affairs, a prosthodontist may resort to alternative option of removable partial denture, to replace the lost hard as well as soft tissue to reinstate esthetics, phonetics, masticatory function. This removable prosthesis accomplishes the purposes of the rehabilitation by achieving adequate support, stability, and retention for the removable prosthesis. It will not only restore the esthetics but also eases the hygiene maintenance of the grafted tissue for rehabilitation of resected mandible.[55–58]

Development in the field of surgery and reconstruction has upgraded the ability of surgeon to restore facial form and mandibular continuity, which helps to achieve successful esthetic as well as functional outcome. Apart from that, use of dental implants

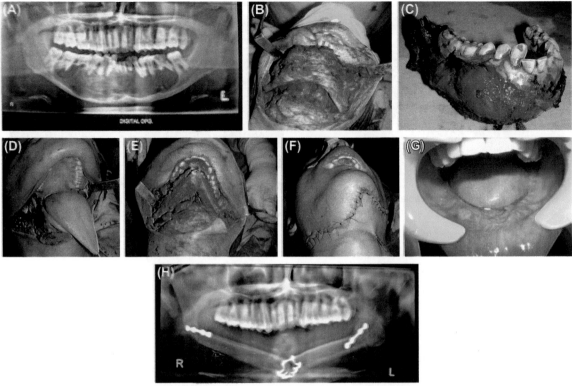

FIG. 6.24 (a) Radiograph showing mandible with extensive radiolucency due to ameloblastoma. (b) Excessively increased dimensions of mandible due to ameloblastoma. (c) Resection of affected portion of mandible due to ameloblastoma. (d) Residual mandible after resection of ameloblastoma. (e) Reconstruction of mandible with free fibula flap. (f) Closure of surgical site after reconstruction of mandible with free fibula flap. (g) Intraoral view after reconstruction of mandible. (h) Orthopantomograph after reconstruction of mandible. (i) CBCT showing width of bone available for implant placement. (j) CBCT showing height of bone available for implant placement. (k) Surgical as well as radiographic guide for implant placement. (l) Surgical guide used for implant placement. (m) Assessment of implant angulation. (n) Closure of surgical site. (o) Orthopantomograph after implant placement. (p) Attachment for incorporation in prosthesis. (q) Ball abutment for implants. (r) Final prosthesis with retentive components.

increases the probability of efficacious functional rehabilitation for the patient. Several studies have shown that the rate of osseointegration is better with grafted bone due to high vascularity.[59-65] As per the two-phase theory of osteogenesis, few bone cells remain active after transplantation and form the preliminary osteoid during the first phase in random manner.[66] During second phase, osteoid is resorbed and gets replaced by bone, which is derived from cells in the recipient bed. According to the concept of osteoinduction, some factor in the grafted bone causes induction of mesenchymal cells in the surrounding soft tissue bed for transformation into osteoblasts. Such proteins that are responsible for the process of induction are found in organic demineralized bone. Urist has termed

these proteins as bone morphogenetic proteins as per the available documentation.[67] Ellis has described further details regarding biology of the bone grafting.[68]

Among the various autogenous bone grafts used for reconstruction of mandible, the iliac crest is the most common site as compared with other sites such as outer table of cranium, rib, tibia, and fibula. Also graft harvested from tibia can provide abundant volume of bone with minimal postoperative morbidity. Apart from that, bone graft can be harvested successfully under local anesthesia.[69-71] Iliac crest graft provides good amount of either cortical or cancellous bone. Apart from that, harvesting iliac crest bone graft has less morbidity as well as risk. Morbidity related to blood loss, pain, and gait disturbances is less.[72] These

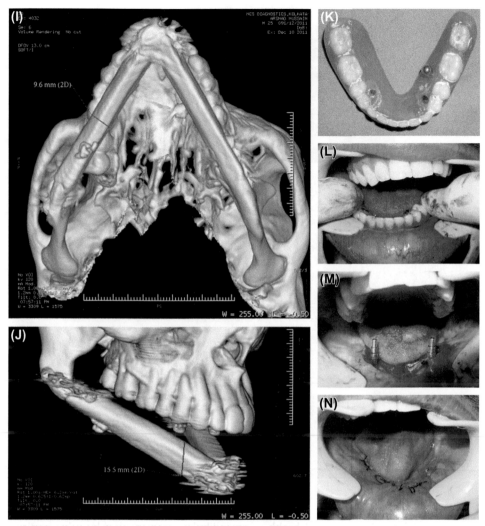

FIG. 6.24 **cont'd.**

technical details regarding surgical techniques for procurement of various autogenous bone grafts have been described by Marx.[73] Dacron-Urethane trays are preferred by some surgeons to hold the harvested autogenous bone graft.[74,75] Apart from that, cadaveric mandible or cadaveric ribs can be bent, shaped, and adapted to hold the compressed autogenous bone graft. Use of cadaveric bone has been suggested to hold the harvested autogenous bone by few clinicians.[76]

Different protocols have been followed by clinicians regarding the timings multiple surgical procedures such as resection of the tumor, reconstruction of the resected site, and dental implant placement for prosthetic rehabilitation. It is essential to weigh the risks as well as

benefits of primary versus delayed mandibular reconstruction. It has been proposed by various clinicians that increased risk of infection occurs at the time of resection followed by immediate reconstruction due to oral communication. Apart from that, chances of recurrence of tumor, radiotherapy, and chemotherapy may lead to loss of graft, which is more problematic as compared with the benefits of immediate reconstruction. Lawson et al. have stated that infection is the major obstacle in immediate reconstruction with bone graft as compared with delayed reconstruction and more than 40% infection rate has been found in grafts, which are having communication with oral cavity.[77,78] Several studies have reported greater success with

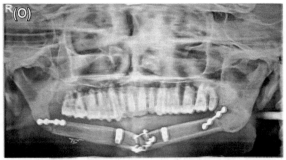

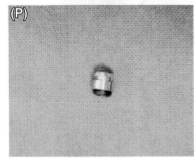

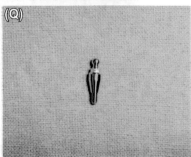

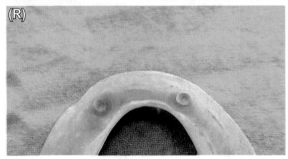

FIG. 6.24 **cont'd.**

delayed reconstruction.[79–81] On the other hand, health-related quality of life (QOL) has demonstrated that better improvement is seen in quality of life after immediate reconstruction and patients prefer immediate reconstruction more as compared with delayed reconstruction.[82–87] Not a single method of reconstruction deals with all variables of mandibular defects in the affected patient.[88–94] But several studies have described regarding use of reconstruction plates with bone grafts for reconstruction of mandible after resection of tumor.[95–103] Various bone substitutes such as autologous free-bone grafts, irradiated or cryopreserved mandible, and alloplastic materials have been used for reconstruction of mandible.[104–112] Kinoshita et al. and several others have found good results toward

mandibular reconstruction by using particulate bone and cancellous marrow.[113–122] In case of fibula graft, devascularization of bone does not happen due to segmental and intraosseous blood supply.[123] Dental implants have higher percentage of osseointegration in viable bone as compared with nonvascular bone graft.[124] Harvesting of autografts leads to morbidity of the donor site. These complications have been documented by Dodson and Kaban[125] and Criccio and Lundgren.[126] Reconstruction with free flaps is considered better in most of the patients including those who are elderly and have compromised health.[127] Surgical guide is used for precise alignment of the graft segment (Fig. 6.28) and repositioning of residual mandibular fragments.[128,129] Cortical property of fibula

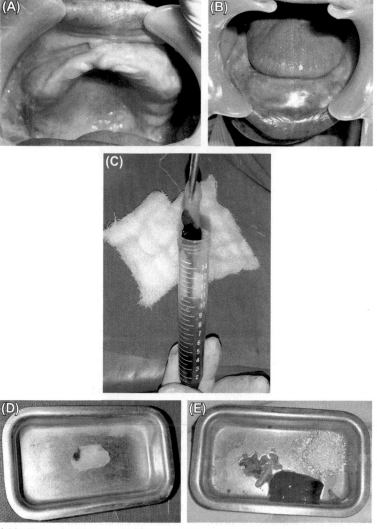

FIG. 6.25 (a) Maxillary edentulous arch. (b) Mandibular arch after reconstruction with fibula graft. (c) PRF used to improve osseointegration of implant in radiated fibula. (d) PRF membrane. (e) Combination of autograft, alloplast, and PRF. (f) Surgical site sutured after placement of implants in fibula graft. (g) Healing abutments placement after debulking/deepthelization of free fibula flap. (h) Frontal view before prosthesis. (i) Frontal view after prosthesis insertion.

and its thickness help for better outcome of the prosthetic rehabilitation with implants with successful osseointegration (Fig. 6.28).[130−134]

MANDIBULAR GUIDING PROSTHESIS
Even though free flaps, myocutaneous flaps, and reconstructive plates are being used for reconstructive surgery, several patients present with discontinuity defect of the mandible. Such kind of situation affects the balance and symmetrical functional pattern of the mandible.[135] There will be change in the envelope of motion. Apart from that several complex and interrelated factors affects the severity of deviation.[136−139]

Cantor and Curtis have classified the mandibular defects into six categories (Chart 6.2).[140]

There is loss of the proprioception affecting occlusion after mandibular resection, which leads to the

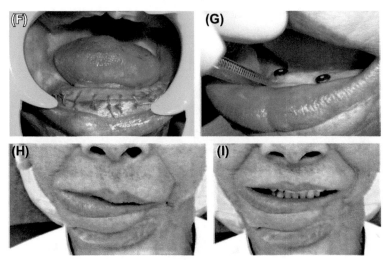

FIG. 6.25 **cont'd.**

uncoordinated mandibular movements. The fundamental idea behind guidance therapy is to train the muscles to restore a satisfactory interocclusal relationship. Guide flange prosthesis (GFP) is a mandibular conventional prosthesis fabricated for those patients who are able to attain a suitable mediolateral movement, leading to maximum intercuspal position of the mandible without significant efforts so that the patient will be able to repeat this position constantly to correct the deviation of mandible and perform acceptable mastication.[141–143] Whenever delayed reconstruction procedures such as secondary osseous grafting are scheduled, it is mandatory for the clinician to wait until complete healing of the graft takes place. Apart from that, the lesion may take additional time to heal due to radiotherapeutic effects to subside the clinical signs as well as symptoms. Once the graft is healed properly, the planning for a definitive prosthesis can be executed. Guidance prosthesis must be inserted in patient's mouth to correct the deviation of mandible due to unilateral muscular pull.[144–153] Also every patient is not willing for second surgery, i.e., reconstructive surgery, so definitive prosthesis is not possible or needs to be delayed. Guide flange prosthesis is a very important part of treatment planning for such patients. It is on interim basis until acceptable occlusal relationships

and proper proprioception are reestablished. Rehabilitation of defects involving resection of mandible along with some part of floor of mouth and tongue is extremely challenging.[154] The functional disabilities of tongue–mandible resections are principally dependent on the amount of tongue resected, method of closure, and amount of deviation of mandible. Subsequent to resection of mandible, the part of the bony mandible as well as teeth that remains has to articulate with normal structures of maxilla, and this function is facilitated by guide flange prosthesis. When a part of mandible has been resected, the movements of the mandible in the functional range and occlusal proprioception differ from that normal mandible. The residual mandibular segment will retrude and deviate toward the surgical site. During mastication, entire envelope of motion occurs on the surgical defect side. The normal hinge movement parallel to the sagittal plane is lost, and guide flange prosthesis helps to redevelop the normal hinge movement.

Goals in rehabilitation of mandibular discontinuity defects with guide bite prosthesis:
1. To restore lower facial contour
2. To restore as occlusal relationship
3. To maintain maximum tooth to tooth contact
4. To prevent postradiotherapy deviation

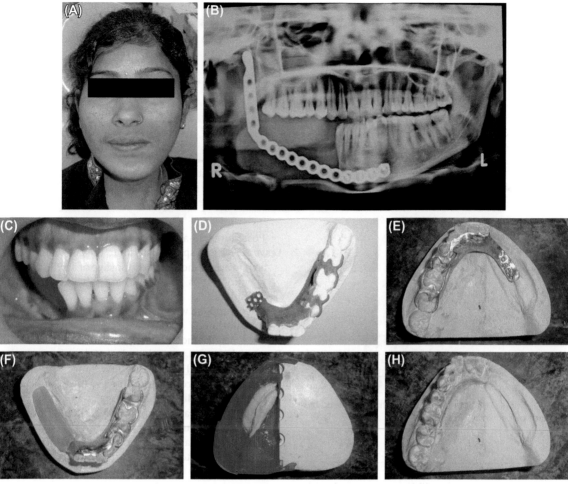

FIG. 6.26 (a) Frontal view after reconstruction of resected mandible with reconstruction plate. (b) Orthopantomograph after reconstruction of resected mandible with reconstruction plate. (c) Intraoral view. (d) Cast framework pattern. (e) Cast framework. (f) Cast framework with custom tray for functional impression. (g) Boxing of final impression to prepare altered cast. (h) Final cast.

a. Palatal Origin (One Piece)

Most common type.

Indicated in patients with normal or reduced mouth opening (trismus).

Benefits of one-piece guide flange prosthesis:
  Simple to fabricate

Easy to adjust
Cost-effective
Require less number of patient visits
More comfortable as compared with two-piece prosthesis
Restores occlusion in more precise manner
Can be prescribed in patients with trismus

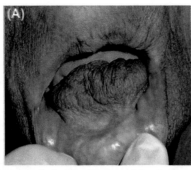 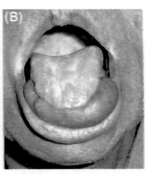

FIG. 6.27   (a) Excessive bulk of free fibula graft leading to compromised esthetics due to lack of debulking. (b) Excessive bulk of free fibula graft affects the functional movements during prosthetic rehabilitation.

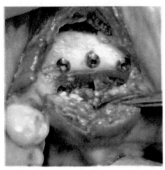

FIG. 6.28   Fibula graft contoured in the shape of mandible for implant placement.

More acceptance in mandible reconstructed with fibular flap

Procedure to fabricate one-piece guide flange prosthesis (Fig. 6.29):

V bend—Occlusal extent of bend with respect to buccal cusps of maxillary teeth should be at the junction of occlusal and middle one third.

Zig-zag form:

Increases flexibility.

Prevents rotation of the buccal plate.

Extent of zig-zag form should be shorter than the distal aspect of posterior most tooth.

Posterior wrap-around last tooth in the arch:

Leave 0.5—1 mm space posterior to the last tooth in the arch to accommodate for shrinkage of acrylic around retention loops and also to act as a leeway during activation.

After complete wire bending.

Acrylization.

Clear acrylic buccal/labial plate:

Protects the maxillary teeth and gingiva.

Provides reciprocal support to pink flange by resisting forces of arch contracture in view of dynamic dislodging pull following resection.

Contour of palatal ramp: concave, should not traumatize tongue.

Pink acrylic palatal surface with guidance ramp extends onto lingual surfaces of mandibular teeth.

Planning of Guide Flange Prosthesis

If the patient able to achieve occlusion with manual manipulation of the mandible, activation of guide flange prosthesis is done with the help of V loop.

If fibrosis and intercuspation are not achievable, plan sequential guidance therapy starting with flange at an obtuse angle to maxillary teeth, which is then adjusted periodically by chair-side addition of acrylic on the inside surface of the ramp till the occlusion is achieved. This needs to be communicated to the lab technician at the beginning.

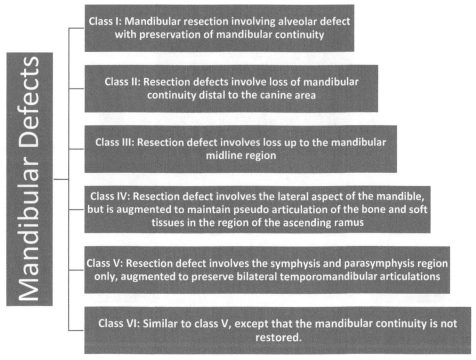

Mandibular Defects

Class I: Mandibular resection involving alveolar defect with preservation of mandibular continuity

Class II: Resection defects involve loss of mandibular continuity distal to the canine area

Class III: Resection defect involves loss up to the mandibular midline region

Class IV: Resection defect involves the lateral aspect of the mandible, but is augmented to maintain pseudo articulation of the bone and soft tissues in the region of the ascending ramus

Class V: Resection defect involves the symphysis and parasymphysis region only, augmented to preserve bilateral temporomandibular articulations

Class VI: Similar to class V, except that the mandibular continuity is not restored.

CHART 6.2   Classification of mandibular defects.

Timing of Guide Flange Prosthesis Fabrication

1. Fabrication of guidance prosthesis can be done on preoperative models prior to surgery after determination of extent of resection and prosthesis fitted immediately after postsurgical sequelae have subsided.
2. After 15 days postsurgery (ideal time 2–4 weeks) and definitely before initiation of radiation therapy.
   Definitive guide flange prosthesis: Definitive prosthesis prescribed after careful assessment of the clinical findings and history related to radiotherapy (Figs. 6.30 and 6.31).
   Definitive guide flange prosthesis with cast metal framework can be prescribed after precise clinical

assessment and history of the patient. Proper designing and utilization of support area is necessary for definitive guide flange prosthesis with cast metal framework so that the mandibular guidance appliance will not exert excessive forces on the residual mandible and other tissues (Fig. 6.32).

Some patient, however, may carry on for the foreseeable future with a guide flange, and for this reason, stress generated to the remaining teeth must then be carefully supervised. It is advisable to advocate use of guide flange prosthesis as early as possible after surgery, so that it will guide the muscles and residual mandible in proper position so as to establish intimate occlusion. Delayed use of guide flange prosthesis makes the

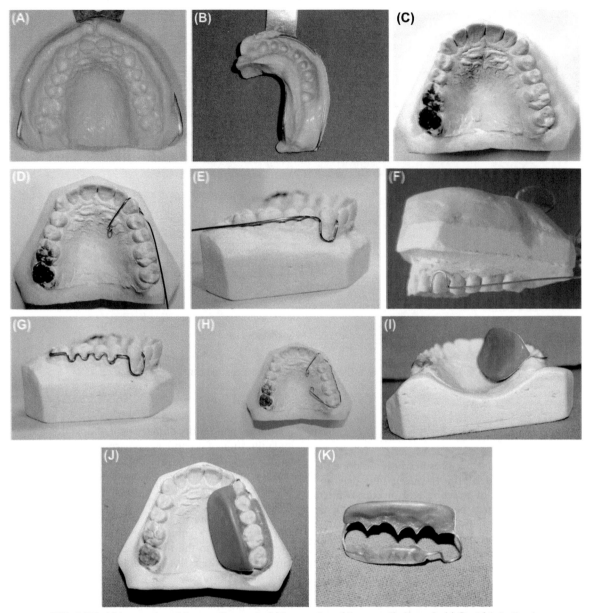

FIG. 6.29   (a) Impression of the maxillary arch. (b) Impression of the mandibular arch. (c) Cast fabrication by using the impressions. (d) Adaptation of wire in the interproximal area. (e) Preparation of U loop. (f) Preparation of V bend. (g) Preparation of zig-zag bend. (h) Occlusal view after final wire bending. (i) Palatal flange of the prosthesis. (j) Final guide Flange prosthesis. (k) Finished and polished guide Flange prosthesis.

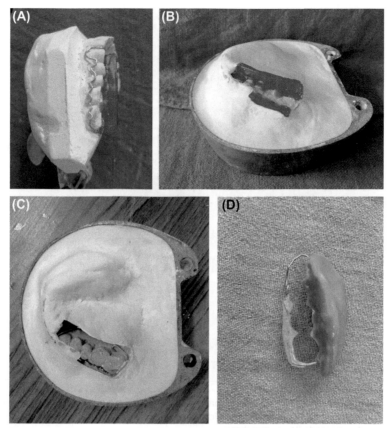

FIG. 6.30 (a) Wax up for guide flange prosthesis. (b) Flasking of guide flange prosthesis. (c) After dewaxing. (d) Final guide flange prosthesis.

correction of occlusion very difficult due to contracture in the resected region. If the patient has undergone radiotherapy treatment, then it will worsen the prognosis of treatment outcome with guide bite prosthesis (Fig. 6.33).

Once deviation is corrected definitive prosthesis in the form of partial denture, implant-supported prosthesis can be given (Figs. 6.34—6.38).

b. Mandibular Origin (Two-Piece) Guide Flange Prosthesis

This type of guide flange prosthesis can be prescribed in patients with adequate mouth opening. This prosthesis relatively less acceptable as compared with one-piece guide flange prosthesis. Using two-piece prosthesis creates some discomfort immediately after insertion in patient's oral cavity.

Resembles a partial denture base fitting on the mandibular teeth with a ramp extending upward 7—10 mm from the buccal aspect of premolars and molars of the unaffected sites.

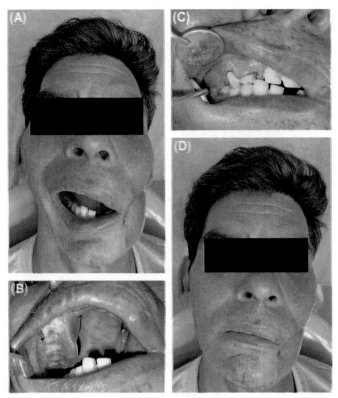

FIG. 6.31 (a) Disfigured face due to deviation of mandible to the resected side. (b) Guide flange prosthesis inserted. (c) Intercuspal position achieved due to guide flange prosthesis. (d) Disfigurement of face corrected after insertion of guide flange prosthesis.

The buccal ramp engages the maxillary teeth during mandibular closure and guides the deviated mandible into its correct occlusal position.

A maxillary framework with a buccal plate is incorporated in the design to prevent trauma to maxillary teeth and gingiva from the guidance ramp (Fig. 6.39).

Management of Completely Edentulous Mandibular Arch

1. Precludes use of guide flange prosthesis
2. Correction of mandibular deviation entirely depends on the exercise program

Treatment planning

Set of complete dentures with maxillary complete denture having additional row of artificial teeth on palatal aspect of normally arranged teeth on the unaffected side.

Lower posterior teeth occlude with the inner additional row due to deviated closure.

Missing teeth

If posterior teeth are missing in either of the arch on the normal side, jaw relation to be recorded.

Acrylic occlusal table to be given in area of missing teeth (Fig. 6.40).

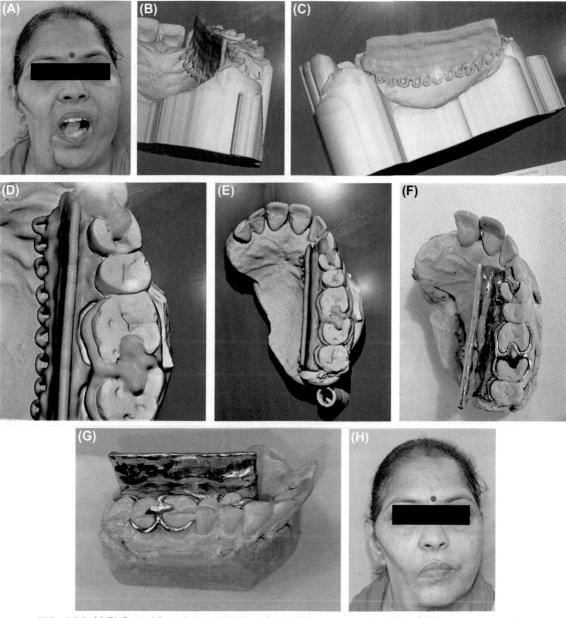

FIG. 6.32 (a) Disfigured face due to deviation of mandible to the resected side. (b) Virtual planning of the palatal side of guide flange prosthesis inserted. (c) Virtual planning of the retentive meshwork of guide flange prosthesis inserted. (d) Virtual planning of the occlusal aspect of guide flange prosthesis inserted. (e) After complete virtual planning of guide flange prosthesis inserted. (f) Occlusal aspect of definitive guide flange prosthesis. (g) Buccal aspect of definitive guide flange prosthesis. (h) Disfigurement of face corrected after insertion of guide flange prosthesis.

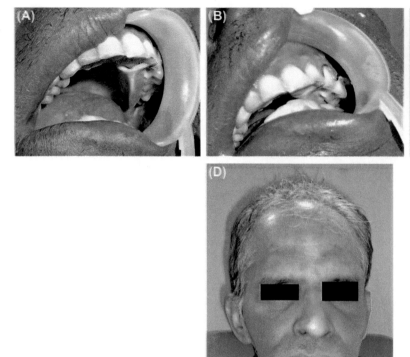

FIG. 6.33 (a) Guide flange prosthesis inserted. (b) Guide flange prosthesis needs to be modified in a stepwise manner for patients having severe trismus. (c) Intercuspal position achieved with guide flange prosthesis. (d) Facial deviation corrected with guide flange prosthesis.

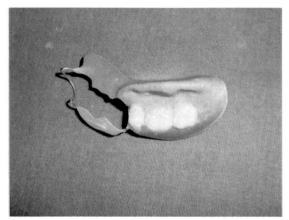

FIG. 6.34 Combination of guide flange prosthesis and removable partial denture.

Manual correction of mandibular deviation when residual coronoid interferes during impression making helps to record the buccal vestibule and distal aspect of last tooth (Fig. 6.41).

Postinsertion instructions

Guide flange prosthesis to be worn continuously.
This should be supported by exercise program
  2 weeks after surgery, several times a day.
Correction will be seen after 2—3 weeks.
To be worn for 3—6 months.
Gradually weaning can be advised to the patient by
  reducing the duration and frequency.

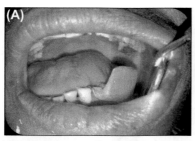
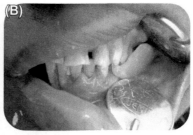

FIG. 6.35 (a) Guide flange prosthesis for mandibular arch. (b) Intercuspal position achieved with guide flange prosthesis.

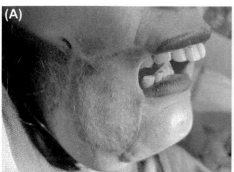
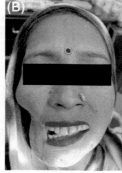
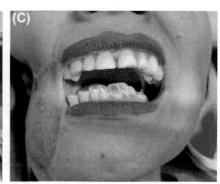

FIG. 6.36 (a) Severe fibrosis of the flap due to radiotherapy. (b) Facial deviation due to radiotherapy related fibrosis. (c) Severe trismus leading to restricted mouth opening.

Used only at night to reinforce corrected maxillomandibular relationship.[155–160] Weaning-related instructions depend on the following factors:

a. Patient's comfort
b. Amount of resections
c. Patient's dependency on the prosthesis

If the anatomy permits, we can give definitive partial denture after a certain follow-up period.[161–164] Aramany and Myers have reported the use of gunning splint in completely edentulous patients to correct the deviation by maxillomandibular fixation.[165] Once the maxillomandibular fixation is removed, only few patients can establish sufficient deviation for preparation of palatal guidance restoration. Otherwise most of the edentulous patients get satisfactory correction of the mandibular deviation by maxillomandibular fixation. It is considered as one of the cost-effective techniques to establish intercuspal position of maxilla and mandible.[166] Gunning splint is prescribed in elderly patients who have compromised medical condition and various contraindications for the surgical treatment.[167,168]

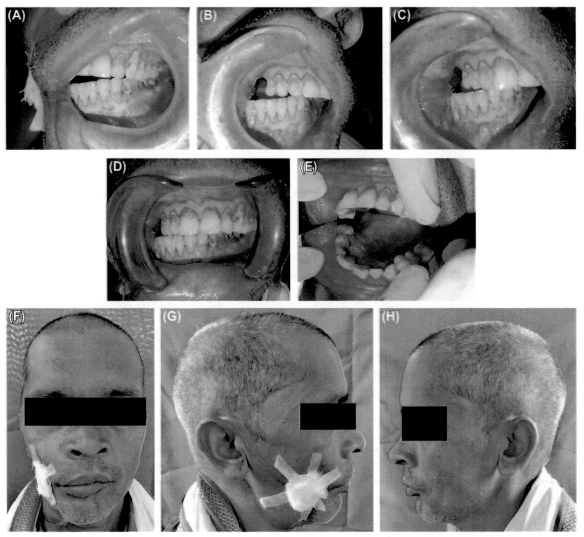

FIG. 6.37 (a) Frontal plane rotation after mandibular resection. (b) Excessive deviation after mandibular resection. (c) Increased overjet after mandibular resection. (d) Disturbed balance and intercuspal position. (e) Severe trismus leading to restricted mouth opening. (f) Affected esthetics due to primary closure after resection. (g) Dehiscence of the wound at the site of primary closure. (h) Lateral profile affected due to primary closure after mandibular resection.

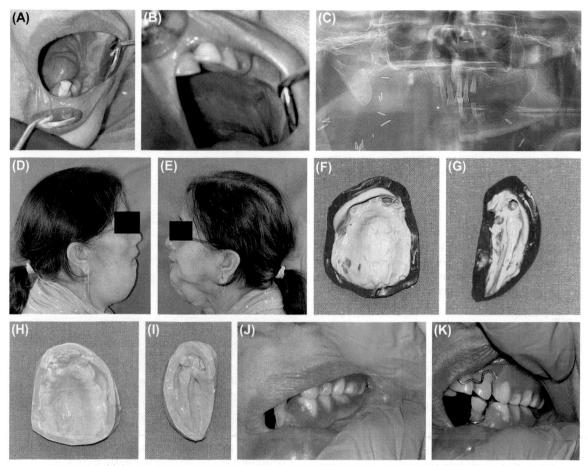

FIG. 6.38 (a) Intraoral view of mandible after mandibular resection. (b) Intraoral view of maxilla. (c) Orthopantomograph after resection of mandible. (d) Right lateral profile view affected due to lack of mandibular reconstruction. (e) Left lateral profile view. (f) Maxillary impression made with rubber base. (g) Mandibular impression made with rubber base. (h) Maxillary cast. (i) Mandibular cast. (j) Try-in of the prosthesis. (k) Insertion of the final prosthesis.

Application of guide flange prosthesis can be considered as a directive type of prosthesis after mandibular resection without continuity.[169–171] If the patient is able to achieve the occlusal relationship precisely, the prosthodontist may ask the patient to conclude with the guide flange prosthesis.[172–178]

However, in a long-standing case, definitive mandibular guidance prosthesis will act as savior to alleviate the occlusion efficaciously to correct the deviation as well as accomplish satisfactory occlusion for usual mandibular function.[52,179–194]

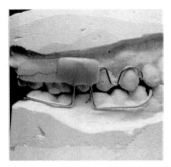

FIG. 6.39 Two-piece guide flange prosthesis.

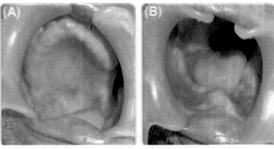

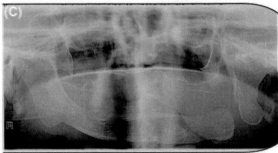

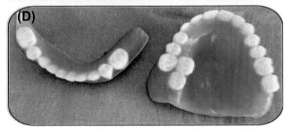

FIG. 6.40 (a) Edentulous maxillary arch. (b) Edentulous mandibular arch after segmental mandibulectomy. (c) Orthopantomograph showing edentulous mandibular arch after segmental mandibulectomy. (d) Maxillary prosthesis with additional palatal row of teeth.

If prosthetic management is required to correct the deviation of mandible after radiotherapy, additional precaution needs to be taken to manage the side effects of radiotherapy in surrounding tissues. Excessive fibrosis after radiotherapy treatment may worsen the deviation, leading to difficulty in manipulation of tissues while planning for mandibular guidance therapy.[195–197]

Management of Traumatic Mandibular Defects

Intermaxillary fixation by using gunning splints with an arch wire requires extreme meticulousness in removal, which may turn precarious while managing an emergency condition, which is life-threatening.[198–200] Frequent follow-up visits should be scheduled without fail to assess whether the patient is regularly wearing the prosthesis so that it will help the mandible to achieve centric occlusion without guidance prosthesis in future. It will help the patient to maintain the capability to slide smoothly into centric position once the use of guiding prosthesis is stopped. Once the patient is able to attain best possible occlusion in addition to regular function without the assistance of the guiding prosthesis, definitive guidance prosthesis with the incorporation of a cast partial framework can also be planned. If required, guidance prosthesis can be incorporated in the design of the definitive prosthesis (Fig. 6.42).[201–204]

The prognosis of a prosthetic management is relentlessly influenced by the significant involvement of bony as well as soft tissues, loss of sensory and motor innervations, and scar tissue formation due to primary closure after hemimandibulectomy. Retraining the muscles for consistent occlusal approximation is one of the major goals of prosthetic treatment.[3,205–211]

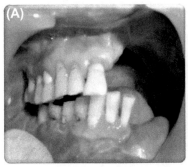
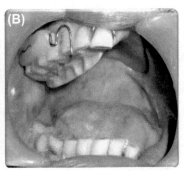
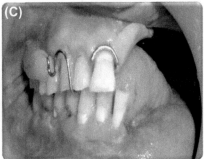

FIG. 6.41 (a) Maxillomandibular relation after manual manipulation of mandible. (b) Guide flange prosthesis insertion. (c) Intercuspal position achieved after guide flange prosthesis insertion.

Speech and Swallowing Assessment

Speech and swallowing assessment needs to be done before the surgery, after the surgical reconstruction, before as well as prosthetic rehabilitation. Both subjective and objective assessments of speech and swallowing should be done whenever possible. Dr. Speech software has been used very effectively to assess speech as well as swallowing during several clinical trials. During every follow-up appointment, speech and swallowing assessment can be repeated to figure out if any modifications are required in the prosthesis.

Summary

For the patient who has undergone segmental or total resection of the jaw, reconstruction with free fibula flap and prosthetic rehabilitation with implants improves quality of life. Altered tissue histology, soft tissue thickness, and radiation with lack of oral hygiene are contributing factors for soft tissue dehiscence and peri-implantitis in grafted jaws. Socioeconomic status plays a significant role in success rate of rehabilitation. Recent progresses in facial reconstructive surgery and osseointegrated endosseous dental implants offer a treatment plan that might be adequate enough to rehabilitate head–neck cancer patients so they can lead healthy as well as productive lives once again after the oncology treatment.

Prosthetic rehabilitation will help to improve the quality of life of oral cancer patients. The functional disabilities related with resection of mandible are basically reliant on the amount of resection and method of surgical closure. Treatment planning by a multidisciplinary team, which includes oncosurgeon, reconstructive surgeon, maxillofacial prosthodontist, and speech therapist, will lead to most precise treatment outcome for managing mandibular defects. Resected part of mandible can be rehabilitated at the time of tumor resection. Suitable flap needs to be selected to restore the lost bulk as well as function of the mandible. Mobility as well as bulk of adjacent tissues should be given equal importance while planning rehabilitation of missing portion of mandible. The soft part of the flaps should be used to restore the lost bulk of adjacent tissues by shaping them properly, whereas bony component of the flap should be used to restore the continuity of the mandible so that appropriate maxillomandibular relation as well as occlusion can be reestablished. Continued efforts are necessary to conduct the clinical trials with adequate sample size to improve the quality of life of patients with mandibular defects. Prosthetic rehabilitation of complex mandibular defects improves masticatory performance, swallowing as well as speech abilities.

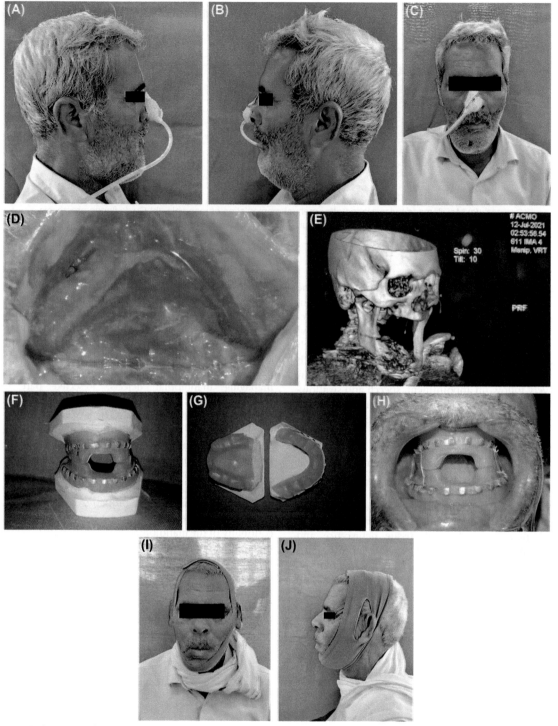

FIG. 6.42 (a) Right profile view with discontinuity of mandible. (b) Left profile view with discontinuity of mandible. (c) Frontal view with discontinuity of mandible. (d) Intraoral view of the mandibular arch. (e) CT scan showing discontinuity of mandible. (f) Gunning splint fabricated with desirable occlusion. (g) Gunning splint with provision to restrict movement. (h) Gunning splint in patient's mouth. (i) Frontal view with chin strap bandage and gunning splint. (j) Lateral view with chin strap bandage and gunning splint.

REFERENCES

1. Munot VK, Nayakar RP, Patil R. Prosthetic rehabilitation of mandibular defects with fixed-removable partial denture prosthesis using precision attachment: a twin case report. *Contemp Clin Dent.* 2017 Jul-Sep;8(3):473−478. https://doi.org/10.4103/ccd.ccd_117_17.
2. Bhochhibhoya A, Shakya P, Mathema S, Maskey B. Simplified technique for the prosthodontic rehabilitation of a patient with a segmental mandibulectomy with a hollow cast partial dental prosthesis: a clinical report. *J Prosthet Dent.* July 2016;116(1):144−146. https://doi.org/10.1016/j.prosdent.2015.12.009.
3. Brown JS, Barry C, Ho M, Shaw R. A new classification for mandibular defects after oncological resection. *Lancet Oncol.* 2016;17(1):e23−e30.
4. Boyd JB, Gullane PJ, Rotstein LE, Brown DH, Irish JC. Classification of mandibular defects. *Plast Reconstr Surg.* December 1993;92(7):1266−1275.
5. Pavlov BL. Classification of mandibular defects. *Stomatologiia (Mosk).* 1974;53:43−46.
6. David DJ, Tan E, Katsaros J, Sheen R. Mandibular reconstruction with vascularized iliac crest: a 10-year experience. *Plast Reconstr Surg.* 1988;82:792−803.
7. Urken ML, Weinberg H, Vickery C, Buchbinder D, Lawson W, Biller HF. Oromandibular reconstruction using microvascular composite free flaps. Report of 71 cases and a new classification scheme for bony, soft-tissue, and neurologic defects. *Arch Otolaryngol Head Neck Surg.* 1991;117:733−744.
8. Iizuka T, Häfl iger J, Seto I, Rahal A, Mericske-Stern R, Smolka K. Oral rehabilitation after mandibular reconstruction using an osteocutaneous fibula free flap with endosseous implants. Factors affecting the functional outcome in patients with oral cancer. *Clin Oral Implants Res.* 2005;16:69−79.
9. Hashikawa K, Yokoo S, Tahara S. Novel classification system for oncological mandibular defect: CAT classification. *Jpn J Head Neck Cancer.* 2008;34:412−418.
10. Baumann DP, Yu P, Hanasono MM, Skoracki RJ. Free flap reconstruction of osteoradionecrosis of the mandible: a 10-year review and defect classification. *Head Neck.* 2011;33:800−807.
11. Schultz BD, Sosin M, Nam A, et al. Classification of mandible defects and algorithm for microvascular reconstruction. *Plast Reconstr Surg.* 2015;135(4):743e−754e.
12. Leong EW, Cheng AC, Tee-Khin N, Wee AG. Management of acquired mandibular defects–prosthodontic considerations. *Singapore Dent J.* December 2006;28(1):22−33.
13. Arden RL, Rachel JD, Marks SC, Dang K. Volume-length impact of lateral jaw resections on complication rates. *Arch Otolaryngol Head Neck Surg.* January 1999;125(1):68−72.
14. Mariani PB, Kowalski LP, Magrin J. Reconstruction of large defects postmandibulectomy for oral cancer using plates and myocutaneous flaps: a long-term follow-up. *Int J Oral Maxillofac Surg.* May 2006;35(5):427−432.
15. Taylor TD. Diagnostic considerations for prosthodontic rehabilitation of the mandibulectomy patient. In: Taylor TD, ed. *Clinical Maxillofacial Prosthetics.* Chicago, IL: Quintessence Publishing; 2000:55−170.
16. Shafer WG, Hine MK, Levy BM, et al. *A Textbook of Oral Pathology.* 4th ed. Philadelphia, PA: WB Saunders; 1993:86−229.
17. Olson ML, Shedd DP. Disability and rehabilitation in head and neck cancer patients after treatment. *Head Neck Surg.* 1978;1:52−58.
18. Curtis DA, Plesh O, Miller AJ, et al. A comparison of masticatory function in patients with or without reconstruction of the mandible. *Head Neck.* 1997;19:287−296.
19. Marunick MT, Mathes BE, Klein BB. Masticatory function in hemimandibulectomy patients. *J Oral Rehabil.* 1992;19:289−295.
20. McConnel FM, Pauloski BR, Logemann JA, et al. Functional results of primary closure vs flaps in oropharyngeal reconstruction: a prospective study of speech and swallowing. *Arch Otolaryngol Head Neck Surg.* 1998;124:625−630.
21. Hsiao HT, Leu YS, Lin CC. Primary closure versus radial forearm flap reconstruction after hemiglossectomy: functional assessment of swallowing and speech. *Ann Plast Surg.* 2002;49:612−616.
22. McConnel FM, Teichgraeber JF, Adler RK. A comparison of three methods of oral reconstruction. *Arch Otolaryngol Head Neck Surg.* 1987;113:496−500.
23. Pauloski BR, Rademaker AW, Logemann JA, et al. Surgical variables affecting swallowing in patients treated for oral/oropharyngeal cancer. *Head Neck.* 2004;26:625−636.
24. Hsiao HT, Leu YS, Chang SH, et al. Swallowing function in patients who underwent hemiglossectomy: comparison of primary closure and free radial forearm flap reconstruction with videofluoroscopy. *Ann Plast Surg.* 2003;50:450−455.
25. Wagner JD, Coleman 3rd JJ, Weisberger E, et al. Predictive factors for functional recovery after free tissue transfer oromandibular reconstruction. *Am J Surg.* 1998;176:430−435.
26. Hidalgo DA. Aesthetic improvements in free-flap mandible reconstruction. *Plast Reconstr Surg.* 1991;88:574−585.
27. Dholam KP, Bachher GK, Yadav P, et al. Assessment of quality of life after Implant retained prosthetic rehabilitation in reconstructed maxilla and mandibles post cancer treatments. *Implant Dent.* 2011;20:85−90.
28. Oh KC, Park JH, Lee JH, Moon HS. Treatment of a mandibular discontinuity defect by using a fibula free flap and an implant-supported fixed complete denture fabricated with a PEKK framework: a clinical report. *J Prosthet Dent.* June 2018;119(6):1021−1024. https://doi.org/10.1016/j.prosdent.2017.07.024.
29. Ntounis A, Patras M, Pelekanos S, Polyzois G. Treatment of hemi-mandibulectomy defect with implant-supported

telescopic removable prosthesis. A clinical report. *J Prosthodont.* August 2013;22(6):501–505. https://doi.org/10.1111/jopr.12012.

30. Wang W, Mao CY, Gu XH. Prosthodontic rehabilitation of malpositioned implants after ameloblastoma followed by mandibulectomy and costal bone graft: a clinical report. *Implant Dent.* February 2013;22(1):16–19. https://doi.org/10.1097/ID.0b013e31827afbb0.

31. Wong TL, Wat PY, Pow EH, McMillan AS. Rehabilitation of a mandibulotomy/onlay/graft-reconstructed mandible using a milled bar and a tooth- and implant-supported removable dental prosthesis: a clinical report. *J Prosthet Dent.* July 2010;104(1):1–5. https://doi.org/10.1016/S0022-3913(10)00095-8.

32. Vecchiatini R, Mobilio N, Barbin D, Catapano S, Calura G. Milled bar-supported implant overdenture after mandibular resection: a case report. *J Oral Implantol.* 2009;35(5):216–220. https://doi.org/10.1563/1548-1336-35.5.216.

33. Siadat H, Khojasteh A, Beyabanaki E. Reconstruction of a mandibular defect with Toronto Bridge following tumor resection and bone graft: a case report. *Front Dent.* 2019 Mar-Apr;16(2):153–157. https://doi.org/10.18502/fid.v16i2.1368.

34. Cakan U, Anil N, Aslan Y. Prosthetic rehabilitation of a mandibular gunshot defect with an implant-supported fixed partial denture: a clinical report. *J Prosthet Dent.* April 2006;95(4):274–279. https://doi.org/10.1016/j.prosdent.2006.01.011.

35. Awadalkreem F, Khalifa N, Ahmad AG, Suliman AM, Osman M. Prosthetic rehabilitation of maxillary and mandibular gunshot defects with fixed basal implant-supported prostheses: a 5-year follow-up case report. *Int J Surg Case Rep.* 2020;68:27–31. https://doi.org/10.1016/j.ijscr.2020.02.025.

36. Wong HH, Pow EH, Choi WW. Management of mandibular rotation after a mandibulectomy: a clinical report. *J Prosthet Dent.* December 2013;110(6):532–537. https://doi.org/10.1016/j.prosdent.2013.04.001.

37. Hayden RE, Mullin DP, Patel AK. Reconstruction of the segmental mandibular defect: current state of the art. *Curr Opin Otolaryngol Head Neck Surg.* August 2012;20(4):231–236. https://doi.org/10.1097/MOO.0b013e328355d0f3.

38. Fang W, Liu YP, Ma Q, Liu BL, Zhao Y. Long-term results of mandibular reconstruction of continuity defects with fibula free flap and implant-borne dental rehabilitation. *Int J Oral Maxillofac Implants.* 2015 Jan-Feb;30(1):169–178.

39. Zou D, Huang W, Wang F, et al. Autologous ilium grafts: long-term results on immediate or staged functional rehabilitation of mandibular segmental defects using dental implants after tumor resection. *Clin Implant Dent Relat Res.* August 2015;17(4):779–789.

40. Kumar BP, Venkatesh V, Kumar KA, Yadav BY, Mohan SR. Mandibular reconstruction: overview. *J Maxillofac Oral Surg.* 2016;15(4):425–441.

41. Jacobsen HC, Wahnschaff F, Trenkle T, Sieg P, Hakim SG. Oral rehabilitation with dental implants and quality of life following mandibular reconstruction with free fibular flap. *Clin Oral Investig.* January 2016;20(1):187–192.

42. Mertens C, de San Jose Gonzalez J, Freudlsperger C, et al. Implant-prosthetic rehabilitation of hemimaxillectomy defects with CAD/CAM suprastructures. *J Craniomaxillofac Surg.* November 2016;44(11):1812–1818.

43. Tripathi A, Gupta A, Gautam V, Anwar M, Arora V. The efficacy of guiding flange appliance in correcting mandibular deviation in the hemi-mandibulectomy patient. A correlative study. *J Prosthodont.* February 2015;24(2):121–126.

44. Goh BT, Lee S, Tideman H, Stoelinga PJW. Mandibular reconstruction in adults: a review. *Int J Oral Maxillofac Surg.* 2008;37(7):597–605. https://doi.org/10.1016/j.ijom.2008.03.002.

45. Ruggiero G, Bocca N, Carossa M, Gassino G. Alterations in surgical interventions to improve the prosthetic prognosis in patients with mandibular defects: a review of the literature. *J Osseointegr.* 2020;12(2):1. https://doi.org/10.23805/JO.2020.12.03.4.

46. Adisman IK. Prosthesis serviceability for acquired jaw defects. *Dent Clin North Am.* 1990;34(2):265–284.

47. Academy of Prosthodontics. Principles, concepts, and practices in prosthodontics—1994. *J Prosthet Dent.* 1995;73(1):73–94.

48. Taylor TD. *Clinical Maxillofacial Prosthetics.* Chicago: Quintessence; 2000:171–188.

49. Desjardins RP. Occlusal considerations for the partial mandibulectomy patient. *J Prosthet Dent.* 1979;41(3):308–315.

50. Martin JW, Lemon JC, King GE. Maxillofacial restoration after tumor ablation. *Clin Plast Surg.* 1994;21(1):87–96.

51. Beumer J, Marunick MT, Esposito SJ. *Maxillofacial Rehabilitation: Surgical and Prosthodontic Management of Cancer-Related, Acquired, and Congenital Defects of the Head and Neck.* Chicago: Quintessence; 2011:123.

52. Dholam K, Kharade P, Bhirangi P. Simple prosthesis for a cancer patient with a segmental mandibulectomy and free fibula flap reconstruction: a clinical report. *Gen Dent.* 2015;61(7):e23–e25.

53. Bakamjian VY. A two-stage method for pharyngoesophageal reconstruction with a primary pectoral skin flap. *Plast Reconstr Surg.* 1965;36:173–184.

54. McGregor IA, Reid WH. The use of the temporal flap in the primary repair of full-thickness defects of the cheek. *Plast Reconstr Surg.* 1966;38:1–9.

55. Cheatham JL, Newland JR, Radentz WH, O'Brien R. The 'fixed' removable partial denture: report of case. *J Am Dent Assoc.* 1984;109:57–59.

56. Mueninghoff KA, Johnson MH. Fixed-removable partial denture. *J Prosthet Dent.* 1982;48:547–550.

57. Jeyavalan MI, Narasimman M, Venkatakrishnan CJ, Philip JM. Management of long span partially edentulous maxilla with fixed removable denture prosthesis. *Contemp Clin Dent.* 2012;3:314–316.

58. Jain AR. A prosthetic alternative treatment for severe anterior ridge defect using fixed removable partial denture Andrew's Bar system. *World J Dent.* 2013;4:282–285.

59. Dodson TB, Smith RA. Mandibular reconstruction with autogenous and alloplastic materials following resection of an odontogenic myxoma. *Int J Oral Maxillofac Implants.* 1987;2(4):227–229.

60. Listrom RD, Symington JM. Osseointegrated dental implants in conjunction with bone grafts. *Int J Oral Maxillofac Surg.* April 1988;17(2):116–118.

61. Keller EE. Mandibular discontinuity reconstruction. *J Oral Maxillofac Surg.* March 1991;49(3):324.

62. Keller EE. Mandibular discontinuity reconstruction with composite grafts. Free autogenous iliac bone, titanium mesh trays, and titanium endosseous implants. *Oral Maxillofac Surg Clin North Am.* 1991;3:877–878.

63. Roumanas ED, Chang TL, Beumer J. Use of osseointegrated implants in the restoration of head and neck defects. *J Calif Dent Assoc.* 2006;34:711–718.

64. Habal MB, Rasmussen RA. Osseointegrated implants in cranial bone grafts for mandibular reconstruction. *J Craniofac Surg.* 1993;4:51–57.

65. Chana JS, Chang YM, Wei FC, et al. Segmental mandibulectomy and immediate free fibula osteoseptocutaneous flap reconstruction with endosteal implants: an ideal treatment method for mandibular ameloblastoma. *Plast Reconstr Surg.* January 2004;113:80–87.

66. Axhausen W. The osteogenetic phases of regeneration of bone; a historial and experimental study. *J Bone Joint Surg Am.* June 1956;38-A(3):593–600.

67. Urist MR. Surface-decalcified allogeneic bone (SDAB) implants. A preliminary report of 10 cases and 25 comparable operations with undecalcified lyophilized bone implants. *Clin Orthop Relat Res.* 1968 Jan-Feb;56:37–50.

68. Ellis E. Biology of bone grafting: an overview. In: O'Ryan F, ed. *Selected Readings in Oral and Maxillofacial Surgery. San Francisco: the Guild for Scientific Advancement in Oral and Maxillofacial Surgery.* 1991:1–28.

69. Kirmeier R, Payer M, Lorenzoni M, et al. Harvesting of cancellous bone from the proximal tibia under local anesthesia: donor site morbidity and patient experience. *J Oral Maxillofac Surg.* November 2007;65(11):2235–2241.

70. Gerressen M, Prescher A, Riediger D, et al. Tibial versus iliac bone grafts: a comparative examination in 15 freshly preserved adult cadavers. *Clin Oral Implants Res.* December 2008;19(12):1270–1275.

71. Walker TW, Modayil PC, Cascarini L, Williams L, Duncan SM, Ward-Booth P. Retrospective review of donor site complications after harvest of cancellous bone from the anteriomedial tibia. *Br J Oral Maxillofac Surg.* 2009;47:20–22.

72. Marx RE, Morales MJ. Morbidity from bone harvest in major jaw reconstruction: a randomized trial comparing the lateral anterior and posterior approaches to the ilium. *J Oral Maxillofac Surg.* March 1988;46(3):196–203.

73. Marx RE. Philosophy and particulars of autogenous bone grafting. *Oral Maxillofac Surg Clin North Am.* 1993;5:599–611.

74. Schwartz H. Mandibular reconstruction in the head and neck cancer patient. In: Kagan R, Miles J, eds. *Head and Neck Oncology.* New York: Pergamon; 1989:142–154.

75. Leake DL. Mandibular reconstruction with a new type of alloplastic tray: a preliminary report. *J Oral Surg.* 1974;32:23–26.

76. Marx RE. Current advances in reconstruction of the mandible in head and neck cancer surgery. *Semin Surg Oncol.* 1991 Jan-Feb;7(1):47–57.

77. Lawson W, Loscalzo LJ, Baek SM, Biller HF, Krespi YP. Experience with immediate and delayed mandibular reconstruction. *Laryngoscope.* January 1982;92(1):5–10.

78. Manchester WM. Immediate reconstruction of the mandible and temporomandibular joint. *Br J Plast Surg.* July 1965;18:291–303.

79. Marx RE, Ames JR. The use of hyperbaric oxygen therapy in bony reconstruction of the irradiated and tissue deficient patient. *J Oral Maxillofac Surg.* 1982;40:410.

80. Marx RE. Mandibular reconstruction. *J Oral Maxillofac Surg.* 1993;51:466.

81. Carlson ER, Monteleone K. An analysis of inadvertent perforations of mucosa and skin concurrent with mandibular reconstruction. *J Oral Maxillofac Surg.* 2004;62:1103.

82. Cordeiro PG, Hidalgo DA. Conceptual considerations in mandibular reconstruction. *Clin Plast Surg.* 1995;22:61.

83. Baker A, McMahon J, Parmar S. Immediate reconstruction of continuity defects of the mandible after tumor surgery. *J Oral Maxillofac Surg.* 2001;59:1333. https://doi.org/10.1053/joms.2001.27825.

84. Li X, Zhu K, Liu F, Li H. Assessment of quality of life in giant ameloblastoma adolescent patients who have had mandible defects reconstructed with a free fibula flap. *World J Surg Oncol.* 2014;12:201. https://doi.org/10.1186/1477-7819-12-201.

85. Netscher DT, Meade RA, Goodman CM, et al. Quality of life and disease specific functional status following microvascular reconstruction for advanced (T3 and T4) oropharyngeal cancers. *Plast Reconstr Surg.* 2000;105:1628. https://doi.org/10.1097/00006534-200004050-00005.

86. Weymuller EA, Yueh B, Deleyiannis FWB, et al. Quality of life in patients with head and neck cancer. *Arch Otolaryngol Head Neck Surg.* 2000;126:329. https://doi.org/10.1001/archotol.126.3.329.

87. Boyd JB, Mullholland RS, Davidson J, et al. The free flap and plate in oromandibular reconstruction: long-term review and indications. *Plast Reconstr Surg.* 1995;95:1018.

88. Havlik RJ. Reconstruction of the pediatric mandible. *Oper Tech Plastic Reconstr Surg.* 1996;3(4):272–288.

89. Gullane PJ, Holmes H. Mandibular reconstruction new concept. *Arch Otolaryngol Head Neck Surg.* 1976;112:714–719.

90. Urken ML. Composite free flaps in oro-mandibular reconstruction. *Arch Otolaryngol Head Neck Surg.* 1991; 117:724–732.

91. Komisar A. The functional result of mandibular reconstruction. *Laryngoscope.* 1990;100:364–374.

92. Peled M, El-Naaj IA, Lipin Y, Ardekian L. The use of free fibular flap for functional mandibular reconstruction. *J Oral Maxillofac Surg.* 2005;63:220–224.

93. Yim KK, Wei FC. Fibula osteoseptocutaneous flap for mandible reconstruction. *Microsurgery.* 1994;15(4): 245–249.

94. Haughey BH, Fredrickson JM, Lerrick AJ, et al. Fibular and iliac crest osteomuscular free flap reconstruction of the oral cavity. *Laryngoscope.* 1994;104:1305.

95. Vuillemin T, Raveh J, Sutter F. Mandibular reconstruction with the titanium hollow screw reconstruction plate (THORP) system: evaluation of 62 cases. *Plast Reconstr Surg.* 1998;82:804.

96. Schusterman MA, Reece KP, Kroll SS, et al. Use of the A–O plate for mandibular reconstruction in cancer patients. *Plast Reconstr Surg.* 1991;88:588–593.

97. Chow J, Hill J. Primary mandibular reconstruction using the A–O reconstruction plate. *Laryngoscope.* 1986;96: 768–773.

98. Poswillo D. Experimental reconstruction of the mandibular joint. *Int J Oral Surg.* 1974;3:400.

99. Guyuron B, Lasa C. Unpredictable growth pattern of costochondral graft. *Plast Reconstr Surg.* 1992;90:880–886.

100. Medra AM. Follow up of mandibular costochondral grafts after release of ankylosis of the temporomandibular joints. *Br J Oral Maxillofac Surg.* 2005;43(2): 118–122.

101. Lata J, Kapila BK. Overgrowth of a costochondral graft in temporomandibular joint reconstructive surgery: an uncommon complication. *Quintessence Int.* 2000;31(6): 412–414.

102. Fernandes R, Fattahi T, Steinberg B. Costochondral rib grafts in mandibular reconstruction. *Atlas Oral Maxillofac Surg Clin North Am.* 2006;14(2):179–183.

103. Caccamese JF, Ruiz RL, Costello BJ. Costochondral rib grafting. *Atlas Oral Maxillofac Surg Clin North Am.* 2005; 13:139–149.

104. Hamaker RC. Irradiated autogenous mandibular grafts in primary reconstructions. *Laryngoscope.* 1981;91: 1031–1051.

105. Leipzig B, Cummings CW. The current status of mandibular reconstruction using autogenous frozen mandibular grafts. *Head Neck Surg.* 1984;8:992–998.

106. Schmoper RR. Mandibular reconstruction using a special plate: animal experiments and clinical appearance. *J Maxillofac Surg.* 1983;11:99–108.

107. Burwell RG. Studies in transplantation of bone. VII. The fresh composite homograft-autograft of cancellous bone; an analysis of factors leading to osteogenesis in marrow transplants and in marrow-containing bone grafts. *J Bone Joint Surg Br.* 1964;46:110–140.

108. Rappaport I, Boyne PV, Nethery J. The particulate graft in tumor surgery. *Am J Surg.* 1971;122(6):748–755.

109. Boyne PJ. Restoration of osseous defects in maxillofacial casualities. *J Am Dent Assoc.* 1969;78(4):767–776.

110. Leake DL, Rappoport M. Mandibular reconstruction: bone induction in an alloplastic tray. *Surgery.* 1972; 72(2):332–336.

111. Cheung LK, Samman N, Tong AC, Tideman H. Mandibular reconstruction with the Dacron urethane tray: a radiologic assessment of bone remodeling. *J Oral Maxillofac Surg.* 1994;52(4):373–380.

112. Cheung LK, Samman N, Chow TW, Clark RKF, Tideman H. A bone graft condensing syringe system for maxillofacial reconstructive surgery. *Br J Oral Maxillofac Surg.* 1997;35:267–270.

113. Kinoshita Y, Kobayashi M, Hidaka T, Ikada Y. Reconstruction of mandibular continuity defects in dogs using poly (l-lactide) mesh and autogenic particulate cancellous bone and marrow: preliminary report. *J Oral Maxillofac Surg.* 1997;55(7):718–723.

114. Louis P, Holmes J, Fernandes R. Resorbable mesh as a containment system in reconstruction of the atrophic mandible fracture. *J Oral Maxillofac Surg.* 2004;62(6): 719–723.

115. Takagi S, Chow LC, Markovic M, Friedman CD, Costantino PD. Morphological and phase characterizations of retrieved calcium phosphate cement implants. *J Biomed Mater Res.* 2001;58(1):36–41.

116. Samman N, Cheung LK, Tideman H. Functional reconstruction of the jaws: new concepts. *Ann R Australas Coll Dent Surg.* 1996;13:184–192.

117. Tideman H, Samman N, Cheung LK. Functional reconstruction of the mandible: a modified titanium mesh system. *Int J Oral Maxillofac Surg.* 1998;27(5): 339–345.

118. Warnke PH, Springer IN, Wiltfang J, et al. Growth and transplantation of a custom vascularised bone graft in a man. *Lancet.* 2004;364(9436):766–770.

119. Celeste AJ, Iannazzi JA, Taylor RC, et al. Identification of transforming growth factor beta family members present in bone-inductive protein purified from bovine bone. *Proc Natl Acad Sci USA.* 1990;87(24):9843–9847.

120. Moghadam HG, Urist MR, Sandor GK, Clokie CM. Successful mandibular reconstruction using a BMP bioimplant. *J Craniofac Surg.* 2001;12(2):119–127.

121. Herford AS, Boyne PJ. Reconstruction of mandibular continuity defects with bone morphogenetic protein-2 (rhBMP-2). *J Oral Maxillofac Surg.* 2008;66(4):616–624.

122. Clokie CM, Sándor GK. Reconstruction of 10 major mandibular defects using bioimplants containing BMP-7. *J Can Dent Assoc.* 2008;74(1):67–72.

123. Hidalgo DA, Rekow A. Review of 60 consecutive fibula free flap mandible reconstructions. *Plast Reconstr Surg.* 1995;96:585.

124. Hellem S, Olofsson J. Titanium-coated hollow screw and reconstruction plate system (THORP) in mandibular reconstruction. *J Cranio-Maxillo-Fac Surg.* May 1988; 16(4):173–183.

125. Schultz JD, Dodson TB, Meyer RA. Donor site morbidity of greater auricular nerve graft harvesting. *J Oral*

Maxillofac Surg. 1992;50(8):803–805. https://doi.org/10.1016/0278-2391(92)90269-6. In this issue.

126. Cricchio G, Lundgren S. Donor site morbidity in two different approaches to anterior iliac crest bone harvesting. *Clin Implant Dent Relat Res.* 2003;5(3):161–169.

127. Urken MI, Buchbinder D, Constantino PD, et al. Oromandibular reconstruction using composite flaps: report of 210 case. *Arch Otolaryngol Head Neck Surg.* 1998;124:46–55.

128. Markowitz BL, Calcaterra TC. Preoperative assessment and surgical planning for patients undergoing immediate composite reconstruction of oromandibular defects. *Clin Plast Surg.* January 1994;21(1):9–14.

129. Freiberg A, Bartlett GS. Two-team approach to surgery for head and neck cancer. *Can J Surg.* January 1980;23(1):35–38.

130. Swartz W, Janis J. *Head and Neck Microsurgery.* Baltimore: Williams and Wilkins; 1992.

131. Hidalgo DA. Fibula free flap: a new method of mandible reconstruction. *Plast Reconstr Surg.* July 1989;84(1):71–79.

132. Roumanas ED, Markowitz BL, Lorant JA, Calcaterra TC, Jones NF, Beumer III J. Reconstructed mandibular defects: fibula free flaps and osseointegrated implants. *Plast Reconstr Surg.* February 1997;99(2):356–365.

133. Kramer FJ, Dempf R, Bremer B. Efficacy of dental implants placed into fibula-free flaps for orofacial reconstruction. *Clin Oral Implants Res.* February 2005;16(1):80–88.

134. Wu YQ, Huang W, Zhang ZY, Zhang ZY, Zhang CP, Sun J. Clinical outcome of dental implants placed in fibula-free flaps for orofacial reconstruction. *Chin Med J (Engl).* October 5, 2008;121(19):1861–1865.

135. Beumer 3rd J, Curtis TA, Marunick MT. Prosthodontic and surgical consideration. In: *Maxillofacial Rehabilitation.* St. Louis: Ishiyaku Euro America; 1996:113–224.

136. Taylor TD. *Clinical Maxillofacial Prosthetics.* Illunios: Quintessence Publication Co; 1997:171–188.

137. Marathe AS, Kshirsagar PS. A systematic approach in rehabilitation of hemimandibulectomy: a case report. *J Indian Prosthodont Soc.* 2016;16:208–212.

138. Branchi R, Fancelli V, Desalvador A, Durval E. A Clinical Report for Corrective Mandibular Movement Therapy. Last Accessed on 2020 December 25, 2020.

139. Desjardins RP. Relating examination findings to treatment procedures. In: Laney WR, ed. *Maxillofacial Prosthetics.* Littleton: PSG Publishing; 1979:69–114.

140. Fonsica RJ, Davis WH. *Reconstruction Preprosthetic Oral and Maxillofacial Surgery.* 2nd ed. Philadelphia: WB Saunders Company; 1986:1063–1067.

141. Maroulakos G, Nagy WW, Ahmed A, Artopoulou II. Prosthetic rehabilitation following lateral resection of the mandible with a long cantilever implant-supported fixed prosthesis: a 3-year clinical report. *J Prosthet Dent.* 2017;118:678–685.

142. Kadain P. Prosthodontic rehabilitation of a hemimandibulectomy patient. *J Indian Prosthodont Soc.* 2020;20(Suppl S1):26–27.

143. Hazra R, Srivastava A, Kumar D. Mandibular guidance prosthesis: conventional and innovative approach: a case series. *J Indian Prosthodont Soc.* 2021 Apr-Jun;21(2):208–214.

144. Jewer DD, Boyd JB, Manktelow RT, et al. Orofacial and mandibular reconstruction with the iliac crest free flap: a review of 60 cases and a new method of classification. *Plast Reconstr Surg.* 1989;84:391–403.

145. Soutar DS, Widdowson WP. Immediate reconstruction of the mandible using a vascularized segment of radius. *Head Neck Surg.* 1986;8:232–246.

146. Matloub HS, Larson DL, Kuhn JC, Yousif NJ, Sanger JR. Lateral arm free flap in oral cavity reconstruction: a functional evaluation. *Head Neck.* 1989;11:205–211.

147. Garrett N, Roumanas ED, Blackwell KE, et al. Efficacy of conventional and implant-supported mandibular resection prostheses: study overview and treatment outcomes. *J Prosthet Dent.* 2006;96:13–24.

148. McGarry TJ, Nimmo A, Skiba JF, et al. Classification system for partial edentulism. *J Prosthodont.* 2002;11:181–193.

149. Bandodkar S, Arya D, Singh SV, Chand P. Guide flange Prosthesis for management of hemimandibulectomy. *Natl J Maxillofac Surg.* 2021 May-Aug;12(2):289–293.

150. Misra S, Chaturvedi A, Misra NC. Management of gingivobuccal complex cancer. *Ann R Coll Surg Engl.* 2008;90:546–553.

151. Abdulla R, Adyanthaya S, Kini P, et al. Clinicopathological analysis of oral squamous cell carcinoma among the younger age group in coastal Karnataka, India: a retrospective study. *J Oral Maxillofac Pathol.* 2018;22:180–187.

152. Babshet M, Nandimath K, Pervatikar S, Naikmasur V. Efficacy of oral brush cytology in the evaluation of the oral premalignant and malignant lesions. *J Cytol.* 2011;28:165–172.

153. Chaturvedi P. Effective strategies for oral cancer control in India. *J Cancer Res Ther.* 2012;8(Suppl 1):S55–S56.

154. Curtis TA, Cantor R. The forgotten patient in maxillofacial prosthetics. *J Prosthet Dent.* 1974;31:662–680. https://doi.org/10.1016/0022-3913(74)90122-X.

155. Master SB. UICC, Role of the Patient in Post Surgical Rehabilitation of Oral Cancer Patients. Textbook on Cancer Managent by UICC: page 135–154.

156. Jamayet NB, Fard AY, Husein A, Ariffin Z, Alam MK. Combined mandibular guidance therapy in the management of a hemimandibulectomy patient. *Int J Prosthodont (IJP).* 2015 Nov-Dec;28(6):624–626.

157. Krenkel C, Anthofer R, Lixl G. Sagittal splitting with screw fixation in patients with mesial bite wearing dentures—planning surgery and prosthetic design. *Z für Stomatol (1984).* March 1989;86(1):37–48.

158. Rosenquist B, Rune B, Selvik G. Displacement of the mandible after removal of the intermaxillary fixation

following oblique sliding osteotomy. *J Maxillofac Surg.* 1986;14:251–259.

159. Hasanreisoglu U, Uçtasli S, Gurbuz A. Mandibular guidance prostheses following resection procedures: three case reports. *Eur J Prosthodont Restor Dent.* December 1992;1(2):69–72.

160. Susarla S, Gordon PE, Attarpour AR, Winograd JM, Peacock ZS. Use of a mandibular plate to maintain intergonial width in a partially edentulous patient undergoing mandibular symphysis reconstruction. *Craniomaxillofac Trauma Reconstr.* December 2013;6(4):281–284.

161. Krekmanov L. Orthognathic surgery without the use of postoperative intermaxillary fixation. A clinical and cephalometric evaluation of surgical correction of mandibular and maxillary deformities. *Swed Dent J Suppl.* 1989;61:8–62.

162. Aggarwal H, Jurel SK, Kumar P, Chand P. Rehabilitating mandibular resection with guide flange prosthesis. *J Coll Physicians Surg Pak.* May 2014;24(Suppl 2):S135–S137.

163. Harianawala H, Kheur M, Kheur S, Matani J. Management of severe mandibular deviation following partial mandibular resection: a case report. *Gen Dent.* 2015 Jan-Feb;63(1):e24–e27.

164. Hindocha AD, Dudani MT. Detachable palatal ramp of teeth to improve comfort in a completely edentulous patient with a segmentally resected mandible. *J Prosthodont.* July 2017;26(5):474–480.

165. Aramany MA, Myers EN. Intermaxillary fixation following mandibular resection. *J Prosthet Dent.* April 1977;37(4):437–444.

166. Akadiri OA, Omitiola OG. Maxillo-mandibular fixation: utility and current techniques in modern practice. *Niger J Med.* 2012 Apr-Jun;21(2):125–133.

167. Dharaskar S, Athavale S, Kakade D. Use of gunning splint for the treatment of edentulous mandibular fracture: a case report. *J Indian Prosthodont Soc.* December 2014; 14(4):415–418.

168. Fattore L, Marchmont-Robinson H, Crinzi RA, Edmonds DC. Use of a two-piece Gunning splint as a mandibular guide appliance for a patient treated for ameloblastoma. *Oral Surg Oral Med Oral Pathol.* December 1988;66(6):662–665.

169. Prakash V. Prosthetic rehabilitation of edentulous mandibulectomy patient: a clinical report. *Indian J Dent Res.* 2008 Jul-Sep;19(3):257–260.

170. Schneider RL, Taylor TD. Mandibular resection guidance prostheses: a literature review. *J Prosthet Dent.* January 1986;55(1):84–86.

171. Nakajima J. Application of the palatal ramp in a reconstructed mandibulectomy patient. *Nihon Hotetsu Shika Gakkai Zasshi.* July 2008;52(3):388–391.

172. DeSanto LW, Whicker JH, Devine KD. Mandibular osteotomy and lingual flaps. Use in patients with cancer of the tonsil area and tongue base. *Arch Otolaryngol.* November 1975;101(11):652–655.

173. Gerngross PJ, Chambers MS, Martin JW. Oral rehabilitation of a mandibular discontinuity defect: a clinical report. *Tex Dent J.* May 2008;125(5):438–441.

174. Menard P, Germain MA, Kapron AM, Foussadier F, Schwabb G, Bertrand JC. Mandibular reconstruction by a free peroneal transfer. *Rev Stomatol Chir Maxillofac.* 1992;93(2):98–105.

175. Balaji SM. Callus molding in external and internal distraction of mandible. *Indian J Dent Res.* 2015 Nov-Dec;26(6):603–608.

176. Yang Z, Xiang X, Yan Y, Shi P, Wang C. Application of occlusal guide plate combined with intermaxillary fixation screw in mandibular defect repair with free fibular flap. *Zhongguo Xiu Fu Chong Jian Wai Ke Za Zhi.* March 2013;27(3):292–294.

177. Sullivan PK, Fabian R, Driscoll D. Mandibular osteotomies for tumor extirpation: the advantages of rigid fixation. *Laryngoscope.* January 1992;102(1):73–80.

178. Kurtulmus H, Kumbuloglu O, Saygi T, User A. Management of lateral mandibular discontinuity by maxillary guidance. *Br J Oral Maxillofac Surg.* March 2008;46(2):123–125.

179. Nelogi S, Chowdhary R, Ambi M, Kothari P. A fixed guide flange appliance for patients after a hemimandibulectomy. *J Prosthet Dent.* November 2013;110(5):429–432.

180. Abler A, Roser M, Weingart D. On the indications for and morbidity of segmental resection of the mandible for squamous cell carcinoma in the lower oral cavity. *Mund Kiefer Gesichtschir.* May 2005;9(3):137–142.

181. Koumjian JH, Firtell DN. An appliance to correct mandibular deviation in a dentulous patient with a discontinuity defect. *J Prosthet Dent.* June 1992;67(6):833–834.

182. Nielsen A, Poulsen H. The surgical and prosthetic treatment of a central epidermoid carcinoma of the mandible: a clinical report. *J Prosthet Dent.* November 1995;74(5):446–448.

183. Kobayashi T, Takebe J, Nitanai H, Furukawa K, Ishibashi K. Functional recovery with prosthetic management for segmental resection of the mandible without reconstruction. *Nihon Hotetsu Shika Gakkai Zasshi.* January 2006;50(1):10–15.

184. Kent J, Reid R, Hinds EC. Use of acrylic splint without intermaxillary fixation for anterior alveolar osteotomy. *J Oral Surg.* January 1969;27(1):11–14.

185. Moore DJ, Mitchell DL. Rehabilitating dentulous hemimandibulectomy patients. *J Prosthet Dent.* February 1976;35(2):202–206.

186. Marunick M, Mathes BE, Klein BB, Seyedsadr M. Occlusal force after partial mandibular resection. *J Prosthet Dent.* June 1992;67(6):835–838.

187. Simunović-Soskić M, Juretić M, Kovac Z, et al. Implant prosthetic rehabilitation of the patients with mandibular resection following oral malignoma surgery. *Coll Antropol.* March 2012;36(1):301–305.

188. Andrä A, Hildebrandt H, von Schwanewede H. Prosthetic aids in the resection of the middle portion of the mandible. *Stomatol DDR.* May 1975;25(5):332–335.

189. Bergman SA, Elias EG, Didolkar MS, Morris DM. Maintenance of function and esthetics after partial mandibulectomy without bone grafting. *J Oral Surg.* June 1981;39(6):421–425.

190. Bhattacharya SR, Majumdar D, Singh DK, Islam MD, Ray PK, Saha N. Maxillary palatal ramp prosthesis: a prosthodontic solution to manage mandibular deviation following surgery. *Contemp Clin Dent.* March 2015;6(Suppl 1):S111–S113.

191. Monaghan AM, Bear AS. A simple appliance to correct mandibular deviation following hemimandibulectomy. *Br J Oral Maxillofac Surg.* December 1990;28(6):419–420.

192. Watanabe Y, Yamada T, Miyamoto K, et al. Consideration on the shift of the mandibular bone fragments during intermaxillary fixation following sagittal split osteotomy. *Hiroshima Daigaku Shigaku Zasshi.* December 1988;20(2):329–333.

193. Cheng AC, Leong EW, Tee-Khin N, Shu YC, Wee AG. Prosthodontic management of acquired partial mandibulectomy discontinuity defects: a clinical report. *Singapore Dent J.* December 2006;28(1):47–53.

194. Judy KW, Robertson E, Chabra D, Ogle O, Aykac Y. Prosthetic rehabilitation with HA-coated root form implants after restoration of mandibular continuity. *Int J Oral Implantol.* 1991;8(1):25–28.

195. Oelgiesser D, Levin L, Barak S, Schwartz-Arad D. Rehabilitation of an irradiated mandible after mandibular resection using implant/tooth-supported fixed prosthesis: a clinical report. *J Prosthet Dent.* April 2004;91(4):310–314.

196. Singh B, Sinha N, Sharma R, Parekh N. Non surgical correction of mandibular deviation and neuromuscular coordination after two years of mandibular guidance therapy: a case report. *J Clin Diagn Res.* November 2015;9(11):ZD07–9.

197. Sakai T. Case of mandibular deviation with tongue habits treated with occlusal reconstruction]. *Nihon Hotetsu Shika Gakkai Zasshi.* January 2008;52(1):91–94.

198. Midis GP, Feuer A, Bergman SA, Elias EG, Lefor AT, Didolkar MS. Immediate mandibular stabilization following resection of advanced oral cavity carcinoma using the Joe Hall Morris external fixation device. *J Surg Oncol.* May 1992;50(1):22–26.

199. Mohanani K, Bhat S, Maiya R, Kamath G. Novel approach for intermaxillary fixation of fractured mandible using gunning splints for easy disengagement: a case report. *Gerodontology.* December 2021;38(4):449–451.

200. Leeb DC, Friedlander AH, Mazzarella Jr L. Mandible stabilization between ablative and reconstructive surgery. *Head Neck Surg.* 1979 Sep-Oct;2(1):67–70.

201. Adaki R, Shigli K, Hormuzdi DM, Gali S. A novel speech prosthesis for mandibular guidance therapy in hemimandibulectomy patient: a clinical report. *Contemp Clin Dent.* 2016 Jan-Mar;7(1):118–121.

202. Lingeshwar D, Appadurai R, Sswedheni U, Padmaja C. Prosthodontic management of hemimandibulectomy patients to restore form and function—a case series. *World J Clin Cases.* October 16, 2017;5(10):384–389.

203. Babu S, Manjunath S, Vajawat M. Definitive guiding flange prosthesis: a definitive approach in segmental mandibulectomy defect. *Dent Res J.* 2016 May-Jun;13(3):292–295.

204. George A, Shetty S, Subash A, Kudpaje A, Rao VUS. Modified compartmental resection-is mandibulotomy access justified? *Oral Surg Oral Med Oral Pathol Oral Radiol.* January 2021;131(1):139–140.

205. Kusugal P, Kalaivani VN, Patil A, Krishnamurthy S, Ruttonji Z. An innovative technique for the fabrication of fixed removable guide flange prosthesis for lateral mandibular resection. *Dent Res J.* January 21, 2020;17:80–83.

206. Pandey S, Kar S, Sharma NK, Tripathi A. An innovative approach to the prosthodontic management of Class III mandibular defect. *Natl J Maxillofac Surg.* 2018;9:90–95.

207. Gupta SG, Sandhu D, Arora A, Pasam N. The use of mandibular guidance prosthesis to correct mandibular deviation following hemimnadibulectomy—case reports. *Indian J Dent Res Rev.* 2012;2:71–73.

208. Mathew A, Thomas S. Management of a hemimandibulectomy defect with a definitive guiding flange prosthesis. *Pushpagiri Med J.* 2012;3:132–134.

209. Sahu SK. Mandibular guide flange prosthesis following mandibular resection; a clinical report. *J Clin Diagn Res.* 2010;4:3266–3270.

210. Agarwal S, Praveen G, Agarwal SK, Sharma S. Twin occlusion: a solution to rehabilitate hemimandibulectomy patient-a case report. *J Indian Prosthodont Soc.* 2011;11:254–257.

211. Nair SJ, Aparna IN, Dhanasekar B, Prabhu N. Prosthetic rehabilitation of hemimandibulectomy defect with removable partial denture prosthesis using an attachment-retained guiding flange. *Contemp Clin Dent.* 2018;9:120–122.

CHAPTER 9

Treatment Planning and Prosthetic Management of Ocular Defects

DEEKSHA ARYA, MDS • HIMANSHI AGGARWAL, MDS • SAUMYENDRA V. SINGH, MDS

LEARNING OBJECTIVES

1. Describe gross morphology of the natural eye.
2. Explain the etiology of ocular defects.
3. Perform steps of fabrication of an ocular prosthesis.
4. Make a conformer.
5. Explain the purposes of (1) conformer and (2) prosthesis fabrication.

INTRODUCTION

Loss or absence of an eye either due to congenital or acquired causes (anophthalmia) leads to severe esthetic disfigurement of face besides affecting the individual's physical, psychological, emotional, and social wellbeing. The goal of ocular rehabilitation is to replace the missing tissues with artificial substitutes (implant/ocular prosthesis) and restore facial symmetry and normal appearance. This chapter provides an overview of anatomy of eye, etiology and classification of ocular defects, conformers, ocular implants, and steps in fabrication of a prosthetic eye, with its care and maintenance. The readers should get to know the importance of an ocular prosthesis, and complications of not wearing one.

According to GPT 9, ocular prosthesis is defined as a maxillofacial prosthesis that artificially replaces an eye missing as a result of trauma, surgery, or congenital absence. This prosthesis does not replace missing eyelids or adjacent skin, mucosa, or muscle. It is also known as an artificial eye or prosthetic eye. Ocular prosthesis is different from an interim ocular prosthesis, which is also known as a conformer (see description in section Conformers of this chapter) and orbital prosthesis (separate chapter in this book).

The estimated total population of prosthetic eye wearers in the world is approximately 5 million, with maximum ocular prosthesis cases in China followed by India and the United States. This data clearly suggests that anophthalmia is not uncommon, and provision of ocular prosthesis is an important health issue globally.

History of Ocular Prosthesis

Since centuries, ocular prostheses have been used for esthetic replacement of missing eyes. Timeline for various types of ocular prosthesis used since predynastic period is as follows:

Prosthetic Rehabilitation of Head and Neck Cancer Patients. https://doi.org/10.1016/B978-0-323-82394-4.00002-1

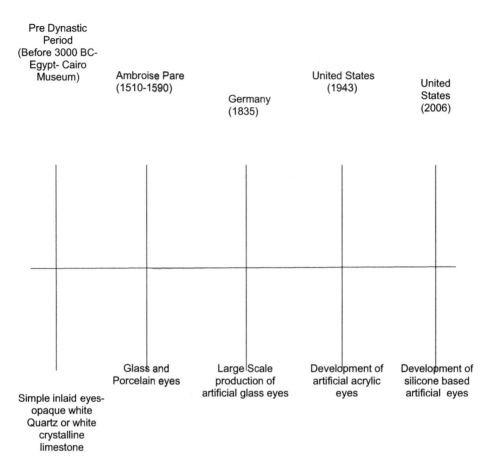

Pre Dynastic Period (Before 3000 BC- Egypt- Cairo Museum)

Ambroise Pare (1510-1590)

Germany (1835)

United States (1943)

United States (2006)

Glass and Porcelain eyes

Large Scale production of artificial glass eyes

Development of artificial acrylic eyes

Development of silicone based artificial eyes

Simple inlaid eyes- opaque white Quartz or white crystalline limestone

ANATOMY OF EYE

The basic knowledge of ocular morphology is essential to successfully manage ocular defects (Figs. 9.1 and 9.2).

Important Terminology

1. Canthus—the outer or inner corner of the eye, where the upper and lower lids meet.
2. Caruncle—the small, pink, globular nodule at the medial canthus of the eye consisting of skin, hair follicles, sebaceous glands, sweat glands, and accessory lacrimal tissue.
3. Ciliary zone (of the iris)—part of the iris that extends between the collarette and limbus.
4. Collarette (of the iris)—the region of the iris immediately surrounding the pupil that separates the pupillary zone from the ciliary zone.
5. Conjunctiva—mucous membrane of the eye that lines the inner surfaces of the eyelids or palpebræ and is reflected over the sclera and cornea.
6. Cornea—transparent part of the eye that covers the pupil (the opening at the center of the eye), iris (colored part of the eye), and anterior chamber of the eye.
7. Ectropion—condition in which eyelid is turned outward, leaving the inner surface exposed.
8. Entropion—condition in which eyelid, usually lower one, is turned inward.

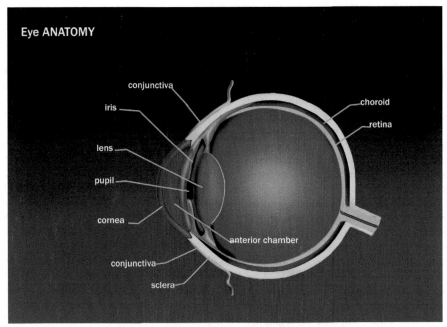

FIG. 9.1 Anatomy of eye (cross-sectional view).

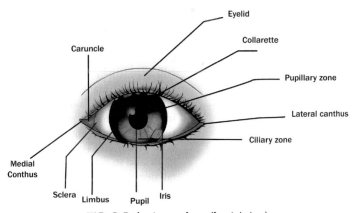

FIG. 9.2 Anatomy of eye (frontal view).

9. Enophthalmos—posterior displacement/sunken appearance of the eyeball with in the orbit.
10. Extraocular muscles—the six muscles (four recti and two oblique) that move the eye.
11. Fornix (fornices)—narrow junction where epithelial tissue lining the eyelids joins epithelium covering the globe.
12. Iris—thin, annular structure in the eye, responsible for controlling diameter and size of the pupil and thus the amount of light reaching the retina. It defines eye color.

13. Limbus—the border of the cornea and sclera.
14. Palpebrae/eyelids—thin fold of skin that covers and protects an eye.
15. Palpebral fissure—the oval aperture between the open eyelids.
16. Pupillary zone (of the iris)—inner region of the iris whose edge forms the boundary of the pupil.
17. Retina—the layer of light-sensitive nerve tissue that lines the inside of the back of the eye.
18. Sclera—the outer white part of the eye that surrounds the cornea.

ETIOLOGY OF DEFECTS

Ocular defects can be due to congenital or acquired causes. The most common congenital defects include congenital anophthalmia and congenital microphthalmia—nanophthalmia. Acquired defects can be surgical or traumatic.

Congenital anophthalmia, a rare developmental defect, is characterized by the complete absence of the eye. It is often seen in conjunction with microphthalmia/nanophthalmia. Its prevalence is approximately 0.2—3.0/10,000 births. Various infections during pregnancy such as rubella or toxoplasmosis have been associated with this anomaly.

Diminished growth of the microphthalmic/anophthalmic orbits results in microorbitism or bony orbital hypoplasia, conjunctival sac atresia, reduced length of the palpebral fissures, shrunken eyelids, and poor function due to atrophy of orbicularis and levator muscles. The diagnosis of this condition is clinical, obtained by ophthalmological examination demonstrating complete absence or decreased size of the globe relative to contralateral eye. Ultrasound, computed tomography, and magnetic resonance imaging tests are routinely performed in such patients to rule out syndromic associations (Fig. 9.3).

Early orbital rehabilitation with use of endogenous and exogenous materials, which act as artificial orbitofacial growth stimulators, is generally recommended

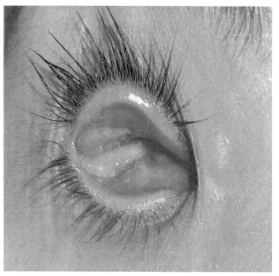

FIG. 9.3 Congenital anophthalmia (acorn shaped socket).

for patients with severe microphthalmia or anophthalmia, without potential vision. (For more details, see description in sections Treatment Planning for Enucleation and Conformers of this chapter.)

Causes of acquired defects are as follows:
1. Surgical defects: Enucleation, evisceration, and exenteration.
2. Traumatic defects: Physical trauma, chemical insult, thermal injury, surgical insult, etc.

Enucleation (Fig. 9.4a here) consists of the removal of entire globe of the eye, muscles, and a portion of the optic nerve normally excluding extraocular muscles. Trauma is the leading cause of eye loss, resulting in enucleation in 41% of cases. Enucleation due to neoplastic disease results in 24% of cases. Other precipitating factors include glaucoma, a blind and painful eye, corneal disease, infection, and uveitis. The leading cause of enucleation in pediatric age group is retinoblastoma, which is a cancer that starts in the retina and may occur in one or both eyes. Retinoblastoma can be of heritable and nonheritable form. Signs of retinoblastoma include redness, swelling, eye that appear to be looking in different directions and a white color in the center circle of the eye (pupil) when light is shown in the eye.

Evisceration (Fig. 9.4b here) involves removal of the contents of the globe leaving the sclera, extraocular muscles, optic nerve, and occasionally the cornea. The knowledge of surgical procedure performed is important as prosthetic treatment plan and option for eviscerated defects may be different from enucleated ones. One reason for this is the presence of cornea may result in sensitivity to the prosthesis.

Exenteration (Fig. 9.4c here) is the most radical surgical procedure, which involves removal of the entire globe and its surrounding structures including muscles, fat, nerves, and eyelids. In these cases, orbital prosthesis rather than an ocular prosthesis is indicated. (Refer to chapter on orbital prosthesis.)

Eyes, being sensitive structures, exhibit profound inflammatory response to various noxious and irritating stimuli. Several traumatic injuries (physical, chemical, thermal), failed surgical procedures (cataract, glaucoma), infections and inflammation (keratitis, uveitis, endophthalmitis), avitaminosis A, and intraocular malignancies (choroidal melanoma, retinoblastoma) and systemic diseases (diabetes, hypertension) may result in an ocular condition known as phthisis bulbi (term derived from the Greek word phthiein or phthinein, meaning shrinkage-shrunken globe). Rehabilitation

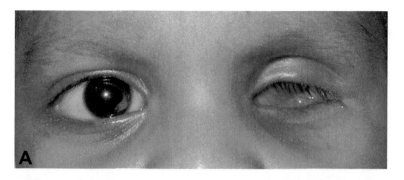

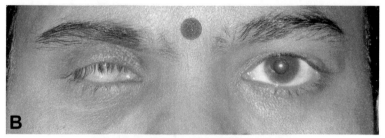

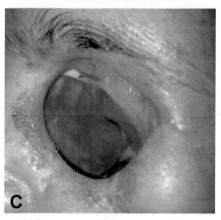

FIG. 9.4 (a) Enucleation. (b) Evisceration. (c) Exenteration.

over the residual phthisical eye is discussed in section Special Considerations and Advancements of this chapter. Traumatic etiology may also be need to be managed by surgical interventions as described before.

CLASSIFICATION

Ocular defects have been classified depending upon the etiology of the defect as discussed in the previous section. However, these etiological or morphological classifications do not facilitate the decision-making process in prosthetic rehabilitation of anophthalmic patients.

Krishna et al. classified ocular sockets into five grades for the sake of convenience in management:

Grade-0: Socket is lined with healthy conjunctiva and normal palpebral aperture and has deep and well-formed fornices.

Grade-I: Socket is characterized by shallow lower fornix or shelving of the lower fornix. Here the lower fornix is converted into a downward sloping shelf, which pushes the lower lid down and out,

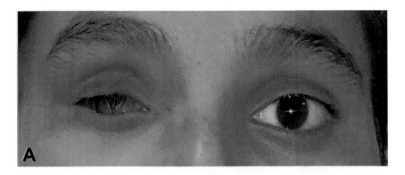

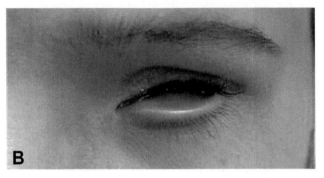

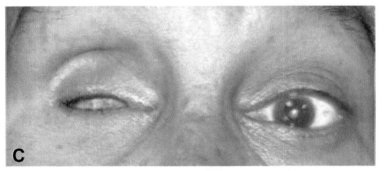

FIG. 9.5 (a) Grade I. (b) Grade II. (c) Grade III. ((b) Pic Courtesy—Dr Abhay Dixit.)

preventing retention of the artificial eyes (Fig. 9.5a here).

Grade-II: Socket is characterized by loss of upper and lower fornices (Fig. 9.5b here).

Grade- III: Socket is characterized by loss of the upper, lower, medial, and lateral fornices (Fig. 9.5c here).

Grade-IV: Socket is characterized by loss of all fornices, and reduction of palpebral aperture in horizontal and vertical dimensions (Fig. 9.6 here).

Grade-V: In some cases, there is recurrence of contraction of the socket after surgical reconstruction.

TREATMENT PLANNING FOR ENUCLEATION
Evaluation of the Patient

Prior to treatment initiation, detailed consultation and physical and psychological evaluation of the patient including his/her desires, expectations, and concerns, related to various aspects of prosthetic rehabilitation, are of utmost importance as it provides insight into the prognosis. History taking should include the surgery done (enucleation or evisceration) and whether an implant was placed at the time of operation. Patients should be sensitized about the expected

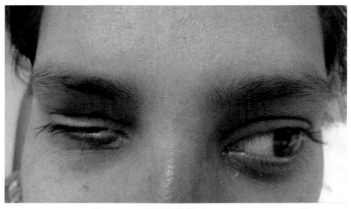

FIG. 9.6 Features of PESS. (Pic Courtesy—Dr Jyotsna.)

outcome, and their role during and after the treatment phase should be emphasized. History taking should also encompass radiation and chemotherapy, which sometimes accompanies ocular ablation to manage malignancies. Prolonged prosthetic procedures may be avoided if the patient has undergone radiotherapy till about 6 months have elapsed, considering the depleted condition of surrounding tissues. A conformer can suffice in the meanwhile.

There are different ways in which the patient can present. Usually, they report with either the conformer or an existing prosthesis in place, or unrehabilitated when coming for treatment for the first time. For the examination of the former, the existing conformer or prosthesis should be removed and given a thorough examination for its adequacy in adapting to the socket, supporting the lids and contour with reference to the normal eye. A lot of pointers for improvement in the new prosthesis can be obtained here. The prosthesis is then removed and followed by a thorough defect examination. Extent of inflammation/healing signs/lack of irritation from the existing prosthesis or conformer, implant exposure should be carefully recorded. If needed, topical application of a steroid/antibiotic/secretion reducing combination (e.g., Atrochlor D or Ocupol D) and for consultation by an ophthalmic surgeon should be made. In case of irritation from the existing prosthesis or conformer, adjustment and polishing should be carried out. The ocular impression for the new prosthesis should be made only after the socket has adequately healed.

The following features should be observed:
1. Relationships of palpebral fissure in an open and closed position.
2. Muscular control, contour, and tonus of the palpebrae.

3. Amount of orbital adipose tissue, development of concerned orbit *vis a vis* the normal one.
4. Internal anatomy of socket (in resting position and during full excursive movements—up, down, left, right—especially mobility of the posterior wall of the tissue bed; also presence/absence of ocular implants).
5. Condition of the conjunctiva and socket lining—any inflammation, excess secretion.
6. Depth of the fornices and presence of cul de sacs (that may improve motion of the artificial eye).
7. Presence of any abnormalities in the tissue, adhesions, muscle attachments, etc.

All the aforementioned features have the potential to influence the prosthetic outcome, and therefore mandate a careful observation before proceeding with treatment. It is important to evaluate the palpebral fissure and eye lid contours before prosthesis fabrication, to judge whether these need any alteration before prosthesis fabrication. Certain contours of the prosthesis can also be changed to alter eyelid contours and position, and palpebral aperture. Depressed orbital region or malformed lids call for preprosthetic plastic surgery to improve prognosis or change of treatment plan to an orbital prosthesis.

One must convey clearly to the patient (and understand as well) that the artificial globe can only transmit muscle movements. Also, the impression must record these movements, to avoid an unstable prosthesis. Any inflammation, abnormality, or irritation of lining tissues has to be managed in conjunction with the ophthalmologist before initiating fabrication. Lack of forniceal depth and tonus creates major issues in prosthesis appearance and retention. Management is discussed later (PESS subsection).

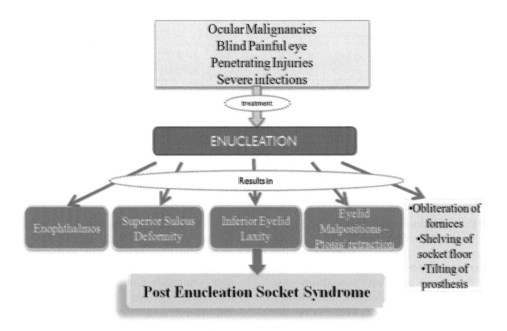

Ocular implants/intraorbital implants

Intraorbital implant was placed for the first time by Mules in 1885 following evisceration and by Frost in 1886 after enucleation, as it was found that following enucleation/evisceration, there was orbital fat atrophy and upper eyelid ptosis (drooping of upper eyelid), sulcus deformity, and lower lid laxity, which together were termed in the postenucleation/postevisceration socket syndrome (PESS). This contributes to producing an enophthalmic appearance.

The contracted eye socket can result from microphthalmos, irradiation of the socket as after enucleation in some cases of retinoblastoma (rare now), severe socket infections, faulty or nonwearing of the artificial eye, keloid-like mass formation in the socket, tissue loss due to injury, and scarring of the conjunctiva.

Primary placement of ocular implants significantly improves prognosis and prosthetic outcome. Secondary implant placement, although recommended, is considered more difficult and demanding, so it is done less often.

The various benefits of placing an intraorbital implant include the following:

1. stimulation of intraorbital growth,
2. enhancement of prosthetic outcome,
3. reduced potential of socket contracture,
4. restoration of lost intraorbital volume, and
5. prevention of PESS.

Various materials have been used as intraorbital implants such as cartilage, coral, bone, cork, rubber, silver, ivory, acrylics, silicone, quartz, glass, different metals, and alloys. Current practice employs intraorbital implants made of nonporous silicone, hydroxyapatite, or PMMA porous polyethylene.

Porous implants (synthetic HA, porous polyethylene, aluminum oxide) were very popular for a time because they provided excellent motility by allowing fibrovascular ingrowth from the socket into the implant. However, they have an increased risk of exposure due to damage or dehiscence of the overlying conjunctiva and socket complications such as granulomas. Porous implants therefore fell.

Nonporous implants may have reduced mobility due to less fibrovascular ingrowth of the surrounding tissues into the implant. This implant is placed into the socket and the Tenon's capsule and conjunctiva sewn over the top.

An ideal ocular prosthesis that corrects volume deficit, matches appearance of fellow eye, exerts minimal pressure upon intraorbital tissues, and achieves an acceptable movement in all gazes can only be fabricated when an ideal socket exists, with an implant placed in it.

An ideal socket can be defined as one with adequately deep fornices, volume loss not exceeding 4.2 mL, having a well-centered intraorbital implant with quiet conjunctiva, and absence of any adverse characteristics such as granulomas, blepharoptosis (abnormal low-lying upper eyelid margin with the eye in primary gaze), eyelid malpositioning or laxity, sulcus deformity, socket contracture, or lagophthalmos (inability to close the eyelids completely).

Formula for selecting ideal implant size was given by Kaltraider and Lucarelli:

Implant diameter (-1 mm for eviscerated eye) $=$ axial length of the contralateral eye $-$ 2 mm.

Choosing an adequately sized implant is as critical as is its precise positioning, so as to facilitate rather than complicate prosthetic rehabilitation (Fig. 9.7) (Table 9.1).

CONFORMERS

Though this forms a different subsection in the chapter, it is an intrinsic part of treatment planning for ocular prosthesis for pediatric and compromised socket patients.

As per GPT-9 definition, a conformer is an interim ocular prosthesis\syn, CONFORMER, OCULAR CONFORMER made usually of PMMA or soft silicone.

Surgical Conformers

Conformer can be a clear acrylic shell fitted after enucleation or evisceration. The use of a conformer is important here in maintaining deep conjunctival fornices and avoiding contracture. Such a conformer may be placed under sutured lids for a while after surgery. It maintains the shape of the eye and protects the suture line from blinking of eyelids. This type of conformer is worn up to 6–8 weeks after surgery till the eye socket is prepared for placement of an ocular prosthesis (though the lid sutures are removed within a week). These conformers are transparent, so that the wound can be easily

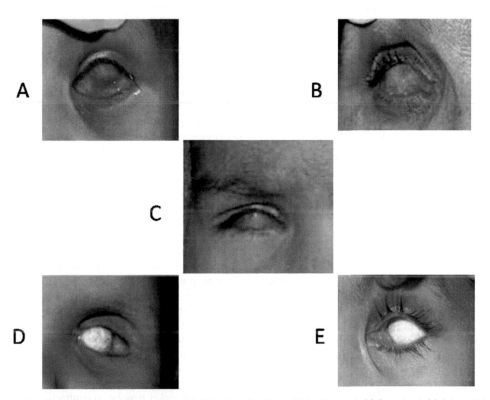

FIG. 9.7 Presentation of different intraorbital implant situations. (a) Undersized. (b) Oversized. (c) Adequately sized embedded. (d and e) Migrated and exposed.

| TABLE 9.1 Intraorbital Implant Situations with Prosthetic Outcomes/Implications | |

Different Intraorbital Implant Situations	Prosthetic Outcome/ Implication and Solutions
1. Adequately sized embedded intraorbital implant	- Best prosthetic outcome—adequate orbital growth stimulation
2. Undersized intraorbital implant	- Compromised esthetic outcome - Inadequate orbital growth stimulation - Enophthalmic appearance of prosthesis - Repeat implant placement
3. Oversized intraorbital implant	- Poor prosthetic outcome - Exophthalmic appearance with inadequate prosthesis bulk - Restricted movement of prosthesis - Increased risk of implant extrusion - Repeat implant placement
4. Exposed intraorbital implant	- Vaulted ocular prosthesis relieving any pressure on exposure site - Patch grafting
5. Migrated intraorbital implant	- Difficulty in ideal prosthesis placement - Repeat implant placement

monitored by the clinician. However, transparent prostheses can cause embarrassment to patients on account of unsightly visualization of the underlying socket. The patient may opt to cover or patch the eye. Surgical conformers have holes that allow easy flow of secretions during the postoperative period to prevent wound from infection (Fig. 9.8a).

Esthetic Conformers

Also called prosthetic or cosmetic conformers, these are painted like a natural eye with an iris component.

Fenestrations for drainage may be present. Esthetic conformers decrease psychological impact of enucleation, yet achieve goals of an ideal conformer. Children may be more comfortable with this conformer type as it avoids the use of patches for camouflage (Fig. 9.8b).

Stock and Custom Conformers

Conformers can also be classified as stock or custom. Postsurgical conformers are stock conformers. These conformers came in different dimensions, and there is no specificity for left or right eyes. Customized conformers need an impression of the concerned defect (similar to impression for prosthesis—next section) and are used for the management of PESS, congenital anophthalmia, pediatric patients, and progressive enlargement of contracted ocular socket.

The relationship of PESS and intraorbital implants has been discussed in the previous section. PESS is the most common late complication of enucleation and occurs if a patient does not wear conformer prosthesis after surgery, wears an ill-fitting or stock ocular prosthesis, or in case of pediatric patients, does not get regular remakes commensurate with growth of orbital region. PESS encompasses shallow anterior fornix, atrophy of orbital tissue, symblepharon (partial or complete adhesion of the palpebral conjunctiva of the eyelid to the bulbar conjunctiva of the eyeball), lower eyelid laxity, ptosis, and entropion or ectropion of the lower lid. These result in orbital depression, palpebral aperture reduction, prosthesis dislocation or troubled insertion, facial deformation and hypoplastic facial bones, depending on the age of occurrence.

This happens because the prosthetic eye does not just have an esthetic function. It also forms the nucleus for support and growth of orbital and associated facial region. If this nucleus does not restore the ocular defect accurately, complications such as contracted socket or PESS are likely to occur. Ocular implants, use of conformers, and well-fitting ocular prosthesis can prevent these complications. PESS is primarily managed surgically, consisting of dermal fat grafting along with fornix deepening sutures. A technique for prosthetic management with custom conformers and bandaging is described under Special considerations and Advancements point 4.

Congenital anophthalmia/microphthalmia (Fig. 9.9) is a common cause of contracted sockets and occurs as a consequence of the missing globe. If not rehabilitated, fornices, eye lids, and orbital region suffer from retarded growth. The socket may be so contracted as to make an ocular impression difficult, let alone retention or placement of a prosthesis. Even if a prosthesis is made, it looks

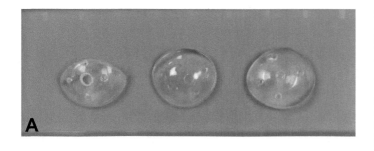
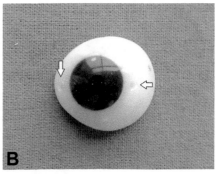

FIG. 9.8 (a) Surgical conformers. (b) Esthetic conformer.

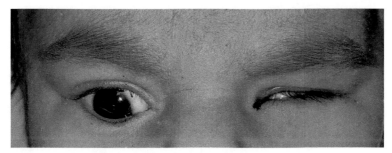

FIG. 9.9 Microphthalmia. (Pic Courtesy—Dr Aditi Verma.)

disproportionately small to the normal eye. This condition needs long-term team commitment. Contracted sockets offer problems for the prosthodontist and plastic/ophthalmic surgeon. The most effective prosthetic approach is fabrication of custom-designed progressively larger conformers used sequentially till enough space is created for fabrication of a normal sized prosthesis (Fig. 9.10).

This "expansion therapy" consists of a custom conformer for the patient, ensuring that it extends well into the fornices and supports the palpebrae. After a period of 2 weeks, fresh impressions are made of a slightly expanded socket and another custom conformer (or the same one relined with a soft liner) is delivered. This procedure is continued for at least three progressive conformer sizes, or till an esthetic symmetric prosthetic eye can be fabricated. The concept is to place the ocular defect connective tissue to achieve the final outcome.

Surgical reconstruction of the contracted socket requires creating a stable socket with adequate fornix depth established by increasing the surface area with the use of graft materials such as conjunctiva, mucous membrane, hard palate mucosa, skin, muscle flaps, temporalis fascia, dermis fat graft, polytetrafluoroethylene, and amniotic membrane.

Surgical procedures depend upon the extent of socket contraction. For mild contraction, autogenous dermal fat grafting and fornix deepening sutures have been advocated. For moderate contraction, mucous membrane graft has been employed. Severely contracted sockets warrant the use of skin grafts. A surgical conformer needs to be kept in the socket as described earlier to prevent recurrence of contracture.

TECHNIQUE AND MATERIALS
Stock Versus Custom Prosthetic Eyes

Stock eyes are prefabricated and do not provide exact color matching with the contralateral eye or custom-fit in the ocular defect. They often lead to complications of PESS. Custom eyes are fabricated in conformance to the individual socket, matching normal, scleral, and iris color and contour. Esthetics, function, prognosis of prosthesis, and surrounding region are naturally superior to the stock prosthesis.

It is assumed that all procedures discussed in treatment planning and conformers sections have been attended to before prosthesis fabrication is initiated. Ocular prosthesis fabrication can be divided according to required appointments:

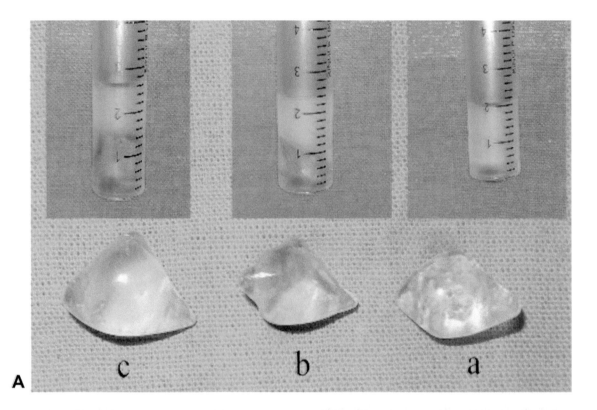

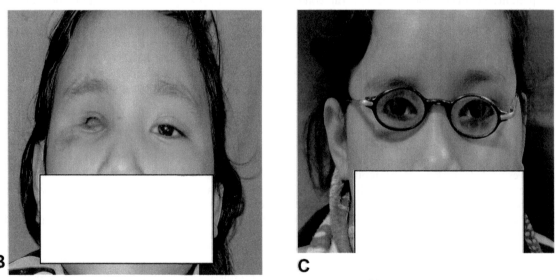

FIG. 9.10 Progressive "éxpansion" therapy for contracted ocular sockets. (a) Progressive increase in size of conformers. (b) Socket before using conformer. (c) Socket size increased after wearing conformer.

First appointment—Examination of socket and impression.

Second appointment—Adjusting the wax pattern, and iris positioning.

Third appointment—Delivery of prosthesis.

Further appointments are needed for follow-up. The multiple laboratory and clinical steps of fabrication are described in the following.

Impression

After examination of the socket as described in treatment planning, the next step is to make an impression of the enucleated socket. For the impression-taking procedure, the patient should be seated upright with head supported with headrest.

Impression Materials and Trays

a. Alginate
b. Ophthalmic alginate
c. Nonaqueous elastomeric impression material

Alginate is the most inexpensive and easily available impression material. Flow of the material is good, it records fine details, but dimensional stability is not good and material distorts early.

Ophthalmic alginate is specifically formulated for this purpose, with increased flow and a neutral pH to prevent irritation to the ocular socket. It is less readily available in a dental setup and is costlier.

Nonaqueous elastomeric impression material is one of the most suitable materials because of being self-supportive, moldable, not distorting easily, and having high tear resistance. Polyvinyl siloxane is the material of choice. A disadvantage of the material is higher cost.

Impressions can be made with a perforated stock/prefabricated ocular tray/conformer or in a customized ocular impression tray. Ocular impression trays are available in various sizes (Factor 2 and Technovent).

Prefabricated trays came with either a long stalk or short stalk. Stalk is the hollow tube part of the ocular tray, for attaching a syringe to inject impression material into the socket. Long stalks may be better suited for alginate impressions and short one for polyvinyl siloxane impression materials (Fig. 9.11).

Customized ocular trays can be made with conformers and syringes. First an appropriate size of conformer has to be selected by trying it in the socket to ensure that it is aligned properly and not over extended. The conformers can also be adjusted according to the size of the ocular socket. A 5−10 mL syringe with plunger may be used after removing the needle and attaching the hub or tip to the central hole/stalk in the selected conformer tray. It should be ensured that the hub/tip is positioned in the center of the ocular defect (pupillary region), so that impression material flows uniformly all around the defect (Fig. 9.12a and b).

Impression Technique

Tray positioning should be rehearsed before the impression. Remove the plunger from the syringe barrel, insert the mixed impression material, and insert the plunger back. Then the tray is loaded approximately with 5 mL of impression material following manufacturer instructions and ensuring no bubbles. When inserting the tray, conformer, or prosthesis into the socket, the patient should be relaxed and trained not to constrict the lids. If the eyelashes are long, they may be trimmed or lubricated. First, the upper eyelid is lifted and the tray rotated in, followed by pulling the lower lid down and maneuvering the lower end in. Ensure that the tray is

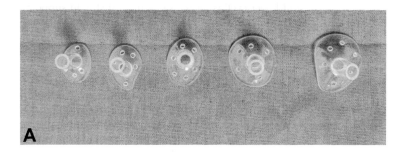
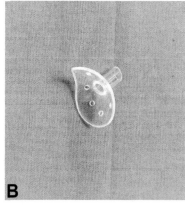

FIG. 9.11 Prefabricated trays of various sizes.

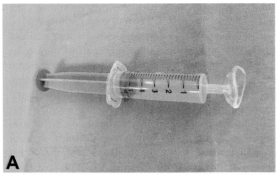 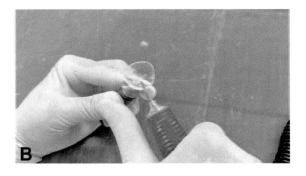

FIG. 9.12 (a) Tray conformer adjustment. (b) Syringe attached to conformer.

positioned properly. Initially the patient should be looking straight ahead (about 6 feet), followed by rotating gaze in all directions, to record movements of the tissue bed. It should be ensured that impression material flows out of the tray perforations as this indicates proper flow of the material.

Wiggle out the tray after material sets. Impression should be examined for any voids/bubbles and confirm that the fornices were recorded properly. Repeat impression if required after necessary adjustments.

A good impression extends fully into the fornices without overstretching the conjunctiva and accurately records the shape of the posterior aspect of the socket. An overextended impression may restrain movements of the prosthetic eye or create instability in movement while one that is underextended may result in a prosthesis that does not support the orbital region (Fig. 9.13).

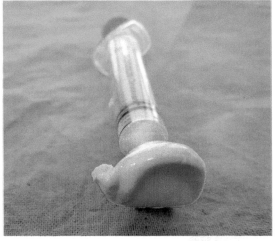

FIG. 9.13 Impression with ocular tray.

Scleral pattern

Trim excess impression material from the tray. For pattern fabrication, ocular waxes can be used as well as mixture of three parts carving wax and one part yellow sticky wax (by weight) produced by heating the two together on direct flame in a metallic container till they turn liquid. Take care as this can splatter.

In the meanwhile, pour about half to three-quarters of a paper cup with alginate impression material and embed the ocular impression while the mix is setting. On setting, the alginate mold is cut vertically into two halves, to facilitate ocular tray removal. The two halves are joined back by adhesive or elastics. The molten wax is now poured directly into mold slowly, as the wax contracts while solidifying. After cooling, pattern is ready for modification in the socket, where it is inserted to check fit, contours, and adaptation. Initially, the eye may water, but this diminishes with habituation. If pattern insertion is uncomfortable for the patient, the pattern may be slightly lubricated or topical anesthesia applied sparingly in the socket. The pattern should be adjusted so as not to bulge or weigh down the upper and lower eyelids; at the same time, it should support the eyelids to their normal contour and position. Wax pattern should not protrude too far out and neither be too flat. The normal eye and its lids provide a ready reckoner for gauging the correct pattern dimension. Adjust pattern as needed (Fig. 9.14).

The starting point for comparing the two eyes should be with the patient gazing ahead in a relaxed manner, and then the comparison is to be made moving the eyes all around. Displacement of pattern indicates overextension. For example, if the patient looks down and the pattern is displaced, it means that the superior forniceal extension of the pattern needs to be thinned or shortened. The pattern should also be left in the socket a few minutes and checked. Displacement by rebound in such cases indicates that the tissue bed aspect needs

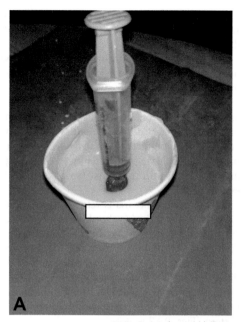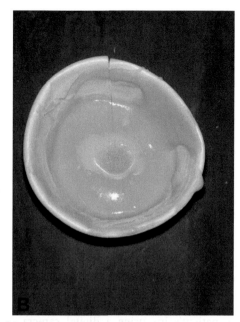

FIG. 9.14 (a and b) Pattern fabrication in alginate mold.

relief. Special care of lower margin extension needs to be taken when there is lower lid laxity to reduce shelving and improve stability. A ptotic upper lid can often be compensated by increasing the pattern contour just above the palpebral aperture. Scar tissue or an exposed implant on the tissue bed needs to be relieved in the pattern creating a vaulted prosthesis. The pattern stage is a good time to estimate how much mobility the final prosthesis will have.

Iris

The pattern is now ready to accept the iris component. Common techniques for iris creation are iris disc painting, digital imaging, and retrieval from stock eye.

Iris painting is done on premanufactured iris discs, which come in different sizes. A rod of sticky wax is attached to an appropriately size-matched iris disc so that it can be easily handled during painting. Oil pigments may be used to paint the iris mixed with monomer–polymer syrup to facilitate rapid drying. The color of the limbus area is mixed first and applied as a base layer, over which the colors of the collarette and stroma are applied; working from the center outwards in multiple layers (Figs. 9.15 and 9.16). This method is artistically demanding but has the most esthetic results.

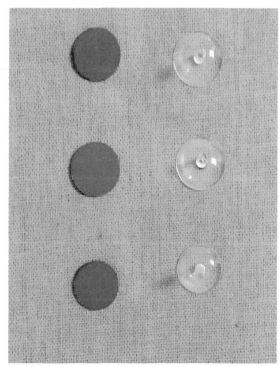

FIG. 9.15 Iris discs and corneal buttons of various sizes.

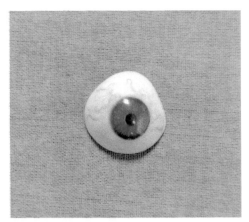

FIG. 9.16 Ocular prosthesis with painted iris.

The use of digital imaging presents several advantages to the conventional iris painting technique, as it provides acceptable esthetics result with minimal artistic skill requirement. Here, a digital photograph of the patient's iris using a digital camera with macrolens and ring flash is taken. Graphic software can be used for adjustment of slight differences.

Iris is printed and attached to an iris disc with monopoly syrup or cyanoacrylate adhesive. This method may be slightly costlier.

The stock eye/shell retrieval technique is less time-taking, inexpensive, easy to use, and less demanding of artistic or technological skills. Its disadvantages are less than perfect iris match with normal eye at times (size, color), and difficulty in adjusting the iris disk in very thin patterns (small defect volume, evisceration).

In this technique, iris is retrieved from a stock eye. Color and size of the iris should match with the normal eye (diameter of iris can be measured with gauges, divider, and scale). The matched iris portion should be cut out from the stock eye using acrylic trimmers, discs, and burs, taking special care of the border in the limbus region. The disc can also be thinned from its posterior surface for better positioning in the scleral pattern (Figs. 9.17 and 9.18).

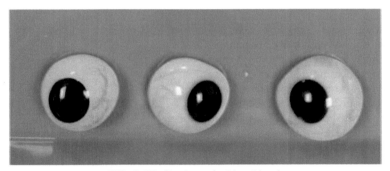

FIG. 9.17 Stock eye for iris retrieval.

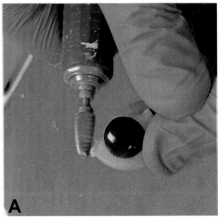

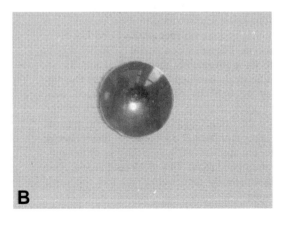

FIG. 9.18 (a) Trimming the iris out from stock eye. (b) Retrieved iris.

Iris positioning

Precise positioning of the iris in the pattern is key to a natural looking ocular prosthesis. There are varied techniques to do this using a plastic strip template, Boley's gauge, millimeter ruler, pupillometer, window light or light reflection viewed symmetrically in the eyes, ocular locator with fixed caliper, inverted anatomic tracings, transparent graph grid, computer simulation approach with optical scanning technique and CAD, customized scale for assessing the position of the ocular prosthesis, etc.

Roberts in 1969 introduced the pupillometer for iris positioning, with the pupil as a fixation point and two plastic rotatable discs having scale markings on the bridge of the nose. Dasgupta et al. took a good quality digital facial photograph from a digital single lens reflex camera, such that the flashlight reflected at the pupil of the normal eye. Different measurements were then recorded for positioning the iris accurately. This did not require complex armamentarium and patient cooperation. However, additional knowledge and skills for using this method were needed. Bi et al. used a three-dimensional scanning (CAD/CAM) system to record patients' faces to form a 3D facial model. The measurements of normal iris were recorded and then mirrored on the defect area to position the iris. The advantage of this technique was short length of clinical appointment.

Whatever the means, the end should be a prosthetic iris and pupil, which simulates the natural one in superoinferior, mediolateral, and anteroposterior position. The glabella, bridge of the nose, eye brows, medial and lateral canthi, and upper and lower lids are adjacent anatomical landmarks, which lend themselves well to estimate this placement.

After making necessary measurements with a scale and divider and transferring them to the pattern, wax from the pattern of approximately the size of the iris disc is removed from the marked area with a hot spoon-shaped spatula. The iris is then seated so that the contours of the pattern are undisturbed (Figs. 9.19 and 9.20).

For painted iris disk method, transparent corneal buttons with attached stalks are available. This is carefully joined to the iris disc, once the colors have dried, using monopoly syrup (10 parts of heat cure acrylic resin monomer to one-part clear acrylic resin polymer by weight), ensuring that the button center coincides with the pupillary position. The button–disc combination is embedded in the scleral pattern as described before.

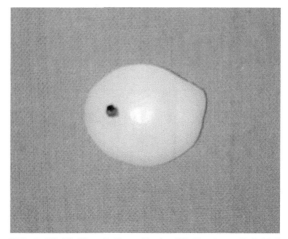

FIG. 9.19 Markings for iris positioning. (Pic Courtesy—Dr Rohini.)

Try-in

After iris positioning, final pattern try-in is done. The patient is seated upright with no head support, and looking directly ahead at a distance of about 6 feet, in a relaxed manner. This position is preferred as it is the normal gaze in a social setting, and the iris is located in the center while looking here. This gives a good starting point for comparison with the normal eye. Often because of surgery, trauma, or contracture, the palpebral aperture space becomes larger than the normal side. In such cases, camouflage has to be done to prevent the prosthetic eye from looking bulbous by reducing the contour of the pattern. If the palpebral aperture is smaller than the contralateral eye, a slightly smaller iris size than normal may be selected to make the disparity less pronounced (Fig. 9.21).

Mold

After the try-in is perfected, mold preparation has to be done. First, a self-cure PMMA stalk (approx. 2 mm diameter and 4 mm length) is attached to the iris, to prevent its displacement while packing the mold with resin under pressure. This step is not required for corneal button-painted iris disc assembly, as this already has the stalk attached.

An ocular flask (small brass flask specially use for curing ocular prosthesis) may be used for mold preparation. White dental stone is mixed and poured in the first half of the flask. This is preferred because it provides a suitable background for scleral characterization. The wax pattern is half embedded in the half pour,

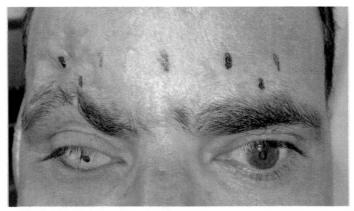

FIG. 9.20 Pupil mark on the pattern. See that this is not necessarily at the center of the pattern.

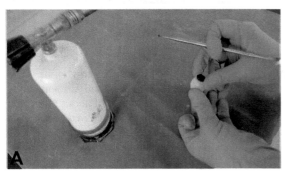

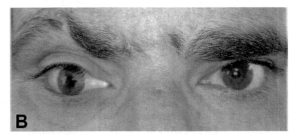

FIG. 9.21 (a) Iris positioned on the scleral wax pattern. (b) Final pattern try-in.

while ascertaining there is no undercut in this pour. After setting, separating media is applied, the second pour is done, and two flask halves are approximated. The flask is clamped under hand pressure and dewaxed. Dewaxed mold is cleaned well with soap and hot water (Fig. 9.22a and b).

Scleral coloration

The mold is ready now for packing with characterized scleral resins. Scleral acrylics are marketed for the purpose but are costly. Equally effective results can be obtained with tooth-colored heat-polymerized polymethyl methacrylate (PMMA). They have good flow, are color stable, and have color variability from yellow—white—gray. They can be combined with each other and with easily available acrylic colors by trial and error, to produce different scleral shades. The polymer—monomer—acrylic color combined is placed thinly between two layers of cellophane sheet and compared with the scleral color of the patient. Different scleral colors may have to be achieved, for example, the

caruncle region is pink to red, sclera of pediatric patients is normally blue—grey and that of older adults is yellow to brown. The effect of veins can be simulated by placing tiny red cotton/wool/rayon flockings, wisps, or fibers at requisite places in the mold. These are made to adhere to their position by lightly painting PMMA monomer on them. Some specialists make customized scleral shade tabs or guides based on precalculated polymer—acrylic color weight ratios for ease and precision (Figs. 9.23a,b and 9.24).

Processing, finishing, and insertion

After applying separating media, appropriately colored PMMA is manipulated as per manufacturer's instructions and packed in the mold in the dough stage, making sure there are no air bubbles in the mix. Trial closure and flash removal make packing more predictable. After bench curing, the flask is placed in a hot water bath for polymerization at 100°C for 1 h. After cooling, the prosthesis is extricated from the mold taking care to preserve the mold (for adding the corneal layer). Surfaces are

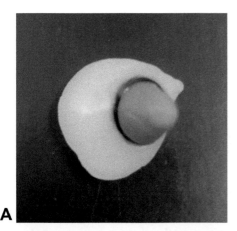

A

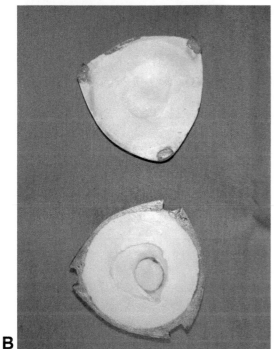

B

FIG. 9.22 (a) Acrylic stalk for indexing. (b) Mold after dewaxing.

checked for porosities, nodules, or irregularities. Excess material and stalk is trimmed off, and the prosthesis is finished and polished. If corneal button was used, then further processing for adding the corneal layer is not required (Fig. 9.25).

If the scleral color is lighter or less characterized, than the normal eye, minor extrinsic corrections can be done at this stage and sealed with monopoly syrup.

For the iris retrieval from scleral shell method, a corneal layer has to be added after finishing and polishing of prosthesis. This helps mimic normal ocular anatomy. The mold is scraped with a blunt rounded instrument (like a round coin) in the region housing the iris by 0.5−1 mm and finished with find sand paper. The created space is then packed with transparent autopolymerizing polymethyl methacrylate, and the finished eye is carefully seated back into the mold. The second half of the mold is closed, clamped, and put in a pressure pot as per instructions. The prosthesis is retrieved with the corneal portion and polished with a pumice paste. Polishing has to be done carefully, so as not to fracture or crack the prosthesis (Fig. 9.26).

Insertion and Removal of Prosthesis

The patient should be well versed with prosthesis removal and insertion at the end of this appointment. The specialist has to be patient in instructions specially to the old and very young patients. Watering and irritation can be expected at this appointment, which peters off with adaptation. Major corrections are ordinarily not needed in the prosthesis at this time. Esthetics, retention, and mobility of the eye should be reassessed.

The patient should be able to close his lids with the prosthesis in place. At best with the help of ocular implants and active extra ocular muscles, the movement of the natural and artificial eye should be similar. At worst, the irises of both eyes should be similarly located when the patient looks at a spot about 6 feet directly ahead. To escape easy detection, patients with limited ocular movement should be instructed to turn their face toward the object of interest rather than their eyes. The patient should be advised to remove prosthesis by pulling down the lower eyelid, and slipping out the prosthesis. Removal from the socket may be aided by suction tips (Fig. 9.27).

CARE AND REFABRICATION OF PROSTHESIS

Prosthetic eye should not be removed frequently. It should be removed for cleaning once every 2−4 weeks as frequent removal can introduce foreign material and bacteria into the socket and damage the prosthesis.

However, maintenance of socket hygiene is important. The prosthesis should be considered as normal eye during face washing and bathing. Any scratches on the prosthesis need repolishing by the prosthodontist. Frequent touching of the prosthesis is not allowed. Hands should be washed before removing and inserting the prosthesis.

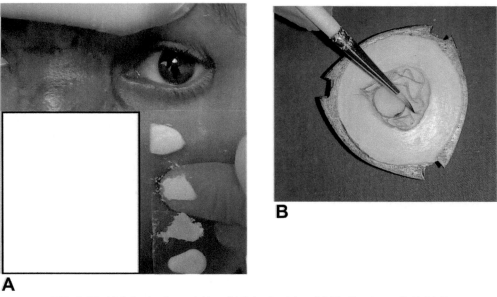

FIG. 9.23 (a) Scleral color matching. (b) Scleral veining. ((a) Pic Courtesy—Dr Rohini.)

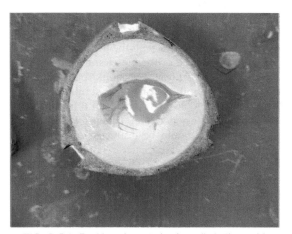

FIG. 9.24 Packing characterized acrylic in the mold.

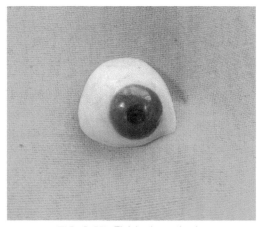

FIG. 9.25 Finished prosthesis.

After the insertion of prosthesis, some amount of discharge is normal, but if this increases, the specialist has to be consulted. Excessive discharge may be because of prosthesis creating pressure on the socket or rough surfaces causing mechanical irritation. Environmental irritants may also cause irritation. To prevent this, the patient should wear protective spectacles, more so to protect the lone natural eye from chance damage.

Topical antibiotics, steroids, and secretion reducers may be indicated for reduction of any inflammation present in socket. If there is dryness, artificial tears or lubricants may be used. Ocular prosthesis should be replaced every 3—5 years in adult patients due to tissue changes, bacterial infiltration, or breakdown of acrylic surface. Children require frequent replacements (4—6 months) due to anatomical growth. If there is a change in appearance, discomfort, or irritation, prosthetic eye can be replaced earlier.

In adults, evaluation of prosthesis is indicated annually, and for the pediatric patient, follow-up appointments should be at 2—4 months intervals on account of growth of the orbital region. Patient should be counseled to keep regular appointments with his ophthalmologist (Fig. 9.28).

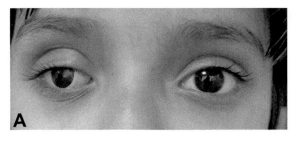 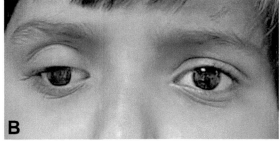

FIG. 9.26 (a) Before placing corneal layer. (b) After placing corneal layer.

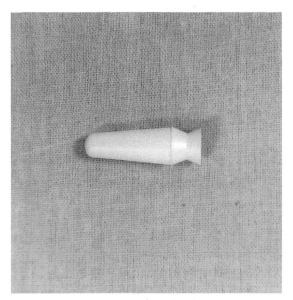

FIG. 9.27 A suction tip.

SPECIAL CONSIDERATIONS AND ADVANCEMENTS

1. Phthisis bulbi or ocular atrophy—Various parameters that influence prosthetic rehabilitation include condition of cornea, contour and color of sclera, degree of enophthalmos, presence of corneal sensitivity, and condition of associated contiguous structures. Whereas enucleation is managed as described in the previous three sections, the management of phthisis bulbi and/or evisceration cases is different as a result of present (albeit shrunken) globe and cornea.

   Based on parameters such as condition of sclera, degree of enophthalmos, and condition of associated surrounding structures, phthisis bulbi defects have been divided into four major classes as mentioned in Table 9.2 and Fig. 9.29.

Corneal sensitivity can be minimized by surgical techniques, which include use of conjunctival flaps to cover the sensitive cornea, but have their own complications. Prosthetic management includes use of contact lens and transparent acrylic shells, which cause gradual desensitization and improved esthetic outcome. Contact lens or scleral shells mask the opaque/disfigured eyeball. The retained eye may provide a good foundation for such prostheses, often providing excellent motility. Difference between a shell and normal prostheses is that a shell is 1.5 mm or less in thickness (Fig. 9.30a and b).

2. CAD-CAM technology has been used for the fabrication of ocular prosthesis. An impression mold of the patient's anophthalmic socket is first optically scanned using a 3D scanner to produce a 3D model. The ocular prosthesis is then produced via a digital light processing 3D printer using biocompatible photopolymer resin. Subsequently, an image of the iris and blood vessels of the eye is prepared by modifying a photographed image of the contralateral normal eye, and printed onto the 3D-printed ocular prosthesis, using a dye sublimation transfer technique. This method has the potential to reduce time and skill required for fabricating a customized ocular prosthesis, though using sophisticated machines and technique.

3. A solid ocular prosthesis in a large socket can be deleterious for the lower fornix and palpebrae. Various techniques have been proposed for fabrication of light weight/pneumatic/hollow prosthesis(which are also more comfortable for the patient) using lost-salt technique, styrofoam, and acrylic shims.

4. In an extremely contracted eye socket, retention of conformer/ocular prosthesis without surgical enlargement is very challenging. Bandaging the custom conformer within a closed eye can be done for a few weeks to retain the prosthesis. Once this

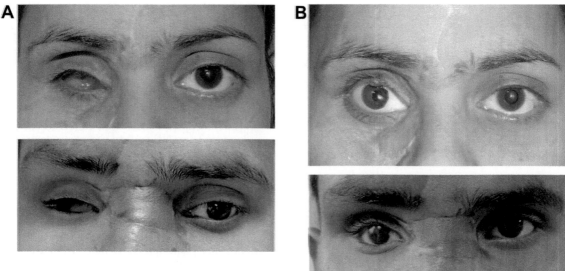

FIG. 9.28 (a) Defect without prosthesis. (b) With ocular prosthesis.

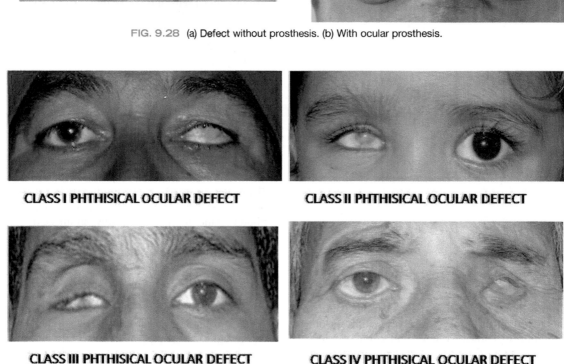

CLASS I PHTHISICAL OCULAR DEFECT

CLASS II PHTHISICAL OCULAR DEFECT

CLASS III PHTHISICAL OCULAR DEFECT

CLASS IV PHTHISICAL OCULAR DEFECT

FIG. 9.29 Classification of phthisis bulbi.

conformer is retentive by selective placement of soft tissues, a larger one can be bandaged in place till desirable enlargement of socket is achieved (Fig. 9.31a,b and c).
5. If unfortunately a patient loses both his eyes, it is entirely his choice, whether he wants an ocular prosthesis or not.

6. A bionic eye (visual eye) is intended to restore functional vision in those suffering from partial or total blindness with the help of image sensors, microprocessors, receivers, radio transmitters, and retinal chips.
7. In case a patient has allergy to acrylic, a silicone eye may be fabricated.

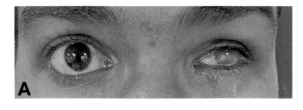
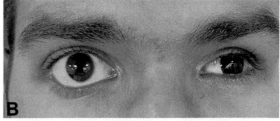

FIG. 9.30 (a) Phthisis bulbi patient. (b) After wearing cosmetic lens. ((a) Pic Courtesy—Dr Neeti Solanki.)

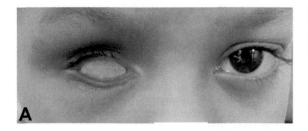
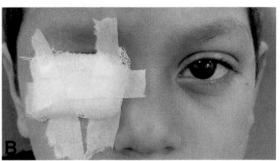
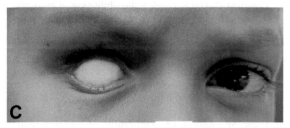

FIG. 9.31 (a) Before. (b) Bandaging. (c) After. ((a) Pic Courtesy—Dr Neeti Solanki.)

TABLE 9.2
Phthisis Bulbi Classification

Class	Condition	Treatment
I a	Corneal opacity with no enophthalmos and normal sclera without corneal sensitivity	Cosmetic lens
I b	Corneal opacity with no enophthalmos and normal sclera with corneal sensitivity	Cosmetic lens after reducing corneal sensitivity
II a	Corneal opacity with mild enophthalmos and normal sclera without corneal sensitivity	Transparent acrylic resin or silicone sclera shell
II b	Corneal opacity with mild enophthalmos and normal sclera with corneal sensitivity	Clear or transparent acrylic resin or silicone sclera shell after reducing the corneal sensitivity
III	Moderate enophthalmos with disfigured sclera	Ocular prosthesis or scleral shell
IV	Severe enophthalmos with disfigured sclera and loss of orbital fat/depressed orbit	Ocular prosthesis or scleral shell after performing additional procedures such as dermal lid fillers or eyelid surgeries/orbital prostheses/grafting in periorbital region

8. Management of pediatric patients and infants may need special training in dealing with this age group.

CONCLUSION

Intraorbital implants and conformers have a crucial role to play in the health of the enucleated socket and surrounding region. The prosthodontist should be well acquainted with them. A well-fitting esthetic custom ocular prosthesis is integral to the health of the periorbital area and socket, along with playing an integral role in improving the patient's quality of life. Creating a beautifully matched eye is a work of art, as much or more than it is a science. Newer technologies are making this process less demanding for those less gifted with artistic skills.

BIBLIOGRAPHY

1. Aggarwal H, Kumar P, Singh RD. Prosthetic management of congenital anophthalmia- microphthalmia patient. *Arch Med Health Sci.* 2015;3:117−120.
2. Aggarwal H, Singh RD, Kumar P, Gupta SK, Alvi HA. Prosthetic guidelines for ocular rehabilitation in patients with phthisis bulbi: a treatment based classification system. *J Prosthet Dent.* 2014;111:525−528.
3. Aggarwal H, Kumar P, Eachempati P, Alvi HA. Different intra-orbital implant situations on ocular rehabilitation. *J Prosthodont.* 2016;25(8):687−693.
4. Aggarwal H, Shah V, Singh SV, Arya D. Volumetric expansion of ocular defect with progressive conformers: an objective assessment. *Natl J Maxillofac Surg.* January−June 2019;10(1):123−125.
5. Aggarwal H, Singh SV, Kumar P, Kumar Singh A. Prosthetic rehabilitation following socket reconstruction with blair-brown graft and conformer therapy for management of severe post-enucleation socket syndrome − a clinical report. *J Prosthodont.* June 2015;24(4):329−333.
6. Ainbinder DJ, Haik BG, Mazzoli RA. Anophthalmic socket and orbital implants. Role of CT and MR imaging. *Radiol Clin North Am.* 1998;36:1133−1147 (xi).
7. Andres CJ, Haug SP. *Clinical Maxillofacial Prosthetics.* 1st ed. Chicago: Quintessence Publishing Co, Inc; 2000: 265−276.
8. Artopoulou II, Montgomery PC, Wesley PJ, Lemon JC. Digital imaging in the fabrication of ocular prostheses. *J Prosthet Dent.* April 2006;95(4):327−330.
9. Ashworth JL, Rhatigan M, Sampath R, et al. The hydroxyapatite intra-orbital implant: a prospective study. *Eye.* 1996;1029−1037.
10. Avisar I, Norris JH, Quinn S, et al. Temporary cosmetic painted prostheses in anophthalmic surgery: an alternative to early postoperative clear conformers. *Eye (Lond).* 2011; 25:1418−1422.

11. Beumer J, Marunick MT, Esposito SJ. *Maxillofacial Rehabilitation.* 3rd ed. Chicago: Quintessence Publishing Co, Inc; 2011:255−314.
12. Brett J. Creating a treatment plan for enucleation or evisceration surgery. *J. Ophthalmic Prosthetics.* 2000;5:45−48.
13. Chalian VA, Drane JB, Standish SM. *Maxillofacial Prosthetics, Multidisciplinary Practice.* Baltimore: The Williams & Wilkins Company; 1971:l−2.
14. Chintagumpala M, Chevez-Barrios P, Paysse EA, et al. Retinoblastoma: review of current management. *Oncol.* 2007; 12:1237−1246.
15. Christmas NJ, Gordon CD, Murray TG, et al. Intra-orbital implants after enucleation and their complications: a 10-year review. *Arch Ophthalmol.* 1998;116:1199−1203.
16. Chowdhury AR, Singh SV, Chand P, Aggarwal H, Arya D. Novel technique for fabrication of pneumatic ocular prosthesis. *Cont Lens Anterior Eye.* October 2018;41(5): 469−470.
17. Custer PL, Kennedy RH, Woog JJ, et al. Intra-orbital implants in enucleation surgery: a report by the American Academy of Ophthalmology. *Ophthalmol Times.* 2003; 110:2054−2061.
18. Dasgupta D, Das K, Singh R. Rehabilitation of an ocular defect with intraorbital implant and custom-made prosthesis using digital photography and gridded spectacle. *J Indian Prosthodont Soc.* 2019;19:266−271.
19. Hadjistilianou T, Francesco S, Marconcini S, Mastrangelo D, Galluzzi P, Toti P. Phthisis bulbi and buphthalmos as presenting signs of retinoblastoma: a report of two cases and literature review. *Eur J Ophthalmol.* 2006;16:465−469.
20. Haug SP, Andres CJ. Fabrication of custom ocular prostheses. In: Taylor TD, ed. *Clinical Maxillofacial Prosthetics.* Chicago: Quintessence Publishing; 2000: 265−267.
21. Kaltreider SA, Lucarelli MJ. A simple algorithm for selection of implant size for enucleation and evisceration: a prospective study. *Ophthal Plast Reconstr Surg.* 2002;18: 336−341.
22. Kavlekar AA, Aras MA, Chitre V. An innovative and simple approach to fabricate a hollow ocular prosthesis with functional lubricant reservoir: a solution to artificial eye comfort. *J Indian Prosthodont Soc.* 2017;17(2):196−202. https://doi.org/10.4103/0972-4052.194946.
23. Krishna G. Contracted sockets -I (Aetiology and types). *Indian J Ophthalmol.* 1980;28:117−120.
24. Kumar P, Singh SV, Aggarwal H, Chand P. Incorporation of a vacuum-formed polyvinyl chloride sheet into an orbital prosthesis pattern. *J Prosthet Dent.* 2015;113(2): 157−159.
25. Kumar P, Aggrawal H, Singh RD, et al. A simplified approach for placing the iris disc on a custom madeocular prosthesis: report of four cases. *J Indian Prosthodont Soc.* 2014;14:124−127.
26. Llorente-González S, Peralta-Calvo J, Abelairas-Gómez JM. Congenital anophthalmia and microphthalmia:

epidemiology and orbitofacial rehabilitation. *Clin Ophthalmol.* 2011;5:1759–1765.

27. Nunnery WR, Ng JD, Hetzler KJ. Enucleation and evisceration. In: Spaeth G, ed. *Ophthalmic Surgery: Principles and Practice.* 3rd ed. Philadelphia: Elsevier; 2003:485–507.

28. Osborn KL, Hettler D. A survey of recommendations on the care of ocular prostheses. *Optometry.* 2010;81:142–145.

29. Pavaiya A, Singh SV, Singh RD, Chand P. Fabrication of an ocular prosthesis for a pediatric retinoblastoma patient by a simplified technique. *IntJ Clin Pediatric Dent.* 2010;3:97–99.

30. Pine KR, Sloan BH, Jacobs RJ. Clinical ocular prosthetics. In: *The Anophthalmic Patient.* Switzerland: Springer; 2015:1–22.

31. Dias RB, Carvalho JCM, Rezende JRV. Light-weight ocular prosthesis. *Braz Dent J.* 1994;5:105–108.

32. Roberts AC. An instrument to achieve pupil alignment in eye prosthesis. *J Prosthet Dent.* 1969;22:487–489.

33. Shenoy KK, Nag PV. Ocular impressions: an overview. *J Indian Prosthodont Soc.* 2007;7:5–7.

34. Shetty PP, Chowdhary R, Yadav RK, Gangaiah M. An iris positioning device and centering approach: a technique. *J Prosthet Dent.* 2018;119:175–177.

35. Stefani FH. Phthisis bulbi-an intraocular fluoride proliferative reaction. *Dev Ophthalmol.* 1985;10:78–160.

36. Sykes LM, Essop AR, Veres EM. Use of custom-made conformers in the treatment of ocular defects. *J Prosthet Dent.* 1999;82:362–365.

37. The glossary of prosthodontic terms: ninth edition. *J Prosthet Dent.* May 2017;117(5S):e1–e105. https://doi.org/10.1016/j.prosdent.2016.12.001.

38. Tucker SM, Sapp N, Collin R. Orbital expansion of the congenitally anophthalmic socket. *Br J Ophthalmol.* 1995;79:667–671.

39. Vincent AL, Webb MC, Gallie BL, Héon E. Prosthetic conformers: a step towards improved rehabilitation of enucleated children. *Clin Experiment Ophthalmol.* 2002;30:58–59.

CHAPTER 10

Prosthetic Rehabilitation of Orbital Defects

SAUMYA KAPOOR, MDS • SAUMYENDRA V. SINGH, MDS • DEEKSHA ARYA, MDS

LEARNING OBJECTIVES

1. Describe applied orbital anatomy and evaluate orbital defects for fabrication of prosthesis.
2. Perform various steps involved in fabrication of orbital prosthesis.
3. Apply various retentive aids to making orbital prosthesis.
4. Explain prosthesis maintenance.
5. Modify prosthesis fabrication as per complexity of case.

INTRODUCTION

The eye has immeasurable importance, not only for vision but for esthetics and exhibition of our emotions as well. Loss of such a vital organ and its associated structures has a devastating effect on the psyche of the person and overall health of the individual, underlining the importance of rehabilitation. Causes include ablative surgeries to manage malignant neoplasms and trauma. Surgical reconstruction falls short in restoring the eye (which always has to be done prosthetically). Often, such invasive surgery is not desirable for a systemically depleted patient. Grafting tissues creates a defect at the donor site and also inhibits regular inspection of orbital resection site for recurrence of disease. Orbital rehabilitation is a complex patient-specific process requiring experience and artistic skill. Orbital prosthesis rehabilitates the defect using various biocompatible, maxillofacial materials. A definitive prosthesis is normally fabricated after complete healing of the site. Success of such prosthesis is dependent on factors such as patient cooperation, complexity of the defect, tissue bed, clinician's skill, and material properties.

Fabrication of orbital prosthesis follows similar steps to that of other facial prosthesis, impression or moulage, making the pattern, creating a mold, and processing the prosthesis. Pattern sculpting and prosthesis coloration usually need artistic skill and experience. Such prosthesis can be fabricated from different materials, such as poly(methyl methacrylate), polyurethane elastomer, silicone elastomer, or urethane-backed medical grade silicone. Silicone elastomer is the most widely used material. These prostheses require excellent retention for success and acceptance by patients. Equally important is mimicking the skin color and merging prosthesis margins with natural tissue.

APPLIED ANATOMY

The orbit grossly comprises of walls of the orbit, eyelids, eyeball, and muscles.

Bony Orbit

Shape—four-sided pyramid, with its apex situated posteriorly and its base anteriorly.

Walls of the orbit

Four walls: a roof, lateral wall, floor, and medial wall (Fig. 10.1).

Roof

Bones: frontal and sphenoid bones.

Houses the fossa for the lacrimal gland anterolaterally.

The optic canal lies in the posterior part of the roof.

Lateral wall

Bones: zygomatic and sphenoid bones; demarcated by the superior and inferior orbital fissures.

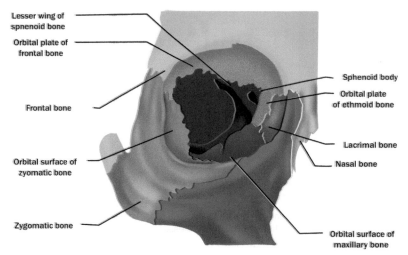

FIG. 10.1 Bones forming the orbit.

The lateral walls of the two orbits are set at approximately right angles to one another, whereas the medial walls are nearly parallel to each other.

Floor

Bones: maxilla, zygomatic, and palatine bones.

Presents the infraorbital groove.

Medial wall

Bones: ethmoid, lacrimal, and frontal bones. It is papyraceous (paper-thin).

Eyelids. The eyelids (palpebrae) are musculofibrous folds in the anterior part of each orbit.

Function—Shade the eyes during sleep, protect the eyes from excessive light and foreign objects and reflex blinking spreads lubricating secretions over the eyeballs and prevents drying of the cornea.

The upper eyelid, more extensive and mobile, meets the lower at the medial and lateral angles (canthi).

The free margin of each lid possesses hair termed eyelashes (cilia).

ETIOLOGY AND CLASSIFICATION

Etiology

1. Resection of tumors originating from the orbital contents. Like basal cell carcinoma, retinoblastoma, malignant melanoma, squamous cell carcinoma of the conjunctiva, and rhabdomyosarcoma.
2. Resection of tumors spreading from paranasal sinuses, palate, nasal cavity, overlying skin, or intraoral mucosa.
3. Midfacial trauma associated with orbital fractures and damage to the orbital contents, with related surgeries.
4. Congenital malformations.
5. Infections such as mucormycosis or untreatable painful glaucoma (exacerbated by immunocompromise).

Surgical procedures in the removal of eye are classified into three categories: by Peyman, Saunders and Goldberg:

1. Evisceration
2. Enucleation
3. Exenteration

Enucleation and evisceration are rehabilitated by ocular prosthesis. Exenteration needs orbital prosthesis. Exenteration is the removal of the entire contents of the orbit, including the extraocular muscles. The eyelids may or may not be involved. When the eyelids are involved, they must be removed during the surgical procedure.

If the size of the defects is large, then also the eyelids must be removed because the resultant large orbital defect will have a relatively small external opening. Such a defect may lead to drainage and infection problems plus difficult prosthetic rehabilitation. A classification of the orbital exenterations based on extensions is given in Fig. 10.2.

TREATMENT PLANNING

Exenteration defects in some instances may be allowed to heal by secondary intent, but adequate space must remain in the resultant defect to allow the prosthesis

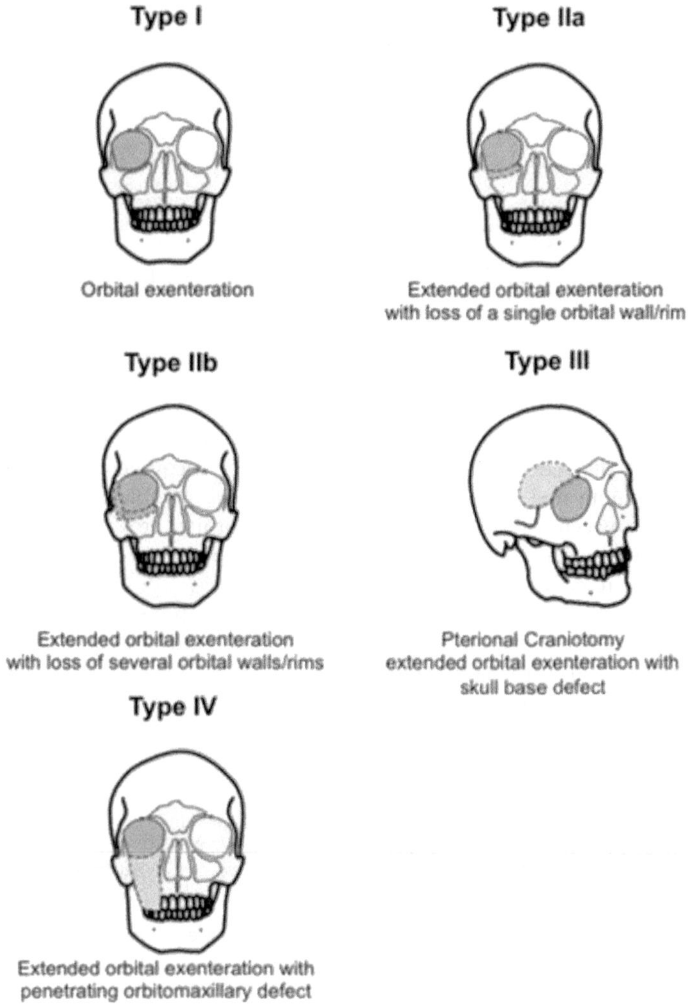

Type I

Orbital exenteration

Type IIa

Extended orbital exenteration
with loss of a single orbital wall/rim

Type IIb

Extended orbital exenteration
with loss of several orbital walls/rims

Type III

Pterional Craniotomy
extended orbital exenteration with
skull base defect

Type IV

Extended orbital exenteration with
penetrating orbitomaxillary defect

FIG. 10.2 Classification of orbital exenteration.

to be positioned for a good cosmetic appearance. As a rule, the prosthodontist would want a defect lined with a split thickness skin graft for the prosthesis to lie against.

Rehabilitation of orbital defects is a challenge for the surgeon as well as the prosthodontist. The surgeon is limited by the availability of tissue, compromise of the local vascular bed by radiation in tumor patients, need for periodic visual inspection of an oncologic defect, and physical condition of the patient. The prosthodontist is limited by the properties of the materials available for restoration, mobility of soft tissues surrounding the defect, difficulty of establishing retention for prostheses, and patient's ability to accept the outcome (Fig. 10.3).

Any patient would want a rehabilitation, which is "natural and fixed," and at the same time would not want to go through the expense, procedure, and invasiveness of surgical reconstruction. There are numerous local and systemic factors in such debilitated patients, which preclude surgery. Radiotherapy for one creates a poor vascular bed for accepting a graft. About 6 months should elapse after radiation treatment to consider any surgical procedure (including implants). A good option is to place implants at the time of the resection surgery itself.

Prosthetic options include interim and definitive conventional adhesive, undercut or implant-retained prostheses. Benefits and limitations of prosthetic intervention should be reviewed with the patient. Success

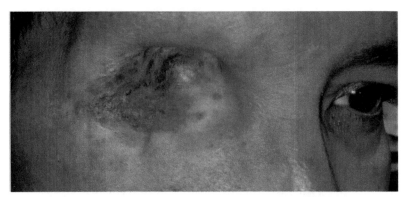

FIG. 10.3 An unfavorable defect. (Pic Courtesy—Dr Rani Ranabhatt.)

with a prosthesis beyond the physical limitations of the defect and materials is highly dependent on sincere commitment by an informed, motivated patient.

The planning often starts between a team of prosthetist/prosthodontist, resecting surgeon, reconstructive surgeon, and patient before the resective surgery. It includes planning implants (time of placement, number, location), defect extent (what all will be rehabilitated by surgeon and by prosthetists, what to keep and remove—eye frame shadow for example provides a good place for camouflage), defect lining, preservation of undercuts (many prosthesis maybe retained this way—more economical and convenient than adhesive or implant retained), and timing of giving the prosthesis. Unfortunately, a lot of prosthetic planning has to take place after the surgeon has done his job and referred the patient, by when the only options in front of the prosthodontist are to select the mode of retention and extent of prosthesis.

Acceptance of facial prostheses by patients has improved dramatically since the introduction of osseointegrated implants. Retention provided by osseointegrated implants allows the use of large prostheses on movable tissues because the margins can be made thinner and more flexible. Acceptance by patients is significantly enhanced because of the quality of retention, improved esthetics, and accurate and repeatable positioning of prosthesis.

Whatever the mode of rehabilitation, the patient should be fully informed of future problems, limitations, and expected quality of the final result. Unesthetic prosthesis creates more psychological trauma than no prosthesis at all. Resections that are confined to removal of the orbital contents only are easier to rehabilitate. As the surgical margins extend beyond the confines of the orbit, prostheses are less esthetic because of the inability to camouflage the lines of juncture between skin and prosthesis. Additionally, as the

prosthesis extends beyond the orbit, movable tissue beds may be encountered, resulting in further exposure of the junction. Table 10.1 outlines the principles for successful orbital prosthetic rehabilitation.

Fabrication of an orbital prosthesis involves four stages:
1. Moulage impression and model fabrication
2. Sculpting and making of the pattern

TABLE 10.1 Basic Principles of Prosthetic Rehabilitation for Successful Orbital Prosthesis		
Form	**Surface Texture**	**Junction Lines**
Size and shape similar to resected tissue	As natural appearing as possible	Least discernible and as thin as possible
Perfect contralateral symmetry not required	Varies with age	Blend with adjacent tissue
Blend with remaining natural structures	In pattern this should be more pronounced as some details are lost during processing	Camouflaged with spectacles or folds or creases of skin
		Cast should be scored lightly (0.5–1 mm) in areas of displaceable tissue such as cheeks

3. Mold fabrication
4. Processing and coloration

IMPRESSIONS—MATERIALS AND TECHNIQUES

An ideal impression material should have the ability to record the defect, adjacent structures, and engageable undercuts with minimal distortion. To prevent the soft tissue deformation by the weight of the material, the impression material should have low viscosity, be fairly flexible, and be used with minimum bulk.

Impression Materials

Materials used for making moulage impression:
1. Plaster
2. Reversible hydrocolloid
3. Irreversible hydrocolloid or alginate
4. Nonaqueous elastomeric materials
   The material chosen depends on the choice of the operator as well as inherent properties.

Plaster

Advantages:
1. Readily available
2. Inexpensive
3. Can be shaped or molded in its plastic state
   Disadvantages:
1. Lacks elasticity and contouring is difficult
2. Cannot be used in undercuts
3. Relatively short setting time

Reversible Hydrocolloid

Advantage:
1. Accurately reproduce fine details.
   Disadvantages:
1. Greater preparation time and armamentarium needed
2. Warm/hot at time of application
3. Poor tear strength, tendency to tear

Nonaqueous Elastomeric Impression Materials

Advantages:
1. Excellent surface detail reproduction
2. High tear resistance
3. Good flow properties
4. Putty consistency maintains shape/body after setting
5. Distort after long—can be poured later or multiple times
6. Good shelf life

Disadvantages:
1. Short working time
2. Relatively high cost
   Addition silicones and polyether are materials of choice.

Irreversible Hydrocolloid

Advantages:
1. Easy availability, inexpensive, long shelf life
2. Good detail reproduction
3. Adequate physical properties, working time can be adjusted
   Disadvantages:
1. Possible entrapment of air during application to the defect area
2. Possibility for distortion or tearing during removal from large undercuts, does not have much body
3. Distort soon
4. Can normally be poured once only

Impression Technique

1. Table 10.2 summarizes the materials needed for making a standard impression. The purpose is to record the orbital and periorbital tissue bed in least displaced state.
2. Explain the impression procedure and temperature changes which occur while the material sets to the patient, for example: alginate and light body rubber base will feel cold.
3. Acquire history of claustrophobia (fear of confined spaces) and achluophobia (fear of darkness). Assure patient of safety of procedure, especially during full facial moulage impression. If required, they should be allowed to hold hand of their companion.
4. Patient should be draped to prevent soiling of clothes—towels and head cap can be used. Facial hair (eyebrows, mustache, etc.) are protected by a light application of petroleum jelly.
5. Isolate the field—A ring of boxing wax should be built around the area to be impressed, or a custom barrier may be made of cardboard. The height of the box depends on the strength/body of the impression material but should be 45–50 mm. In the more conventional approach, a large area of the face, including the normal orbit, is encircled by this ring. Newer technologies utilize record of the defect with only a narrow region of normal tissues. This preserves material, effort, and cost.
6. Position—The patient should be semiupright to minimize the gravitational effect on tissues,

TABLE 10.2
The Armamentarium Required for Alginate Impression
• Petroleum jelly
• Alginate/nonaqueous elastomer with mixing mechanism
• Cold water
• Large flexible mixing bowls and spatula and/or quart-size vacuum mixer
• Fast-set plaster
• Gauze squares opened to single thickness
• Patient drapes
• Boxing wax/poster board

reducing the displacement of tissue bed. Also it is difficult to contain flow of impression materials when the patient is fully upright.

7. Undesirable undercut and potential entrapment areas should be blocked out with lubricated gauze.

8. Midpupillary location of unaffected side may be marked with a marking pen in the conventional approach.

9. A thin layer of impression material is applied to the defect and adjacent tissues to prevent air entrapment. For alginate, water/powder ratio is adjusted as 1.25 to 1.5 times the normal amount of water to adjust flow properties.

10. In the conventional approach, open gauze strips are placed on the layer of alginate while it is setting to provide mechanical retention for rigid plaster backing. Alternatively, a taller impression ring can be used to support alginate and nonaqueous elastomers all by themselves, without any backing.

11. A layer of fast-setting plaster is applied in sufficient thickness to ensure proper strength with minimal weight, facilitating easy removal of impression without distortion

12. The normal eye should remain closed in a relaxed manner during the procedure.

13. During removal of the impression instruct the patient to wiggle the face. It should be removed gently and inspected for voids or deformation/tear (Fig. 10.4).

14. If a nonaqueous elastomer has been used to record the defect, its light body is used for recording the finer detail followed by adding putty/heavy body. This does not apply to single consistency materials (Fig. 10.4c).

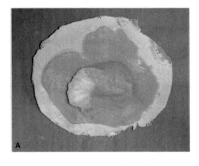
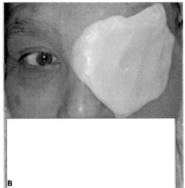
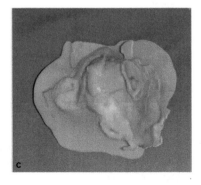

FIG. 10.4 (a) Alginate impression with gauze and plaster backing. (b) Nonaqueous elastomer impression in position. (c) Nonaqueous elastomer impression.

In patients with total maxillectomy accompanying orbital defects, the definitive obturator should be fabricated and positioned before making impressions.

MODEL FABRICATION

1. Most commonly used material—dental stone. A white dental stone is preferred because it is easier to determine color characterization during intrinsic coloring procedures. Die stone is also used for its strength and abrasion resistance.
2. The impression has to be boxed in wax (Fig. 10.5) and poured with a smooth, vacuum mixed stone (Fig. 10.6). After an initial set of 1 cm, remaining material is poured' this prevents distortion of the impression material. Model should be of minimum 2.5 cm thickness in the deepest portion.
3. Epoxy molds can also be prepared. They have greater strength but require a silicone impression material for fabrication.

MAKING/SCULPTING THE PATTERN
Materials Required

Stock eye
Modeling/sculpting clay or wax
Thermoplastic sheet
Gauze
Carving instruments
Burner/water bath

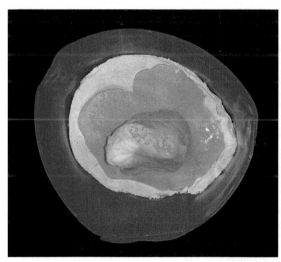

FIG. 10.5 Boxing the impression.

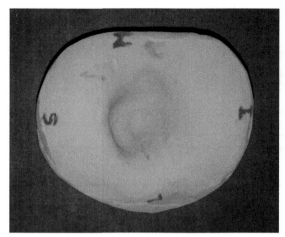

FIG. 10.6 Model poured in die stone.

Technique

1. Unfavorable undercuts are blocked on the model.
2. Stock ocular prosthesis that resembles the normal eye in color, size of the iris and sclera should be selected, or custom ocular prosthesis can be fabricated.
3. A 1 mm thickness PVC thermoplastic sheet is adapted on the cast with a vacuum former machine or a sheet of baseplate wax can also be adapted. The purpose is to form a template for the future pattern. PVC provides a better retaining pattern, while the wax counterpart is more easily made. Template margins should be kept thin and feather edge, for merging prosthesis and tissue margins, and should be slightly extended at this time during trial for easy maneuverability. Check adaptation and extension on the patient. The extended margins can be cut before final pattern finishing on the model/mold.
4. The template should be positioned into the orbital defect, and the patient should be asked to stare in a relaxed manner at a distant point at least 6 feet away, upright, and without any head support.

   A reference mark should be placed at the facial midline, and a Boley gauge can be used to verify medio-lateral placement of ocular component; the pupil of normal eye is used as reference point in this evaluation. Other techniques mentioned in literature for positioning of ocular component include a millimeter ruler, a pupillometer, an ocular locator with fixed caliper, inverted anatomic tracings, transparent graph grid attached to eyewear, digital imaging, and photoediting software to reverse and superimpose the image of normal eye over the defect (Fig. 10.7).

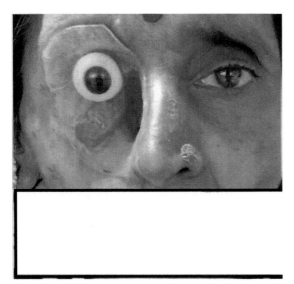

FIG. 10.7 Ocular component positioning. (Pic Courtesy—Dr Siddharth Bandodkar.)

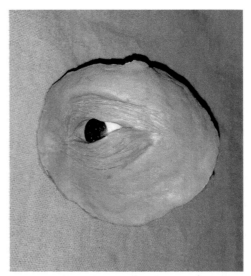

FIG. 10.8 Sculpted prosthesis. (Pic Courtesy—Dr Rohan Grover.)

The artificial eye is placed in the correct position using stalks of softened wax or modeling clay, stabilized on the template. The mediolateral, anteroposterior, and superoinferior positioning should be similar to the normal eye, while being compatible with the periorbital tissue bed. The stalks can be used to adjust the ocular component around.

5. Periorbital tissues are sculpted next. This should be done when the patient is well rested as fatigue and anxiety affect lid contours leading to discrepancy in sculpting. Clay or wax can be used depending on operator preference. While clay is easier to carve and manipulate, it also tends to distort more easily at higher temperatures.

Eyelid contour is created using the normal one as guide, to establish correct aperture. Contour should be established with patient looking ahead in relaxed manner (not staring). Upper lid is carved first and is more difficult. After carving both lids, remaining contours should be built up, merging with lids on one side and normal periorbital tissue margins all around.

The surface contour and skin texture should be similar to periorbital tissue of normal eye (stippling, lines, and wrinkles). Skin texture can be duplicated by using gauze. Multiple try-ins should be done to verify and compare the pattern. The margins should be feather edge and end at eyebrows or under, shadows, wrinkles, creases, bony margins, or eyewear, to camouflage junction lines (Fig. 10.8).

MOLD FABRICATION

1. The model can be directly used as tissue surface or first part of the mold or it may be duplicated and used for this purpose.
2. Small defects can be flasked in a conventional denture flask or Little Giant flask. Large or combination defects need use of freehand stone molds.
3. Pattern is finished and sealed to the model forming base portion of mold, taking care that the margins are thinned out and merged with natural peripheries. These may be scored for better fit (Fig. 10.9).

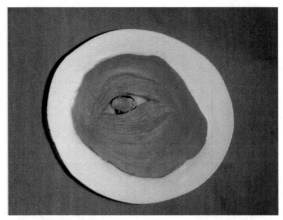

FIG. 10.9 Indexing of ocular segment. (Pic Courtesy—Dr Rohan Grover.)

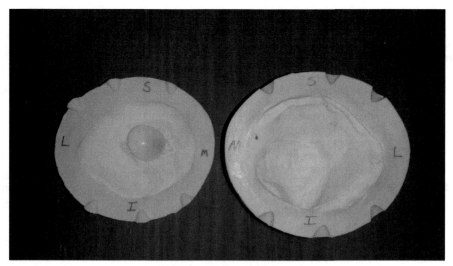

FIG. 10.10 Indexed mold after dewaxing.

4. Indexing should be done to reorient the mold in same position after dewaxing and packing. Size and shape of conical trimming burs lend themselves well to this purpose (Fig. 10.10).

5. Separating medium is applied. The thinner the film, the better it will be.

6. Indexing of the ocular segment is done to secure its position in the mold. This is done with a short acrylic rod, which can be secured to the ocular segment with autopolymerizing resin or monopoly (1:10 polymer to monomer ratio mixed in a water bath and stored at 4°C) (Fig. 10.9). Another method of indexing involves replacement of the eye with its duplicate in dental stone.

7. The second part of the mold is made in white dental stone, for the reason explained previously. It should also be 45–50 mm high. The mold is allowed to set.

8. Mold is then dewaxed completely and cleaned with hot water and detergent (Fig. 10.10)

9. Mold's internal surface should be coated with silicone-releasing agents before packing silicone.

PROCESSING AND COLORATION

Getting acquainted with basic color terminology is important before starting the coloration process (Table 10.3), which should take place in ample natural light around noon. Though intrinsic (placing color in silicone or directly on mold before processing) and extrinsic (applying color on prosthesis after processing) coloration have been identified separately, a combination of the two yields best results. This is because intrinsic coloration gives a more natural appearance, while extrinsic coloration helps in providing the final touches.

1. The first step in intrinsic coloration is to establish the base color of the prosthesis, which is the lightest area of the prosthesis (Table 10.4). Common methods to determine base color are discussed in Tables 10.5 and 10.6.

2. The second step is to characterize the base-colored silicone so as to minutely mimic color and contour variations simulating those in normal counterpart or adjacent tissues (Table 10.3) based on histological and morphological variations.

3. This is done using "laminar glazes," which are portions of the base silicone mixed with antislump (thixotropic) agents. These are painted directly onto the corresponding mold areas in thin quantities. Pigments are used more commonly, while fiber or flock simulates microvasculature without affecting translucency. Too much of pigment leads to opacity of the mix. As you know, the skin is a multilayered, translucent, multicolored structure, which needs to be mimicked as such (Fig. 10.13).

4. Once the individually colored silicones have been layered in, the base-colored bulk of silicone is packed in both halves of the mold (Fig. 10.14). Spatulation technique should be adopted to mix and deair the silicone, which involves spreading the mass thinly onto the slab to remove air bubbles with the help of a thin metal or plastic spatula. A syringe or paint brush can be used to apply silicone in hard to reach areas, without air entrapment. Ensure that both

TABLE 10.3
Color Terminology and Color-Matching Basics

Important Terms	Definition
• Hue	The dimension of color dictated by the wavelength of the stimulus that is used to distinguish one family of color from another as red, green, blue, etc.; white, black, and gray possess no hue.
• Chroma/saturation	(1) The purity of a color, or its departure from white or gray; (2) the intensity of a distinctive hue; saturation of a hue.
• Value	The quality by which a light color is distinguished from a dark color, the dimension of a color that denotes relative blackness or whiteness (grayness, brightness); value is the only dimension of color that may exist alone.
• Opacity	The quality or state of a body that makes it impervious to light.
• Transparency	Quality or state of a body that makes it completely pervious to light.
• Translucency	Having the appearance between complete opacity and complete transparency; partially opaque.
• Pigment loading	Percentage of pigment mixed in silicone. As pigment loading increases, opacity increases, and translucency decreases.
• Metamerism	Pairs of objects that have different spectral curves but appear to match when viewed in a given hue.
• Primary colors: red, yellow, blue Secondary colors: formed by mixing two primary colors. Red + yellow = orange,	Combining all three primary colors or a primary color and its complementary color

TABLE 10.3
Color Terminology and Color-Matching Basics—cont'd

Important Terms	Definition
red + blue = purple, blue + yellow = green Complementary color of red is green, yellow is purple and blue is orange	gives a brown or peach color.
• Color of pigment	Function during characterization
White	Increases opacity and value
Red	Vasculature
Red, yellow, brown	Color of skin in different ratios
Blue, purple	Darken the silicone, simulate shadows
Green	Desaturate the color
Yellow, white	Cartilage
Flocks	Minor color changes without affecting translucency Add surface texture

halves of the mold are completely filled. Air bubbles that rise to the surface can be relieved by gentle vibration or with a pointed instrument.

5. If an acrylic housing is part of the prosthesis (such as: implant retained prothesis), then a thin coat of platinum primer is applied to it as per instructions, before packing the silicone.

6. Mold is reassembled and flash expressed with light pressure to achieve maximum closure. Pressure of 700 kPa is sufficient to ensure good closure. Extra pressure can fracture free hand molds.

7. Silicone is polymerized as per manufacturer's instructions.

8. Bench cool for 1 h before opening the mold.

9. Extra material is trimmed with sharp scissors. Retrieve the prothesis. Replace the stone duplicate with the duplicate of the artificial eye or cut off the acrylic index of the ocular prosthesis and finish the joint portion.

10. Silicone is difficult to finish or polish, and therefore, extra care needs to be taken at the stage of the pattern that all characterization expected in the final prosthesis is already present. Gross trimming

TABLE 10.4
Determining Base Color of Silicone

Determining Base Color for Intrinsic Coloration

Base color forms the bulk of the prosthesis

Generally lighter area is selected, because if required it can be darkened by extrinsic coloration. Reverse cannot happen. Front of tragus, ear lobe, inner forearm, and nape of the neck are common areas to record the base color.

Techniques for color matching to determine the base color:

1. Trial and error mixing
2. Shade guides
3. Colorimeter or spectrophotometer

TABLE 10.5
Trial and Error Method

Trial and Error Method of Preparing Base Colored silicone

1. Subjective method of evaluation.
2. Pigment is added to silicone in small amounts and frequently compared with patients target skin in proper lighting conditions to achieve the desired shade.
3. Color of silicone is matched by placing it in between folded double plastic transparent sheets and comparing it with target skin area (Fig. 10.11). This may be done through a tissue paper window to mask all nonessential areas.
4. Bulk silicone is then prepared using obtained pigment proportion in this shade for packing.
5. Color matching should be done in room with neutral gray walls.
6. Small portions of bulk silicone can also be characterized to represent different areas of the prosthesis—example depressions above the upper eyelid are made to look darker by adding blue or black in the base color (Table 10.3).

can be achieved with stone silicone trimming burs and stones.

11. Prosthesis can be cleaned with mild soap water, followed by iso-propyl alcohol or methanol—to remove surface oils, which may interfere with extrinsic pigmentation silicones.
12. Extrinsic coloration: It helps in minor corrections like a prosthesis with lighter base shade. It involves use of autocatalyzing silicone adhesives into which pigments are added (Table 10.3). This is applied to the surface of prosthesis with brush or gauze taking care not to mask texture of prosthesis. Glossiness due to layer application can be taken care of by dusting the surface with pumice, icing sugar, or kaolin-like fine powders. Cure as per manufacturer's instructions.
13. Eyelashes: Prosthetic eyelashes can be stuck on the undersurface of the upper and lower eyelid.

Natural hair can also be sown on the undersurface of upper eyelid using a thick bore needle, ensuring right direction of emergence (Fig. 10.15). Eyebrows, if required, are sown similarly. These can also be painted. Remember that eyelashes affect the ocular prosthesis contours (narrower appearance).

14. Prosthesis is ready for final insertion (Fig. 10.16). Efforts should be made to preserve the mold and shade match for future remakes.

PROSTHESIS INSERTION, RETENTIVE AIDS, AND MAINTENANCE

- Prosthesis is inserted onto the patient (Fig. 10.17). Retention can be achieved by utilizing favorable mechanical undercuts, tissue adhesives (Table 10.7), or osseointegrated maxillofacial implants with retentive elements (such as bar and clip, or

TABLE 10.6
Spectrophotometry

Spectrophotometry with Computerized Color Evaluation

Objective method of color matching

This computes a pigment formula using color formulation software that matches a measured skin color.

Skin measured with the spectrophotometer yields a spectral curve between 400 and 700 nm (visible range).

Spectrophotometer (Fig. 10.12)

- Handheld device—costly
- Helps in fabricates a nonmetameric prosthesis
- Maintains a record of the shade match, which can be replicated time and again
- View port is on average 5 mm in diameter and denotes the area of skin measured.
- Technique:
1. Device measures skin color and immediately displays on the screen a matching color code from its database.
2. This is fed on the computer software to obtain a pigment recipe, which is a spectral match to patient's target skin area.
3. The pigments and silicone are then weighed on digital balance as per the recipe and weight of prosthesis.
4. They are mixed thoroughly to achieve a homogenous color for base silicone.
5. There is minimal wastage of silicone and pigments.

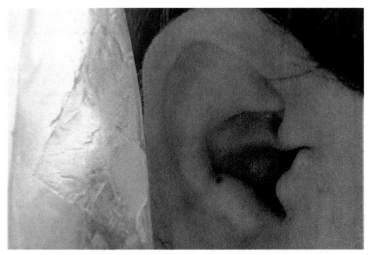

FIG. 10.11 Color matching using cellophane transparent sheet.

magnets). As was emphasized in the treatment planning section, retention aids need to be decided at that preliminary stage.

- The margins should be handled delicately for fear of tearing.
- Spectacles serve for retention as well as camouflage of such prosthesis (Fig. 10.18). Orbital prosthesis can be stuck to the spectacle frame (one piece) with the help of suitably colored acrylic at the nose pad or

bridge, and ear piece. In such a case, the acrylic component must be incorporated at the pattern stage and the spectacle also selected. Then the acrylic part is attached to the silicone prosthesis with primer as discussed during processing. Such a prosthesis can also be two pieces, for example, with the help of magnets placed in the spectacle frame and acrylic housing in the silicone prosthesis. Patient may wear prosthesis with and without spectacles.

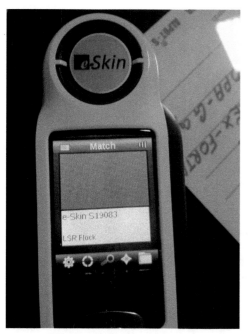

FIG. 10.12 Spectrophotometer.

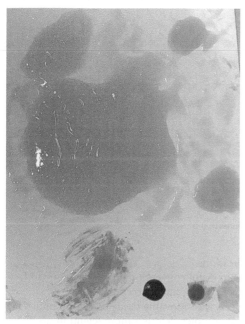

FIG. 10.13 Mixing of silicone with pigments.

- Manufacturer's instructions such as sticking on an adhesive retained prosthesis only after the adhesive loses color should be conveyed to the patient. Risk of marginal tearing with adhesives should be communicated.
- Previous layer of adhesive should be wiped clean before reapplication.
- Patient is advised to turn head for side vision and not just the eye. This reduces noticeability of the prosthesis.
- It should be emphasized that the prosthesis has a life of 2—4 years and that it should be cleaned once a day with gentle soap water and should be protected from harsh climate. Instructions for cleaning bearing tissue surfaces (adhesive or fixture supported) scrupulously with soap water at least once a day are given. This includes clearing off any crusting with a lubricated gauze followed by applying petroleum jelly or an antiseptic as prescribed. Poor hygiene leads to keratin and sebaceous debris accumulation, infection, and implant failure. Area around the bar or implant can be cleaned with periodontal brushes or cotton applicators.
- Patients with implant or adhesive retained prosthesis should visit the expert at least once in 6 months. For other orbital prosthesis, visiting once every year is essential. For implant-supported prosthesis, complications such as loss of retention accompanied by need to replace the clips or magnets may be expected. Once yearly radiograph to monitor the condition of the implants is also needed.
- Prosthesis removal for few hours every day should be advised for tissue rest.

LIMITATIONS OF ORBITAL PROSTHESIS

1. Even the best prosthesis is detachable and takes a long time to feel a part of the body by patient. Environmental and emotional variations on tissues cannot be duplicated in the prosthesis.
2. Facial movement cannot be duplicated.
3. Limited life of prosthesis. Lack of predictability of this life is based on patient variations such as secretions, smoking, and environment.

IMPLANT-RETAINED ORBITAL PROSTHESIS

Introduction of implants to fabrication of orbital prosthesis has led to enhanced retention, reduced bulk of prosthesis (especially at margins), and improved

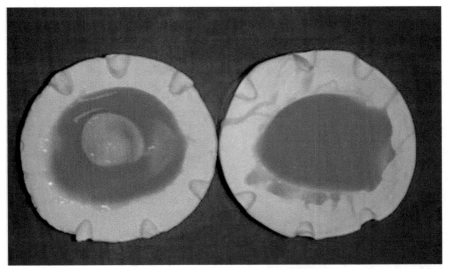

FIG. 10.14 Packing with silicone.

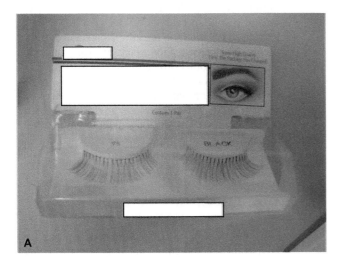

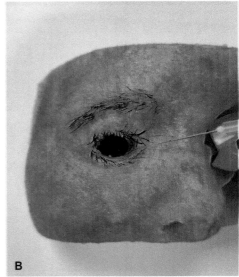

FIG. 10.15 (a) Artificial eye lashes. (b) Insertion of eyelashes.

esthetics, leading to enhanced self-esteem and better quality of life. This is because adhesive-retained prosthesis cannot be too thin at the margins to prevent risk of tearing. Selection of this modality, and the number and size of implants is dependent on the extent of defect and bone quality- and all factors affecting these, therein.

Indications:
1. Unsuccessful conventional prosthesis due to factors such as poor patient acceptance
2. Defects with movable tissue bed or no undercut
3. Large complex defects—more retention needed
   Advantages of implant retained prosthesis:
1. Improved retention and stability of prosthesis

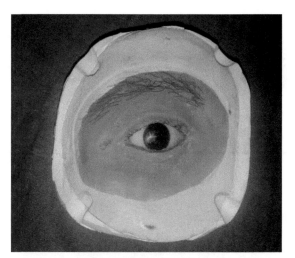

FIG. 10.16 Final prosthesis.

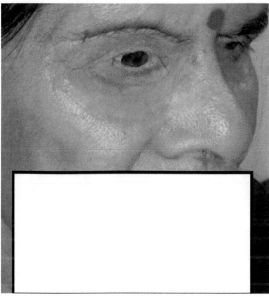

FIG. 10.17 Prosthesis insertion.

2. Elimination of occasional skin reaction to adhesives
3. Improved patient comfort
4. Increased life span of prosthesis
5. Enhanced esthetics as thin junction margins possible

Any systemic or local condition, which precludes surgery, is contraindicated for implant retained prosthesis. Such prosthesis is costlier and needs added training and an integrated interdisciplinary approach.

TABLE 10.7
Tissue Adhesives for Facial Prosthesis
Adhesives
• A material used to adhere external prosthesis to skin and associated structures around the periphery of an external anatomic defect
• Types:
- On dispensing method:
• Sprays—inert silicone base in a propellant
• Pastes—latex based
• Liquids emulsions—mastic gum in fast evaporating silicone
• Double sided tapes
- Acrylic base (water soluble) and silicone base (oil soluble)
• Advantages:
• Ease of application.
• Provide retention for minimum for 12 h daily.
• Easy to remove without harm to underlying tissue
• Disadvantages:
• Patients with poor manual dexterity or coordination may not be able to apply the adhesive or position the prosthesis consistently
• Allergic or irritational responses
• Tendency to tear thin prosthesis margins

Treatment Planning

Radiographic evaluation involves bone site evaluation using computed tomographic scans, subsequent to which number and position of implants is decided. Implant planning software can also be used.

Pretreatment models can be made manually or digitally and used for surgical as well as prosthetic planning and fabrication of surgical stents.

Mobile soft tissue or soft tissue greater in thickness than 5 mm at implant site needs to be removed. Skin graft should be placed if implant site has scar tissue or is denuded. Mobile tissue around implant creates micromovements, causes irritation, and makes hygiene maintenance difficult.

Craniofacial Implants

Craniofacial implants are made of commercially pure titanium. Most commonly used dimensions are 4 mm in length and 5−6 mm diameter. Short length allows

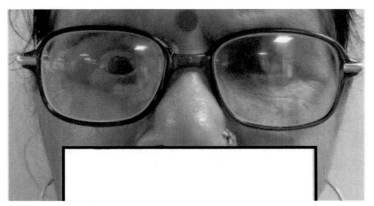

FIG. 10.18 Margins camouflaged by spectacles.

placement in areas with limited bone, and wide diameter provides initial stabilization.

In areas with more bone volume, dental implants may be used; usually, 7 mm implants are placed at an angulation around the rim of the orbit.

The superior orbital rim is considered the primary site for implant placement, and the inferior and lateral bones are secondary sites (Fig. 10.19).

Placement of implants in the orbital region is challenging due to cortical bone and curvature of orbital rim, which requires greater bone removal to countersink the implant, and excessive heat can cause cellular necrosis of the bone. Soft tissue complications are also common.

Retention Systems

Most commonly used retention systems for implant-supported orbital prosthesis are magnetic retention and barclip system. Magnetic abutments are preferred due to ease of insertion and removal by the patient, ease in hygiene maintenance, and rigidity of the bar attachment system, leading to implant overloading. However, magnetic attachment has reduced retention and experiences corrosion after a period of time. Retentive bars with three to four magnets arranged in a triangular or circular fashion are preferable.

Implant Success Rate

Overall, the success rates of implants in the orbital bone reported in literature is between 33.3% and 96.4% in the irradiated bone and between 37.5% and 100% in nonirradiated bone. Failure rate is higher for orbital implants as compared with nasal or auricular implants by three to four times, especially in irradiated bone.

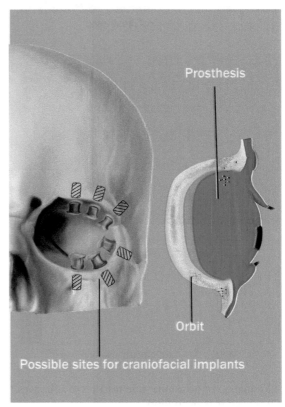

FIG. 10.19 Ideal sites for implant placement and cross-sectional view of orbital prosthesis in the orbit.

Maintaining good hygiene around implants sites is crucial. Debris on abutments is highest in auricular defects followed by orbital defects. Contributing factors to this are location of implants, as access to cleaning is difficult, compromised, and/or monocular vision.

Surgical Phase

Two-stage approach is preferred for orbital implants.

Ideal implant number is three for orbital prosthesis placed in a triangular or circular configuration. Due to high failure rate, spare implants (up to five) can be placed. Improper or outward position/angulation of implants makes placement of substructure difficult and interferes with prosthesis contour. A 3D or conventionally fabricated surgical stent can prevent this.

Seven mm of distance should exist between implants to allow proper hygiene maintenance.

Stage 2 is performed 3−4 months after stage 1 and transcutaneous healing abutments are placed. If implants have not osseointegrated properly or site had irradiated bone, healing time is extended to 6−8 months.

During the second-stage surgery, prior to placement of abutments, soft tissue can be thinned as explained previously.

Prosthetic Phase

Steps involved are as follows.

Impression making

Complexity of impression procedure increases in implant-supported prosthesis due to presence of retentive systems, number, and divergence of implants. Nonaqueous impression materials are preferred.

1. Impression making is done once the site has completely healed after stage 2 surgery.
2. Abutment height should be selected so that abutment extends 1−2 mm above the skin surface.
3. Direction of emergence of implants should be evaluated, and emergence profile should be manipulated to achieve a singular path of placement and removal. This can be done using angulated abutments.
4. Impression can be implant level (preferred) or abutment level.
5. Access holes for impression copings or magnetic keepers must always be kept patent to loosen them once the material sets allowing removal of the impression.

Model fabrication

1. When the impression has been removed, implant or abutment analogs should be secured to the impression copings or magnetic keepers, followed by model fabrication in the regular manner.
2. For magnetic retention, magnets are placed on laboratory keepers in master cast followed by fabrication of autopolymerizing resin substructure. Fit and retention of autopolymerizing resin substructure housing the magnets should be checked.
3. If a bar attachment is to be used, it should be fabricated in wax/autopolymerizing resin and cast, or milled in titanium. Fit of the bar should be passive. This is followed by the fabrication of an acrylic substructure, which houses the clip attachment.

Prosthesis fabrication and delivery

Wax pattern of the orbital prosthesis with stock/custom-made ocular prosthesis is fabricated in similar manner to a conventional orbital prosthesis around the acrylic housing/substructure.

To improve the bond between substructure and silicone, the substructure can be roughened and platinum silicone primers should be used for chemical bonding as described earlier. The margin of the prosthesis can be kept as thin as required for camouflage purposes. The final thinning should be done when the pattern margins have been sealed on the mold model.

COMPLEX DEFECTS

Advanced tumors or certain traumas involve extensive surgical resection of tissues, leading to defects including parts of maxillary, cheek, nose, and orbital region. These are known as midfacial defect. Marunick et al. classified midfacial defects into two major categories: midline midfacial defects, which include the nose and/or upper lip; and lateral defects, which include the cheek and orbital contents. Combinations of these two categories also exist. These defects are rarely rehabilitated by surgical reconstruction alone. However, successful prosthetic outcome is achievable. Rehabilitating speech, swallowing, saliva control, and mastication to improved and acceptable level require multidisciplinary approach, team work, and realistic understanding of the degree of rehabilitation by the patient.

This involves fabrication of the extraoral facial prosthesis such as orbital or nasal prosthesis and an intraoral prosthesis such as an obturator. A major challenge faced in such cases is retention and insertion of the prosthesis due to increased size and weight. Therefore, two-piece prosthesis is preferred here. Intraoral and extraoral prosthesis can be constructed to mutually retain each other using auxiliary retentive aids such as magnets (Fig. 10.20) or attachments.

One-piece prosthesis is preferred in those large defects, which involve orbital, nasal, and cheek region but not lip or oral cavity (Fig. 10.21). Such defects require craniofacial implants for retention.

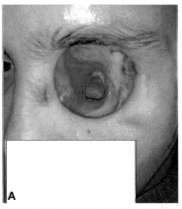
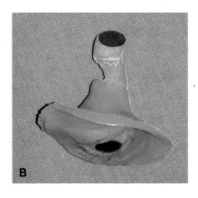
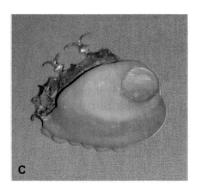

FIG. 10.20 (a) Complex defect. (b) Orbital component of complex prosthesis—magnetic attachment. (c) Obturator component of complex prosthesis—magnetic attachment. ((a) Pic Courtesy—Dr Himanshi Aggarwal. (c) Pic Courtesy—Dr Rohan Grover.)

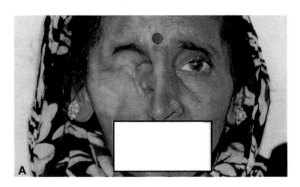
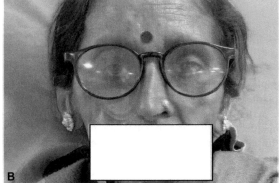

FIG. 10.21 (a) Defect involving orbit, part of nose, and cheek region. (b) Final prosthesis. ((a) Pic Courtesy—Dr Siddharth Bandodkar.)

ADVANCEMENTS

Techniques of imaging such as computer tomography and magnetic resonance imaging have allowed three-dimensional visualization of the defect radiographically. This also improves presurgical treatment planning, especially in defects requiring implants. Three-dimensional computer tomography (CT), computer-aided design (CAD), and stereolithography techniques help in creating orbital models, virtual implant placement and prosthetic planning, and making surgical stents, thus encouraging the surgical procedures to be prosthetically driven.

Digital impressions help record the defect in an undisplaced, nondistorted position and hence can be extremely useful. Even patterns can be rapid prototyped or milled. These are still in developing phase.

Rapid prototyping utilizes the recorded digitalized 3D data to reconstruct a physical model, by using either additive (stereolithography) or subtractive(milling) method. It can involve scanning of subject's face using depth-sensing cameras, laser scanning, or phase measuring profilometry. 3D computer software is used to reconstruct the patient's face from the acquired data, converted to Standard Tessellation Language file (STL) and communicated to a 3D Printer to create a hard copy of the defect or object. Using this data virtual reconstruction of the defect can also be done. However, these methods still cannot accurately reproduce skin texture details, follicular orifices, and thin adaptable margins.

CONCLUSION

Prosthodontic rehabilitation of orbital defects is often preferable to surgical reconstruction due to multiple

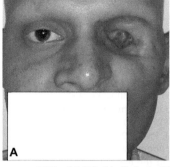
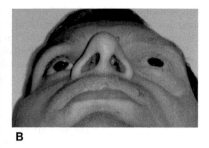
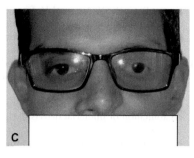

FIG. 10.22 (a) Defect. (b) Prosthesis without spectacles. (c) Prosthesis with spectacles. ((a–c) Pic Courtesy—Dr Rohan Grover.)

factors such as esthetic improvement, patient compliance, feasibility, and low success rate of surgery. It restores patient's esthetics and provides positive psychological reinforcement to the patient. Advancements have led to increased accuracy as well as predictability, leading to better prosthetic outcome and success. There are few outcomes, which can rival the satisfaction of giving a good orbital prosthesis to a patient (Fig. 10.22).

FURTHER READING

1. Aalaei S, Abolhassani A, Nematollahi F, Beyabanaki E, Mangoli AA. Fabrication of an implant-supported orbital prosthesis with bar-magnetic attachment: a clinical report. *J Dent.* 2015;12:932–935.
2. Aerts I, Rouic LL, Gauthier-Villars M, et al. Retinoblastoma. *Orphanet J R,are Dis.* 2006;1:1–11.
3. Beng Z, Dong Y, Zhao Y, et al. Computer-assisted technique for the design and manufacture of realistic facial prostheses. *Br J Oral Maxillofac Surg.* 2010;48:105–109.
4. Beumer III J, Marunick MT, Esposito SJ. *Maxillofacial Rehabilitation: Prosthodontic and Surgical Management of Cancer-Related, Acquired, and Congenital Defects of the Head and Neck.* 3rd ed. Hanover Park IL: Quintessence Publishing Co, Inc; 2011:274–298.
5. Bonanoni MTBC, Almeida MTA, Cristofani LM, Filho VO. Retinoblastoma: a three-year-study at a Brazilian medical school hospital. *Clinics.* 2009;64:427–434.
6. Brignoni R, Dominici JT. An intraoral-extraoral combination prosthesis using an intermediate framework and magnets: a clinical report. *J Prosthet Dent.* 2001;85:7–11.
7. Cheng AC, Leong EW, Khin NT, et al. Osseointegrated implants in craniofacial application: current status. *Singapore Dent J.* 2007;29:1–11.
8. Chintagumpala M, Barrios CP, Paysse EA, Plon SE, Hurwitz R. Retinoblastoma: review of current management. *Oncol.* 2007;12:1237–1246.
9. Davis BK. The role of technology in facial prosthetics. *Curr Opin Otolaryngol Head Neck Surg.* 2010;18:332–340.
10. Dholam KP, Pusalkar HA, Yadav P, Bhirangi PP. Implant retained orbital prosthesis. *J Indian Prosthodont Soc.* 2008; 8:55–58.
11. Goh BT, Teoh KH. Orbital implant placement using a computer-aided design and manufacturing (CAD/CAM) stereolithographic surgical template protocol. *Int J Oral Maxillofac Surg.* 2015;44:642–648.
12. Goiato MC, Fernandes AU, dos Santos DM, Barão VA. Positioning magnets on a multiple/sectional maxillofacial prosthesis. *J Contemp Dent Pract.* 2007;8:101–107.
13. Goiato MC, Santos MR, Pesqueira AA, et al. Prototyping for surgical and prosthetic treatment. *J Craniofac Surg.* 2011;22:914–917.
14. Guttal SS, Patil NP, Nadiger RK, Rachana KB, Dharnendra BN. Use of acrylic resin base as an aid in retaining silicone orbital prosthesis. *J Indian Prosthodont Soc.* 2008;8:112–115.
15. Heckmann M, Zogelmeier F, Konz B. Frequency of facial basal cell carcinoma does not correlate with site-specific UV almol exposure. *Arch Dermatol.* 2002;138:1494–1497.
16. Holgers KM, Ljungh A. Cell surface characteristics of microbiological isolates from human percutaneous titanium implants in the head and neck. *Biomaterials.* 1999; 20:1319–1326.
17. Ihde S, Kopp S, Gundlach K, Konstantinovic VS. Effects of radiation therapy on craniofacial and dental implants: a review of the literature. *Oral Surg Oral Med Oral Pathol Oral Radiol Endod.* 2009;107:56–65.
18. Jebreil K. Acceptability of orbital prostheses. *J Prosthet Dent.* 1980;43:82–85.
19. Kale E, Mese A, Izgi AD. A technique for fabrication of an interim ocular prosthesis. *J Prosthodont.* 2008;17:654–661.
20. Kapoor S, Singh SV, Arya D, Chand P. Technique to prevent fracture of a partial auricular prosthesis mold. *J Prosthet Dent.* May 2020;123(5):769–771.
21. Karakoca-Nemli S, Aydin C, Yilmaz H, Bal BT. A method for fabricating an implant-retained orbital prosthesis using the existing prosthesis. *J Prosthodont.* 2011;20:583–586.
22. Kesting MR, Koerdt S, Rommel N, et al. Classification of orbital exenteration and reconstruction. *J Cranio-Maxillo-Fac Surg.* 2017;45:467–473.

23. Kumar P, Singh SV, Aggarwal H, Chand P. Incorporation of a vacuum-formed polyvinyl chloride sheet into an orbital prosthesis pattern. *J Prosthet Dent.* February 2015; 113(2):157–159.

24. Li S, Xiao C, Duan L, et al. CT image-based computer-aided system for orbital prosthesis rehabilitation. *Med Biol Eng Comput.* 2015;53:943–950.

25. Marunick MT, Harrison R, Beumer 3rd J. Prosthodontic rehabilitation of midfacial defects. *J Prosthet Dent.* 1985; 54:553–560.

26. Nishimura RD, Roumanas E, Moy PK, Sugai T, Freymiller EG. Osseointegrated implants and orbital defects: U.C.L.A. experience. *J Prosthet Dent.* 1998;79: 304–309.

27. Peyman GA, Sanders DR, Goldbeirg MF. *Principles and Practice of Ophthalmology*Vol. 3(2). New Delhi: Jaypee Brothers Medical Publishers (P) Ltd; 1987:2334.

28. Sathe S, Pisulkar S, Nimonkar SV, Belkhode V, Borle A. Positioning of iris in an ocular prosthesis: a systematic review. *J Indian Prosthodont Soc.* 2020;20:345–352.

29. Supriya M, Ghadiali B. Prosthetic rehabilitation of a patient with an orbital defect using a simplified approach. *J Indian Prosthodont Soc.* 2008;8:116–118.

30. Taylor TD. *Clinical Maxillofacial Prosthetics.* Chicago: Quintessence Publishing Co, Inc.; 2000:233–264.

31. The glossary of prosthodontic terms: ninth edition. *J Prosthet Dent.* May 2017;117(5S):e1–e105. https://doi.org/10.1016/j.prosdent.2016.12.001. PMID: 28418832.

32. Toljanic JA, Eckert SE, Roumanas E, et al. Osseointegrated craniofacial implants in the rehabilitation of orbital defects: an update of a retrospective experience in the United States. *J Prosthet Dent.* 2005;94:177–182.

33. Turvey TA, Golden BA. Orbital anatomy for the surgeon. *Oral Maxillofac Surg Clin North Am.* 2012;24:525–536.

CHAPTER 11

Facial Prosthesis

PANKAJ PRAKASH KHARADE, MDS, FJPS • TAPAN KUMAR GIRI, MDS •
ARDHENDU BANERJEE, MDS • SANGEETA AGARWAL, MDS •
PRAVIN BHIRANGI, D. MECH. • AHIRE GORAKH, D. MECH.

The use of facial prostheses such as wax ears has been documented in ancient Egypt. The leading evidence, which has been reported in the history, is from the 16th century where the French surgeon Ambroise Paré has referred to the first nose prostheses fabricated in gold and silver, which were retained to the face by a string tied around the head.[1,2] Apart from that, osseointegrated extraoral implants are extensively prescribed for retention of orbital, ear, as well as nose prostheses. Implants are considered superior as their usage diminishes adhesive-related complications such as discoloration as well as deterioration of the prosthetic material.[3–8] Apart from that, there will be less mechanical and chemical irritation skin as well as mucosal surfaces due to intrinsic mechanical retention, adhesives, or adhesive solvents.[9,10] Maintenance as well as creation of fine feathered margins in addition to simple positioning of an implant-retained craniofacial prosthesis greatly amplify the esthetic qualities of the prosthesis.[11,12] Several clinical trials have concluded regarding the success of implant-retained prosthesis in the form of practical application as well as improvement of patient's quality of life (Fig. 11.1).[13–17]

Several clinical trials have reported that implants have shown intense influence on patient acceptance for facial prostheses.[18,19] Other methods of prosthetic rehabilitation lack the comfort as well as convenience associated with implant-retained facial prostheses.[20,21] The benefits as well as drawbacks of every method of prosthetic rehabilitation should be appraised to the patient. Facial defects create several limitations for surgeon as well as prosthodontist.[22,23] Prosthodontists face challenges related to retention of larger prosthesis, mobility of the tissues surrounding the defects, esthetic outcome of the prosthesis, and selection of suitable material (Fig. 11.2).[24,25]

On the other hand, surgeon faces challenges such as irradiated tissue, leading to compromised blood supply, availability of tissue, and precise evaluation during follow-up visits to assess the recurrence if any.[26,27] Acquired facial defects resulting after radical surgical procedures frequently lead to massive functional, cosmetic in addition to psychological handicap in patients.[28–32] An interdisciplinary approach is essential for rehabilitation of such complex defects,[33] wherever plastic surgical reconstruction of such defects is not possible due to uncomplimentary conditions such as compromised surgical site due to radiotherapy-related hypovascularity and deficient residual soft as well as hard tissues.[34–38] In such situation, rehabilitation of patients with large maxillofacial defects is suitable with prosthesis for acceptable esthetic outcome.[39] The form, shade, and texture of the facial prosthesis must be as undetectable from the surrounding natural tissues to enhance the acceptance.[40–44] Even though physical limitations may restrict the success of the facial prosthesis, use of suitable material for prosthesis fabrication can help to overcome the situation.[45,46] Few trials have also reported that success of implants is not uniform, and the rate of failure is relatively high especially after radiation therapy.[47] Such clinical failures as well as complications seem to be site specific and also depend on the dose of the radiation and time factor.[48,49] Prosthetic rehabilitation can be considered successful only when patients can overcome the fear to attract unwanted attention while appearing in public.[50] A pretreatment planning meeting with the patient as well as multidisciplinary team is very important to show diverse prosthetic options and their maintenance.[51] It is mandatory to explain regarding the expected outcome of the prosthesis and related issues including quality of the prosthesis.[52] It will help to achieve the optimum function as well as esthetics in patients with

Prosthetic Rehabilitation of Head and Neck Cancer Patients. https://doi.org/10.1016/B978-0-323-82394-4.00012-4

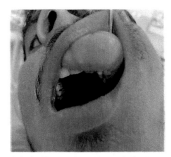

FIG. 11.1 Tumor invading midfacial region.

facial defects (Chart 11.1). Prosthetic rehabilitation of facial defects helps to boost the confidence in addition to positive impact on psychosocial health of the patient (Fig. 11.3).[53]

Different modes of retention for facial prosthesis:
a. Anatomic retention through tissue undercuts
b. Mechanical retention methods such as adhesives, magnets, precision attachments, spectacles, implants, and elastic straps

Most common materials used to fabricate facial prosthesis are acrylic, acrylic copolymer, and medical-grade silicone elastomers.[54–59] There are few limitations of facial prosthesis such as discoloration of prosthesis, lack of bonding with adhesives, tear during removal, changes in mechanical properties, and alteration in surface texture.[60,61] Adhesives are considered as the most widespread form of retention.[62,63]

Adhesives for silicone facial prosthesis are available in the form of sprays, pastes, double-sided tapes, and liquid emulsions.[64,65] Cleaning of the prosthesis is endorsed with water, neutral soap, and chlorhexidine. Adhesives demand use of solvents to clean the skin after removal of the prosthesis.[66,67]

COLORATION OF FACIAL PROSTHESIS

Different types of stains are used for coloration of silicone and other materials.[68,69] Usually, two types of stains are used:
a. Intrinsic stains—These stains are less prone to discoloration. These are more durable.
b. Extrinsic—Extrinsic stains are prone to discoloration. They have short life span.
c. Combination of extrinsic and intrinsic.

Best results are achieved with combination of intrinsic as well as extrinsic coloration.[70,71] Extrinsic stains help to augment the natural appearance of the prosthesis achieved with intrinsic pigments.[72–74] Nowadays, facial prosthesis is fabricated using three different types of pigments, which include silicone, dry earth, and oil.[75]

Coward et al. after a study on effectiveness of computerized color formulation system spectrophotometry to predict pigment formulas of pigmented silicone elastomers to match the skin color of 19 African-Canadian subjects reported that these systems provide a foundation and objectivity for color matching procedures related to facial prostheses.[76]

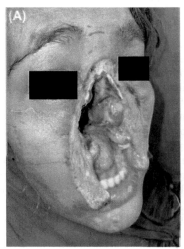
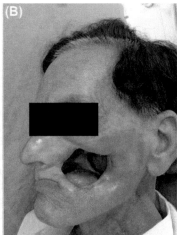
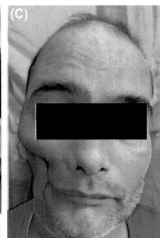

FIG. 11.2 (a) Facial defect after resection of midfacial tumor. (b) Compound facial defect extending to maxilla, mandible, and soft palate. (c) Facial defect due to resection of mandible.

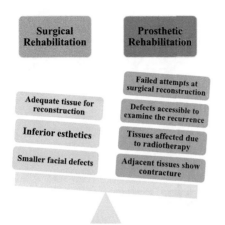

CHART 11.1 Indications of surgical and prosthetic rehabilitation of facial defects.

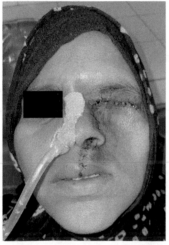

FIG. 11.3 Facial defect after surgical reconstruction leading to compromised esthetics and function.

Color stability of the facial prosthesis is the primary concern for patient as well as clinician. Several color-stable materials have been introduced. Recent research is mostly focused toward invention of techniques to match the color precisely.[77,78] Scientific color matching requires quantitative description of optical properties of colorants being used. Shade of the human skin can be matched precisely by application of these optical properties to mathematical model (Fig. 11.4).[79,80]

PROSTHETIC REHABILITATION OF VARIOUS DEFECTS

Collaboration with the oncosurgeon is very essential for successful rehabilitation of the facial defects. Minimum distortion of the adjacent tissues is required for proper retention as well as camouflage of the facial prosthesis.[81] It is desirable to line the defects with skin grafts to improve the retention by creating favorable undercuts. Hair-containing flaps should be avoided. Hair from the flap makes placement of implants and application of adhesives difficult.[82] It is essential to reproduce natural contours, surface texture, color as well as translucence. Whenever possible, junction of the prosthesis and skin should be placed behind the eye glasses or in the skin folds.[83,84]

ORBITAL PROSTHESIS

The eyes are an important component of personality as well as expression. Eye contact is the primary thing to initiate conversation. Slight discrepancy may immediately come to notice of the observer.[85] Resection of orbital tumors profoundly affects the confidence as well as morale of the patient. Reconstruction after exenteration or resection of large section of orbit surgical reconstruction is complicated, and it is highly cumbersome to restore the esthetics of the patient with surgical reconstruction.[86] Rehabilitation with orbital prosthesis is done most commonly to restore the esthetics as well as psychological status of the patient. It is recommended to line the defect with a split-thickness skin graft to generate the base for the orbital prosthesis.[87] Lining the defect with split-thickness graft makes the surface suitable for application of adhesive.[88] The boundaries of the orbital defect must be stable as well as healthy to prevent the hurdles during impression making.[89] The superior portion should be given prime consideration whenever possible to preserve the position of the eyebrow to improve esthetic outcome of the prosthesis. The material and extensions of the prosthesis are planned by the surgeon in a manner to fulfill the patient's anatomic needs. An orbital prosthesis covers the orbital cavity and helps in prevention of infection by covering the defect. Retention of an orbital prosthesis is most unbeaten after incorporation of osseointegrated implants in the treatment plan. Adhesive retention can be considered for patients with

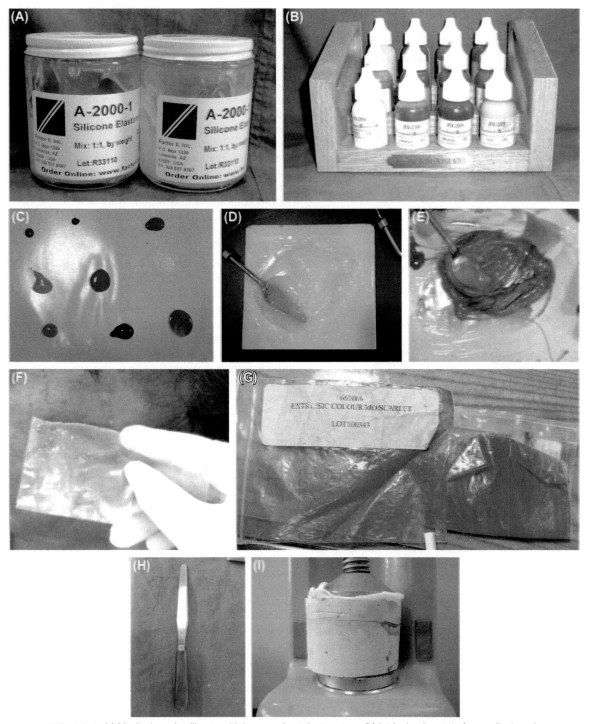

FIG. 11.4 (a) Medical-grade silicone with base and catalyst system. (b) Intrinsic pigments for medical grade silicone. (c) Different shades of intrinsic pigments should be ready before mixing the medical-grade silicone. (d) Medical-grade silicone mixed with equal quantity of the catalyst. (e) Medical grade silicone after addition of intrinsic pigments to achieve the skin shade. (f) Matching of prepared shade with patient's skin shade. (g) Extrinsic stains for shade modifications to give prosthesis life-like appearance. (h) Instrument to mix medical-grade silicone. (i) Silicone packing and pressure applied with Hanau hydraulic press.

incomplete skeletal growth or compromised bone density (Table 11.1).[90] Orbital prostheses can be recommended as a feasible option for rehabilitation after removal of the globe (Figs. 11.5–11.8).

Rehabilitation options for orbital defects are abundant, and the decision rests in the hands of the operator. The operator has to frame a treatment plan taking into concern appropriate parameters such as health, extent of cooperation from the patient, tissue health of the surgical site, the financial constraints of the patient in addition to the operator skill (Fig. 11.9).[91]

NASAL PROSTHESIS

Nasal tumor resection necessitates removal of nasal bone. Retention of the nasal leads to overcontouring of the prosthesis. It will lead to unesthetic outcome due bigger than normal prosthesis. The quality of life after rhinectomy is extremely compromised, which necessitates a proficient surgical or prosthetic device rehabilitation to improve the quality of life. During closure of surgical site after resection of nasal tumor, distortion of lip due to excessive tension should be avoided as it will affect the appearance of prosthesis. In case of partial nasal defects, the margins of the

prosthesis should be placed on the lateral slope of opposite nostril to help in camouflage on the skin and prosthesis junction.[92] Lateral margins of the nasal prosthesis should be planned in such a manner that they should merge with the cheek contours. Apart from that, these margins should be placed behind the eyeglass frames to achieve better camouflage. Primary retention of the nasal prosthesis is achieved through anatomical undercuts.[93] It is necessary to make the prosthesis hollow to reduce the weight and aid in retention of the prosthesis. If tissue undercuts are properly engaged, adhesive may not be required for retention of nasal prosthesis. Surgical reconstruction can be planned wherever possible. Usually, combination of surgical and prosthetic rehabilitation will produce successful outcome. If implant-retained prosthesis is planned, floor of nose is the preferred site. Placement of implants in nasal floor should be judicious as it can traumatize the roots of maxillary anteriors in dentulous patients. The site, size, and etiology of the nasal defect, age, and general medical condition of the patient are the pertinent factors, which will decide the methods of rehabilitation of nasal defect.[94] Complex defects associated with nasal defects may necessitate fabrication of oral and nasal prosthesis, which are connected together with the help of several attachments such as magnetic or precision attachments (Fig. 11.10).

AURICULAR PROSTHESIS

Auricular prosthesis is considered as economical and esthetically acceptable treatment for rehabilitation of missing ear. Apart from that, it supports the spectacles and protects the external auditory meatus from dust and other particulate matter. Whenever surgical reconstruction of resected part of ear is not planned, entire ear should be resected so as to improve the esthetic outcome by creating flat and fixed tissue surface.[95] Lining the tissue bed with pedicle or split-thickness graft will improve the prosthetic outcome. Residual tags of tissue have no value in retention and need removal for better adaptation of auricular prosthesis. Retention of tragus is recommended to camouflage the junction of ear prosthesis and skin. If flaps are used for lining the defects, then they should be without hair to facilitate application of skin adhesives as well as placement of implants for retention. Tissue remnants present as congenital malformation should be resected if surgical reconstruction is not being executed. Implants can be incorporated in the planning for retention of the

TABLE 11.1 Comparison of Anterior and Posterior Indexing Methods

Anterior Indexing Method	Posterior Indexing Method
1. Laborious as it involves many steps	1. Fewer steps
2. More technical procedure and less operator sensitive	2. Less technical procedure and more operator sensitive
3. Custom-matched eye shell is preserved as its duplicate is used during fabrication	3. Color-matched eye shell can get damaged during fabrication
4. Eye shell can be snapped out and replaced easily preserving the prosthesis	4. Eye shell is attached to prosthesis, and as a result, prosthesis has to be remade if eye shell is damaged during use

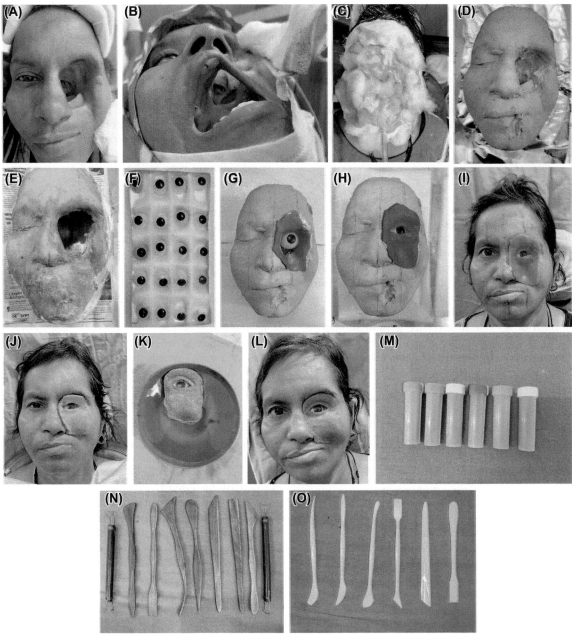

FIG. 11.5 (a) Orbital defect extending to the adjacent part of the face. (b) Orbital defect extending to the oral cavity creating communication. (c) Impression of the orbital defect recorded to fabricate a complete facial moulage. (d) Complete facial moulage fabricated with stone. (e) Complete facial moulage requires blockage of undercuts before fabrication of wax pattern of the prosthesis. (f) Suitable color and size of eye shell should be selected from the set. (g) Orientation of eye shell in accordance with natural gaze. (h) Fabrication of wax pattern for the prosthesis after orientation of eye shell. (i) Fabricated wax pattern is tried on patient's face for assessment of the gaze. (j) Sculpting of wax pattern for the prosthesis using laboratory clay and sculpting instruments. (k) Fabrication of the hollow prosthesis to reduce the weight. (l) Prosthesis completed and inserted in the defect site. (m) Intrinsic stains for prosthesis fabricated in acrylic. (n) Wooden instruments for sculpting of the prosthetic pattern using clay. (o) Plastic instruments for sculpting of the prosthetic pattern using clay.

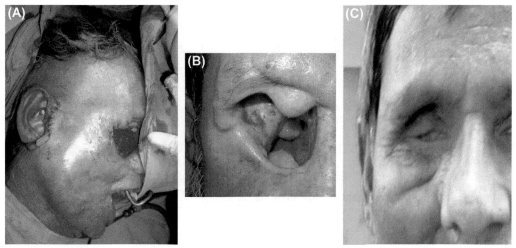

FIG. 11.6 (a) Favorable orbital defect. (b) Favorable orbital defect with retained eyebrow and suitable undercuts for retention. (c) Unfavorable orbital defect.

prosthesis if malignancy is not evident. Placement of implants can be planned immediate or delayed depending on the nature of tumor. Fabrication of auricular prosthesis is a combination of art and science.[96] Fabrication of auricular prosthesis with proper technique helps to improve cosmetic appearance and social and psychological status of the patient. After successful rehabilitation of the auricular defect, the patient can appear in public without fear of attracting unwanted attention. For patients with congenital ear abnormality, prosthetic rehabilitation provides economical and nonsurgical option. Magnets can be used as modes of retention with the help of implants for auricular prosthesis fabrication. Magnets will facilitate precise placement of auricular prosthesis, which may be difficult with other modes of retention due to critical location of ears.

Digital impression of the auricular defect can also be made using phase-measuring profilometry. This is a safe procedure, which employs multiple light sources. It is a very fast procedure. This data generated is used for development of three-dimensional image. Models fabricated using this technology are very precise and very helpful for treatment planning as well as execution. Facial prosthesis can be fabricated with the help of reverse engineering and selective laser sintering as well. These techniques are useful for precise

rehabilitation of unilateral defects in orbital and auricular region (Fig. 11.11).

REHABILITATION OF MIDFACIAL AND COMBINED DEFECTS OF FACE-

Midfacial tumors may require extensive surgical resection for total management of tumors. Usually, it will lead to loss of intraoral and extraoral structures, which will affect the function as well as esthetics tremendously.[97] Along with affected mastication, deglutition, and speech, the overall appearance of the individual leads to poor psychological status of the patient. Disfigurement of face causes drooling of saliva in several cases. Most of the midfacial defects are rehabilitated with prosthetic management as surgical reconstruction will lead to morbidity as well as inferior esthetics. Speech as well as salivary control may improve after prosthetic rehabilitation.

For extensive midfacial defects extending to the oral cavity, prognosis depends on amount of residual hard palate, remaining dentition, condition of the lip, and psychological status of the patient. Reconstruction of upper lip by surgical technique often leads to compromised outcome due to immobility of lip after reconstruction, which also affects the ability to create seal.

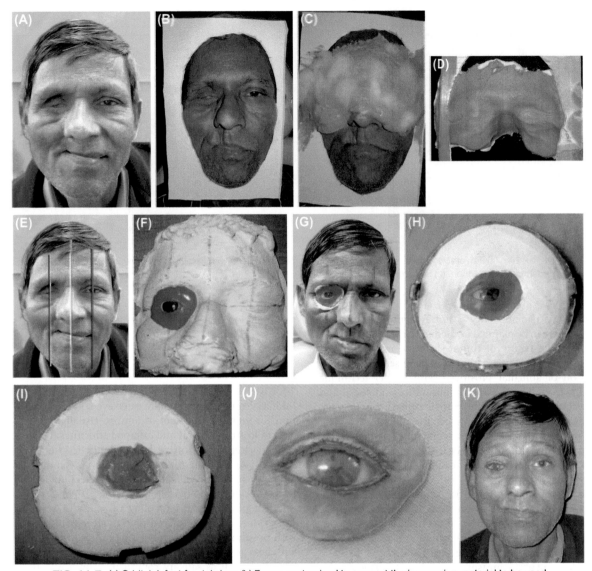

FIG. 11.7 (a) Orbital defect frontal view. (b) Frame customized to support the impression material to be used for orbital defect impression. (c) Impression of the orbital defect recorded with irreversible hydrocolloid. Cotton is applied before final set of irreversible hydrocolloid for retention of supporting plaster. (d) Final impression for facial moulage fabrication. (e) Markings on the face before fabrication of wax pattern of the prosthesis for precise vertical and horizontal placement of eye shell. (f) Fabrication of wax pattern for the prosthesis after orientation of eye shell. (g) Fabricated wax pattern is tried on patient's face for assessment of the gaze. Orientation of eye shell in accordance with natural gaze. (h) Flasking of wax pattern for the prosthesis. (i) Medical-grade silicone packing in the flask after proper shade matching with skin around the orbital defect. (j) Final prosthesis completed after application of extrinsic stains to produce life-like appearance. (k) Final prosthesis placed in the defect area. Prosthesis is retained with adhesive.

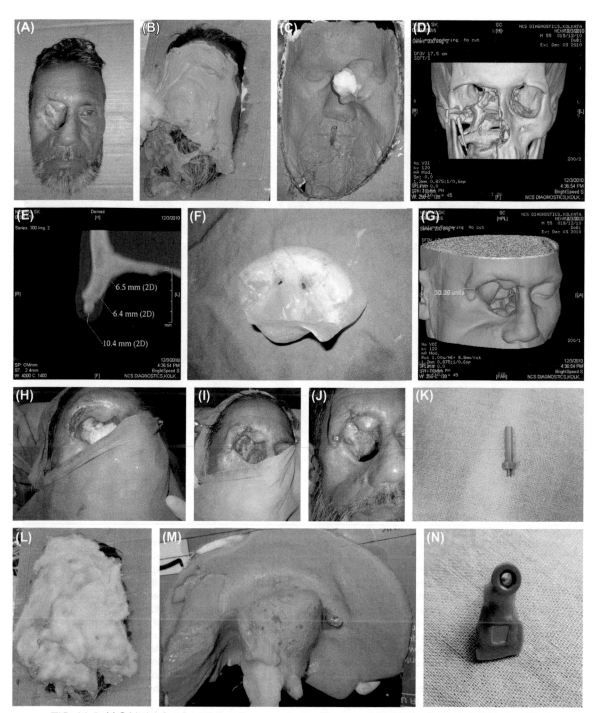

FIG. 11.8 (a) Orbital defect frontal view. Frame customized to support the impression material to be used for orbital defect impression. (b) Impression of the orbital defect recorded with irreversible hydrocolloid. Cotton is applied before final set of irreversible hydrocolloid for retention of supporting plaster. (c) Final impression for facial moulage fabrication. (d) CT imaging to assess the bone available for implant placement. (e) CT imaging to

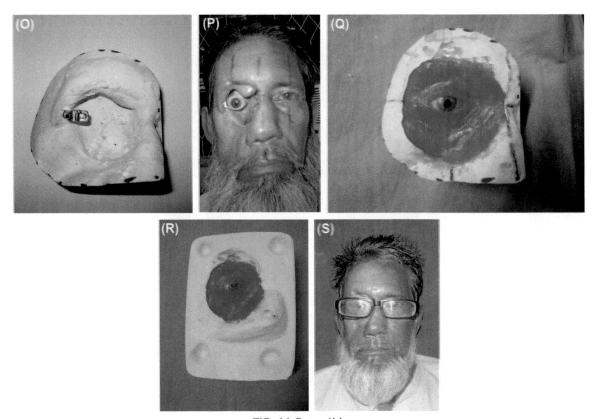

FIG. 11.8 **cont'd.**

assess the mediolateral bone available for implant placement. (f) CT imaging demonstrating 3D reconstruction to assess bone available for implant placement. (g) Surgical guide fabricated for implant placement. (h) Surgical implant placement in the lateral aspect of orbit. (i) Surgical site is sutured. (j) Surgical exposure of implant for placement of prosthetic component. (k) UCLA abutment for attachment to the implant. (l) Impression of the orbital defect to retain the orbital prosthesis with implant. (m) Impression of the orbital defect to with impression coping. (n) Wax pattern of the magnet casing to retain the prosthesis with implant. (o) Moulage fabrication for orbital defect with implant analogue and abutment after casting. (p) Assessment of gaze with the help of eye shell. (q) Markings on the face were used during fabrication of wax pattern of the prosthesis for precise vertical and horizontal placement of eye shell. Wax pattern was fabricated for the prosthesis after orientation of eye shell. Fabricated wax pattern is tried on patient's face for assessment of the gaze. Orientation of eye shell in accordance with natural gaze. (r) Flasking of wax pattern for the prosthesis. Medical-grade silicone packing in the flask after proper shade matching with skin around the orbital defect. (s) Final prosthesis completed after application of extrinsic stains to produce life like appearance. Final prosthesis placed in the defect area. Prosthesis is retained with implants.

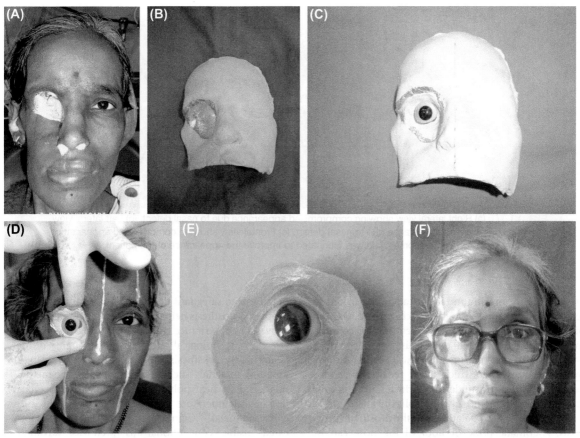

FIG. 11.9 (a) Orbital defect extending to the other part of face-frontal view. Patient had received a radiation dose of 60 Gy. (b) Frame customized to support the impression material to be used for orbital defect impression. Impression of the orbital defect recorded with irreversible hydrocolloid. Cotton is applied before final set of irreversible hydrocolloid for retention of supporting plaster. Final impression for facial moulage fabrication was made. Impression was poured with stone and facial moulage was fabricated. (c) Fabrication of prosthesis pattern with modeling clay after proper orientation of eye shell. (d) Markings on the face before fabrication of wax pattern of the prosthesis for precise vertical and horizontal placement of eye shell. Fabricated wax pattern is tried on patient's face for assessment of the gaze. Orientation of eye shell in accordance with natural gaze. Flasking of wax pattern for the processing of the prosthesis was done. Medical-grade silicone packing in the flask after proper shade matching with skin around the orbital defect. (e) Final prosthesis completed after application of extrinsic stains to produce life-like appearance. (f) Final prosthesis placed in the defect area. Prosthesis was retained with eyeglasses to overcome the side effects of adhesive on the sensitive skin due to radiotherapy.

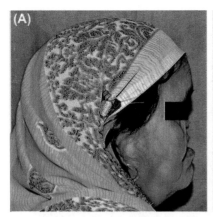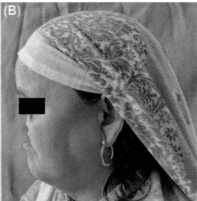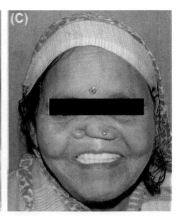

FIG. 11.10 (a) Right lateral view showing compromised appearance due to nasal defect. (b) Left lateral view showing compromised appearance due to nasal defect. (c) Frontal view showing compromised appearance due to nasal defect. Intraoral prosthesis was fabricated to improve the appearance of the patient.

Preservation of maximum teeth is advisable to aid in retention of intraoral as well as facial prostheses. Implants can be considered for retention if retention from teeth and tissue undercuts is not adequate.[98] Fabrication of intraoral prosthesis will restore the primary functions after which facial prosthesis can be planned. Soft tissue undercuts, which are surgically created, should be lined with split-thickness grafts. Resection of the hard palate affects the prosthetic prognosis. Zygomatic bone or floor of the nose can be considered as potential implant placement sites for augmentation of retention of prosthesis. Prosthesis fabricated for large midfacial defects is heavier, and implants will help to bear that load. Depending on the clinical situation, implant placement should be planned at the time of resection to expedite the process of prosthetic rehabilitation. It will also affect the psychological status of the patient to a lesser extent (Figs. 11.12–11.14).

CRANIOFACIAL PROSTHESIS

Various etiological factors for cranial defects include trauma, surgery, congenital defects, or certain diseases. These defects are treated surgically using cranioplasty

prosthesis to safeguard the underlying vital tissue. Cranioplasty prosthesis helps to relieve the pain. It also improves the appearance of patient causing tremendous effect on psychological status as well as quality of life. Cranioplasty prosthesis can be fabricated by using a range of materials such as autopolymerizing methylmethacrylate, heat polymerizing methyl-methacrylate, and high-temperature vulcanizing medical-grade silicone and metal.[99] Cranioplasty prosthesis can be fabricated using conventional as well as advanced techniques. Advanced techniques for fabrication of cranial prosthesis include virtual planning and 3D printing. These materials have their own advantages as well as shortcomings. Certain materials necessitate the use of conventional technique for fabrication of cranioplasty prosthesis. Cranial defect should be recorded precisely to enhance the prognosis of cranioplasty procedure. This chapter deliberates about technical details of cranioplasty prosthesis (Fig. 11.15).

CAD-CAM FOR FACIAL PROSTHESIS

Computer-aided designing and manufacturing (CAD/CAM) is the recent advanced technique being used for fabrication of facial prostheses. It can be used for

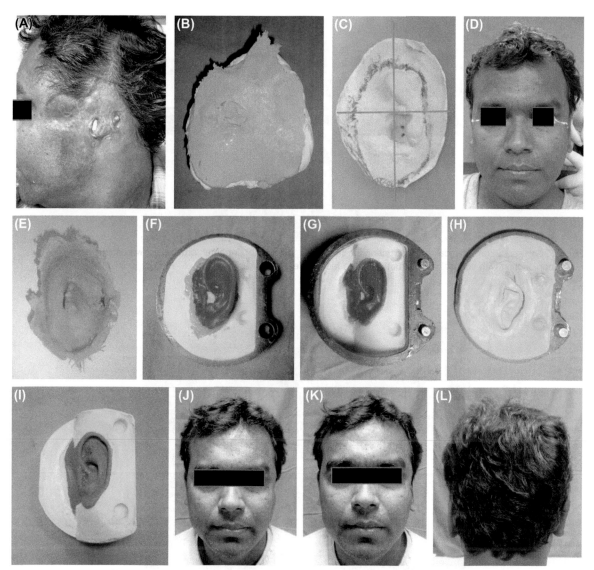

FIG. 11.11 (a) Auricular defect after resection of the ear followed by radiotherapy. (b) Impression of the orbital defect recorded with irreversible hydrocolloid. Cotton is applied before final set of irreversible hydrocolloid for retention of supporting plaster. (c) Impression was poured with stone, and moulage was fabricated. Markings were made for proper orientation of the wax pattern of auricular prosthesis. (d) Fabrication of prosthesis wax pattern after proper orientation. Markings placed in the mastoid region extending toward face before fabrication of wax pattern of the auricular prosthesis. Fabricated wax pattern is tried on patient's face for assessment of the orientation. (e) Relining of the wax pattern of prosthesis after proper orientation for better adaptation. (f) Flasking of wax pattern for the processing of the prosthesis was done. (g) Three-piece mold was fabricated for processing of the auricular prosthesis. (h) Dewaxing was carried out. (i) Medical-grade silicone packing in the flask after proper shade matching with skin around the auricular defect. Final prosthesis completed after application of extrinsic stains to produce life-like appearance. (j) Frontal view without auricular prosthesis. (k) Frontal view with auricular prosthesis. Final prosthesis placed in the defect area. Prosthesis was retained with adhesive. (l) View from the dorsal aspect with auricular prosthesis in position.

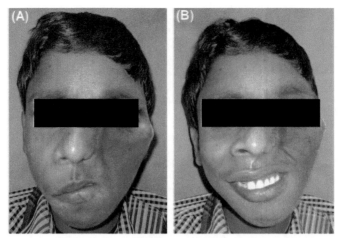

FIG. 11.12 (a) Surgical reconstruction of the facial defect. (b) Intraoral prosthesis was fabricated in conjunction with surgical reconstruction of the facial defect.

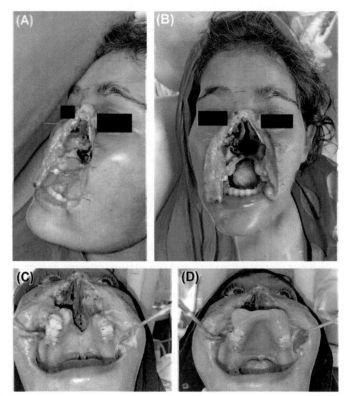

FIG. 11.13 (a) Extensive loss of tissue after resection of tumor in the midfacial region. (b) Defect in the midfacial region showing loss of lip and hard palate leading to oronasal communication. (c) Extensive intraoral defect leading to oro-nasal communication. (d) Intraoral prosthesis was inserted to support feeding. It will also act as partition between oral and nasal cavity.

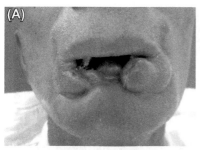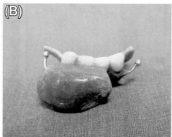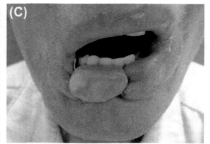

FIG. 11.14 (a) Lip defect due to surgical resection of tumor. (b) Lip prosthesis fabricated with the help of autopolymerizing acrylic resin and intrinsic stains. (c) Lip prosthesis in position leading to improved appearance and proper sealing with the help of upper lip.

superior treatment outcome due to high precision achieved with computerized planning. Laser surface scanning can be done to obtain three-dimensional imaging data related to the patient's facial defect after resection of tumor. The three-dimensional imaging data is transmitted to a CAD/CAM interactive program to process the image.[100] Once the image is processed, it will produce a model for fabrication of the facial prosthesis with the help of mathematical designing. Recent advances in the CAD/CAM technique have the capacity to reduce the efforts required for prosthetic planning. It will simplify the entire laboratory procedure as well. This novel technique is useful for the fabrication of prostheses with superior outcome for the rehabilitation of facial defects. The clinical trials have reported high precision of the facial prosthesis in context with shape, size, and contours of the facial prostheses.[101] The incorporation of rapid prototyping techniques in aggregation with CAD/CAM can be executed as an apposite approach for rehabilitation of facial defects with facial prosthesis (Fig. 11.16).

SUMMARY

Patients with facial defects are not only physically compromised, but it also affects psychological and social health of the patient. Rehabilitation options for these defects are numerous, and the decision rests in the hands of the clinician. The clinician has to formulate a treatment plan taking into consideration pertinent factors such as the health, cooperation level of the patient, tissue health of the surgical site, the financial constraints of the patient, and the operator skill. A multidisciplinary attitude is essential for rehabilitation of facial defects. Collaboration among various specialties prior to surgical procedure will improve the treatment outcome by reducing facial distortion and augmenting the retention-related parameters of facial prosthesis. Implant-retained prostheses are prescribed whenever possible to overcome the drawbacks of adhesive prosthesis. Implants enhance the treatment outcome. Surgical reconstruction can be planned for small defects. Larger defects necessitate prosthetic rehabilitation to achieve an esthetic outcome in addition to less morbidity associated with surgical procedure. Silicone gives life-like appearance to the prosthesis, which has made it material of choice for facial prosthesis. 3D printing and CAD-CAM systems help in precise prosthetic planning with or without incorporating implants for better rehabilitation. Virtual planning with the help of advanced technologies reduces the total number of patient visits and enhances the esthetic outcome. Junction of the prosthesis and surrounding skin should be camouflaged precisely by thinning the margins and proper placement of the prosthesis. Patients who have undergone radiotherapy have poor prognosis due to compromised soft as well as hard tissue bed. Apart from that, shade matching is critical in radiotherapy-treated patients due to changes in the skin tone due to radiation.

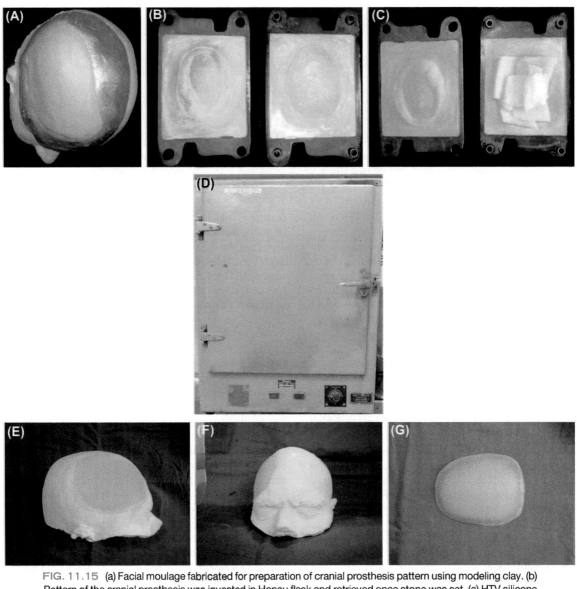

FIG. 11.15 (a) Facial moulage fabricated for preparation of cranial prosthesis pattern using modeling clay. (b) Pattern of the cranial prosthesis was invested in Hanau flask and retrieved once stone was set. (c) HTV silicone MDX-4515 was placed in the mold space and flask was closed. The entire assembly was compressed using hydraulic press. (d) After closure of the flask, they were kept in hot air over for processing of HTV silicone. (e) Lateral view of the moulage showing proper adaptation of cranial prosthesis in the defect region. (f) Frontal view of the moulage showing proper contour of cranial prosthesis on the defect side. (g) Final cranial prosthesis fabricated using HTV silicone. Polishing is done using polishing burs. Dacron mesh is attached for retention of the prosthesis.

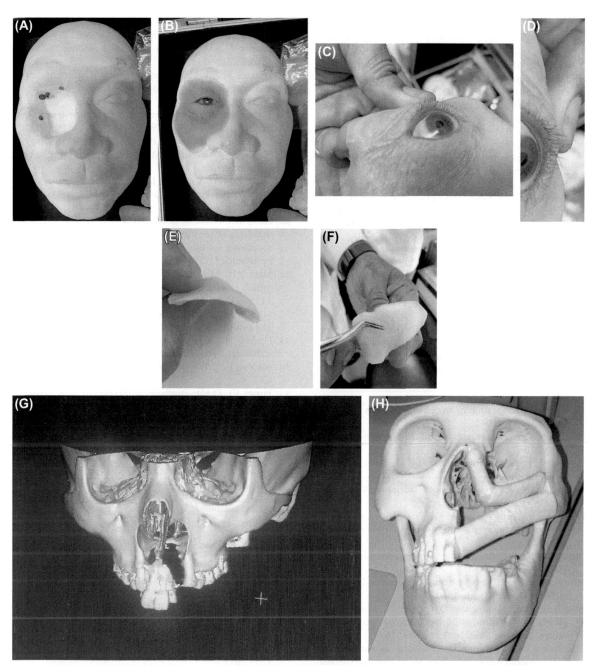

FIG. 11.16 (a) Facial moulage showing magnetic attachments retained with implants in the region of orbital defect. (b) Facial moulage showing orbital prosthesis fabricated using CAD CAM technology. Orbital prosthesis is retained with the help of magnetic attachments attached with implants in the region of orbital defect. Thin margins of the silicone prosthesis help to camouflage the junction of prosthesis and skin. (c) Final orbital prosthesis with life-like appearance. (d) Incorporation of eyelashes augment the esthetics of the prosthesis. (e) Thin margins of the prosthesis are suitable for camouflage making the prosthesis undetectable. (f) Specialized instruments are used for implanting hair in the silicone prosthesis. These hair help for natural appearance of the prosthesis. (g) Scanning of the defect area to fabricate the facial prosthesis using CAD-CAM technology. (h) 3D model of the defect area is fabricated using rapid prototyping and 3D printing technology. It will add precision to the treatment planning especially for placement of implants to retain the prosthesis.

REFERENCES

1. Taylor TD, ed. *Clinical Maxillofacial Prosthetics.* USA: Quintessence Publishing Co, Inc.; 2000.
2. Brown JS, Shaw RJ. Reconstruction of the maxilla and midface: introducing a new classification. *Lancet Oncol.* October 2010;11(10):1001–1008.
3. Hollier Jr LH, Sharabi SE, Koshy JC, Stal S. Facial trauma: general principles of management. *J Craniofac Surg.* July 2010;21(4):1051–1053.
4. Goiato MC, Nicolau EI, Mazaro JV, et al. Mobility, aesthetic, implants, and satisfaction of the ocular prostheses wearers. *J Craniofac Surg.* January 2010;21(1):160–164.
5. Dos Santos DM, Goiato MC, Pesqueira AA, et al. Prosthesis auricular with osseointegrated implants and quality of life. *J Craniofac Surg.* January 2010;21(1):94–96.
6. Abrahamian HA. Maxillofacial prosthetics: an introduction. *Georgetown Dent J.* 1964;31:1–3.
7. Adisman IK. Maxillofacial prosthesis. *Int Dent J.* 1958;8:30.
8. Al-Qudsi FS. *Facial Prosthesis.* Baghdad: Baghdad University Press; 1968.
9. Baker L. An artificial nose and palate. *D Cosmos.* 1905;47:561–562.
10. Barnhart GW. A new material and technic in the art of somatoprosthesis. *J Dent Res.* 1960;39:836–844.
11. Beder OE. *Surgical and Maxillofacial Prosthesis.* Seattle: University of Washington Press; 1959.
12. Braley S. Director, Dow Coming Center for Aid to Medical Research; Personal Communication.
13. Brown KE. Fabrication of an ocular prosthesis. *J Prosthet Dent.* 1970;24:225–235.
14. Bruce GM. Ancient origins of artificial eye. *Ann Med Hist.* 1940;2:10–14.
15. Bryan PL. Consultant Health Care Facilities; Personal Communication.
16. Bulbulian AH. *Facial Prosthesis.* Philadelphia: W. B. Saunders Co.; 1945.
17. Cantor R, Curtis TA, Rozen RD. Prosthetic management of terminal cancer patients. *J Prosthet Dent.* 1968;20:361–366.
18. Cantor R, Hildestad P. A material for epithesis. *Odontol Tidskr.* 1966;74:32–40.
19. Chalian VA. *Maxillofacial Prosthesis.* Houston: University of Texas, Dental Branch; 1960.
20. Chalian VA, Cunningham DM, Drane JB. Maxillofacial prosthetics departments in dental schools and medical centers. *J Prosthet Dent.* 1865;15:570–576.
21. Chalian VA, Thompson LW. *Prosthetic Reconstruction of Facial Disfigurements: Proceedings of the First International Symposium of Plastic and Reconstructive Surgery of the Face and Neck, New York.* Stuttgart: Georg Thieme Verlag; 1970 (in press).
22. Clarke CD. *Facial and Body Prosthesis.* St. Louis: C. V. Mosby Co.; 1945.
23. Dimitry TJ. Story of artificial eye. *Eye Ear Nose Throat Mon.* 1941;21:270–274.
24. Firtell DH, Bartlett SO. Maxillofacial prostheses: reproducible fabrication. *J Prosthet Dent.* 1969;22:247–252.
25. Fonder AC. Maxillofacial prosthetics. *J Prosthet Dent.* 1969;21:310–314.
26. Fonseca EP. The importance of form, characterization and retention in facial prosthesis. *J Prosthet Dent.* 1966;16:338–343.
27. Hawkinson RT. Development of skin surface texture in maxillofacial prosthetics. *J Prosthet Dent.* 1965;15:929–937.
28. Helveston EM. Assistant Professor of Ophthalmology, Indiana University Medical School; personal communication.
29. Kazanjian VH, Converse JM. *The Surgical Treatment of Facial Injuries.* 2nd ed. Baltimore: The Williams & Wilkins Co.; 1959.
30. Laney WR, Drane JB, Rosenthal LE. Educational status of maxillofacial prosthetics: report of the educational survey committee of the American academy of maxillofacial prosthetics. *JADA (J Am Dent Assoc).* 1966;73:647–651.
31. Metz HH. Maxillofacial prosthetic rehabilitation after mouth and facial surgery. *J Prosthet Dent.* 1964;14:1169–1177.
32. Miglani DC, Drane JB. Maxillofacial prosthesis and its use as a healing art. *J Prosthet Dent.* 1959;9:159–168.
33. Nadeau J. Maxillofacial prosthesis with magnetic stabilizers. *J Prosthet Dent.* 1956;6:114–119.
34. Nadeau J. Special prostheses. *J Prosthet Dent.* 1968;20:62–76.
35. Prince JH. *Ocular Prosthesis.* Edinburgh: E. & S. Livingstone, Ltd.; 1946.
36. Riley C. Maxillofacial prosthetic rehabilitation of postoperative cancer patients. *J Prosthet Dent.* 1968;20:352–360.
37. Roberts AC. Facial reconstruction by prosthetic means. *Br J Oral Surg.* 1966;4:157–182.
38. Roberts AC, Penney HD. An Advance in facial and body prosthesis material. *Dent Pract.* 1964;15:7–13.
39. Robinson JE. Prosthetic treatment after surgical removal of the maxilla and floor of the orbit. *J Prosthet Dent.* 1963;13:178–184.
40. Robinson Jr JE, Niiranen VJ, eds. *Maxillofacial Prosthetics: Proceedings of an Interprofessional Conference, Washington, D. C., September, 1966.* Washington, DC: U. S. Public Health Service Publication No. 1950; 1966.
41. Schaaf NG. Color characterizing silicone rubber facial prostheses. *J Prosthet Dent.* 1970;24:198–202.
42. Tashma J. Coloring somatoprostheses. *J Prosthet Dent.* 1967;17:303–305.
43. Welden RB, Niiranen VJ. Ocular pros thesis. *J Prosthet Dent.* 1956;6:272–278.
44. Brown KE. Technique of splint contouring in resected edentulous mandibular reconstruction. *J Prosthet Dent.* 1969;21:532–535.
45. Cook GB, Walker AW, Schewe EJ. The Cerosium mandibular prosthesis. *Am J Surg.* 1965;110:558–572.
46. Grant FC, Norcross NC. Repair of cranial defects by cranioplasty. *Ann Surg.* 1939;110:488–512.

47. Hahn GW. Vitallium mesh mandibular prosthesis. *J Prosthet Dent.* 1964;July-August;14:777−784.
48. Korbicka J, Bechinie E. The carcinogenicity of fine Silon fabrics in animal experiment and the possibilities of using Silon in clinical practice. *Neoplasma (Bratisl).* 1967;14:537−550.
49. Kordan HA. Localized interfacial forces resulting from implanted plastics as possible physical factors involved in tumor formation. *J Theor Biol.* 1967;17:1−11.
50. Lang BR. Constructing mandibular implants during surgery. *J Prosthet Dent.* 1969;22:360−366.
51. Ludwigson DC. Requirements for metallic surgical implants and prosthetic devices. *Metals Eng Quart.* August 1965:1−6.
52. Reeves DL. *Cranioplasty. American Lecture Series 39. American Lectures in Surgery.* Springfield: Charles C Thomas Publisher; 1950:111.
53. Reeves DL. *Neurological Surgery of Trauma.* Washington, DC: Office of The Surgeon General, Department of the Army; 1965:233−256.
54. Roberts AC. A review of materials used for implantation in the human body. *Bio-Med Eng.* 1966;1:397−401.
55. Ross PJ, Jelsma F. Experiences with acrylic plastic for cranioplasties. *Am Surg.* 1960;26:519−524.
56. Spence WT. Form-fitting plastic cranioplasty. *J Neurosurg.* 1954;11:219−225.
57. Szko K. The use of metal prostheses following anterior mandibulectomy and neck dissection for carcinoma of the oral cavity. *Am J Surg.* 1962;104:715−720.
58. Smith Jr E. Maxillo-facial prosthesis. *N Y J Dent.* 1946 Aug-Sep;16:273−276.
59. Mathur PK. Maxillo-facial somato-prosthesis. *J All India Dent Assoc.* September 1965;37(9):296.
60. Ackerman AJ. Maxillofacial prosthesis. *Oral Surg Oral Med Oral Pathol.* 1953;6(1):176−200.
61. Olin W. Maxillofacial prosthesis. *J Am Dent Assoc.* 1954;48(4):399−409.
62. Baima RF. Implant-supported facial prostheses. *J Mich Dent Assoc.* 1996;78(50−4):56−64.
63. Buzayan MM. Prosthetic management of mid-facial defect with magnet-retained silicone prosthesis. *Prosthet Orthot Int.* 2014;38:62−67.
64. Wondergem M, Lieben G, Bouman S, van den Brekel MW, Lohuis PJ. Patients satisfaction with facial prostheses. *Br J Oral Maxillofac Surg.* 2016;54(4):394−399.
65. Dirven R, Lieben G, Bouwman S, Wolterink R, van den Brekel MWM, Lohuis PJFM. Facial prosthetics: grounds and techniques. *Ned Tijdschr Tandheelkd.* 2017;124(9):413−417.
66. Matthews E. Facial prostheses. *Br Dent J.* 1951;90:11−13.
67. Parr GR. Accessory retention for a facial prosthesis. *J Prosthet Dent.* May 1979;41(5):546−547.
68. Vander Poorten V, Meulemans J, Delaere P. Midface prosthetic rehabilitation. *Curr Opin Otolaryngol Head Neck Surg.* 2016;24:98−109.
69. Kantola R, Sivén M, Kurunmäki H, Tolvanen M, Vallittu PK, Kemppainen P. Laser Doppler imaging of skin microcirculation under fiber-reinforced composite framework of facial prosthesis. *Acta Odontol Scand.* February 2014;72(2):106−112.
70. Yoshioka F, Ozawa S, Matsuoka A, Takebe J. Fabricating nasal prostheses using four-dimensional facial expression models. *J Prosthodont Res.* 2021;65:379−386.
71. Andres CJ, Haug SP. Facial prosthesis fabrication: technical aspects. In: Taylor TD, ed. *Clinical Maxillofacial Prosthetics.* Carol Stream: Quintessence; 2000:233−244.
72. Dings JPJ, Merkx MAW, de Clonie Maclennan-Naphausen MTP, van de Pol P, Maal TJJ, Meijer GJ. Maxillofacial prosthetic rehabilitation: a survey on the quality of life. *J Prosthet Dent.* 2018;12:780−786.
73. Strub JR, Rekow ED, Witkowski S. Computer-aided design and fabrication of dental restorations current systems and future possibilities. *J Am Dent Assoc.* 2006;137:1289−1296.
74. Ciocca L, Mingucci R, Gassino G, Scotti R. CAD/CAM ear model and virtual construction of the mold. *J Prosthet Dent.* 2007;98:339−343.
75. Jiao T, Zhang F, Huang X, Wang C. Design and fabrication of auricular prostheses by CAD/CAM system. *Int J Prosthodont (IJP).* 2004;17(4):460−463.
76. Coward TJ, Scott BJ, Watson RM, Richards R. A comparison between computerized tomography, magnetic resonance imaging, and laser scanning for capturing 3-dimensional data from an object of standard form. *Int J Prosthodont (IJP).* 2005;18:405−413.
77. Yoshioka F, Ozawa S, Okazaki S, Tanaka K. Fabrication of an orbital prosthesis using a noncontact three-dimensional digitizer and rapid-prototyping system. *J Prosthodont.* 2010;19:598−600.
78. Matsuoka A, Yoshioka F, Ozawa S, Takebe J. Development of three-dimensional facial expression models using morphing methods for fabricating facial prostheses. *J Prosthodont Res.* 2019;63:66−72.
79. Steyvers M. Morphing techniques for manipulating face images. *Behav Res Methods Instrum Comput.* 1999;31:359−369.
80. Blanz V, Vetter T. A morphable model for the synthesis of 3D faces. In: *Computer Graphics Proceedings of the SIGGRAPH'99.* 26. 1999:187−194.
81. Beumer 3rd J, Zlotolow I. Restoration of facial defects: etiology, disability, and rehabilitation. In: Beumer 3rd J, Curtis TA, Firtell DN, eds. *Maxillofacial Rehabilitation.* St Louis: CV Mosby; 1979:311−371.
82. Kaneko M, Hasegawa O. Processing of face images and its applications. *IEICE Trans Info Syst.* 1999;82-D:589−596.
83. Mehrabian A. *Silent Messages: Implicit Communication of Emotions and Attitudes.* California: Wadsworth; 1971:p76−p77.
84. Patel N, Zaveri M. 3D facial model reconstruction, expressions synthesis and animation using single frontal face image. *Signal Image Video Process.* 2013;7:889−897.
85. Ishikawa T, Morishima S, Terzopoulos D. 3 face expression estimation and generation from 2D image based on a physically constraint model. *IEICE Trans Info Syst.* 2000;EE83-D:251−258.

86. Terzopoulos D, Waters K. Analysis and synthesis of facial image sequences using physical and anatomical models. *IEEE Trans Pattern Anal Mach Intell.* 1993;15:569−579.

87. Ahn S, Ozawa S. Generating another person facial expression based on estimation of muscular contraction parameters from image. *IEICE Trans Info Syst.* 2005;J88-D-2: 2081−2089.

88. Kubon TM. Creating an adaptable anterior margin for an implant retained auricular prosthesis. *J Prosthet Dent.* 2001;86:233−240.

89. Jamayet BN, Abdullah JY, Rajion ZA, Husein A, Alam MK. New approach to 3D printing of facial prostheses using combination of open source software and conventional techniques: a case report. *Bull Tokyo Dent Coll.* 2017;58: 117−124.

90. Jordan-Ribeiro D, Carvalho LML, Vilela R, et al. Development of esthetic prosthesis for a patient with severe stigmatizing facial lesions due to cancer: a pilot study. *Support Care Cancer.* September 2018;26(9):2941−2944.

91. Goiato MC, Zucolotti BC, Mancuso DN, dos Santos DM, Pellizzer EP, Verri FR. Care and cleaning of maxillofacial prostheses. *J Craniofac Surg.* July 2010;21(4):1270−1273. https://doi.org/10.1097/SCS.0b013e3181e1b431.

92. Tessaro YV, Furuie SS, Nakamura DM. Objective color calibration for manufacturing facial prostheses. *J Biomed Opt.* February 2021;26(2). https://doi.org/10.1117/1.JBO.26.2.025002.

93. Ariani N, Visser A, Margot R, et al. Efficacy of cleansing agents in killing microorganisms in mixed species biofilms present on silicone facial prostheses—an in vitro study. *Clin Oral Invest.* 2015;19(9):2285−2293. https://doi.org/10.1007/s00784-015-1453-0.

94. Salazar-Gamarra R, Seelaus R, Lopes da Silva JV, Moreira da Silva A, Lauria Dib L. Monoscopic photogrammetry to obtain 3D models by a mobile device: a method for making facial prostheses. *J Otolaryngol Head Neck Surg.* 2016; 45:33. https://doi.org/10.1186/s40463-016-0145-3.

95. Abdo Filho RC, Oliveira TM, Lourenço Neto N, Gurgel C, Abdo RC. Reconstruction of bony facial contour deficiencies with polymethylmethacrylate implants: case report. *J Appl Oral Sci.* 2011 Jul-Aug;19(4): 426−430. https://doi.org/10.1590/S1678-77572011 000400021.

96. Tanveer W, Ridwan-Pramana A, Molinero-Mourelle P, Forouzanfar T. Systematic review of clinical applications of CAD/CAM technology for craniofacial implants placement and manufacturing of orbital prostheses. *Int J Environ Res Publ Health.* November 2021;18(21):11349. https://doi.org/10.3390/ijerph182111349.

97. Roper MB, Vissink A, Tom D, et al. Long-term treatment outcomes with zygomatic implants: a systematic review and meta-analysis. *Int J Implant Dent.* December 2023;9: 21. https://doi.org/10.1186/s40729-023-00479-x.

98. Cruz RLJ, Ross MT, Skewes J, Allenby MC, Powell SK, Woodruff MA. An advanced prosthetic manufacturing framework for economic personalised ear prostheses. *Sci Rep.* 2020;10:11453. https://doi.org/10.1038/s41598-020-67945-z.

99. Kharade P, Dholam K, Gorakh A. A technique for fabrication of cranial prostheses using high-temperature vulcanizing silicone material. *J Prosthet Dent.* July 2017; 118(1):113−115. https://doi.org/10.1016/j.prosdent.20 16.10.010.

100. Jazayeri HE, Kang S, Masri RM, et al. Advancements in craniofacial prosthesis fabrication: a narrative review of holistic treatment. *J Adv Prosthodont.* December 2018; 10(6):430−439. https://doi.org/10.4047/jap.2018.10.6. 430.

101. Alberga J, Eggels I, Visser A, et al. Outcome of implants placed to retain craniofacial prostheses − a retrospective cohort study with a follow-up of up to 30 years. *Clin Implant Dent Relat Res.* October 2022;24(5):643−654. https://doi.org/10.1111/cid.13106.

CHAPTER 12

Tracheoesophageal Prosthesis

PANKAJ PRAKASH KHARADE, MDS • RAKESH KATNA, MS, FHBNI •
GORAKH AHIRE, D. MECH

Total laryngectomy and total pharyngolaryngectomy have remarkable influence on the quality of life of the patient due to altered physiology of swallowing, respiration as well as speech.[1–3] Total laryngectomy and total pharyngolaryngectomy has been considered as the treatment of choice for advanced pharyngolaryngeal cancer (Figs. 12.1 and 12.2).[4–8]

Even though prosthesis-related complications may alter the quality of life extensively, tracheoesophageal voice is the utmost prevalent treatment preference to restore voice efficiently. Precise knowledge regarding the mechanism of action as well as clinical applications of tracheoesophageal prosthesis will help during surgical resection which in turn will facilitate the speech rehabilitation.[8–15] This technique was developed by Blom and singer in 1980 (Chart 12.1).[16]

Tracheoesophageal prosthesis is fabricated using medical-grade silicone, which is placed in the wall between the trachea and the esophagus.[17–23] The voice prosthesis does not have the characteristics of voice production itself.[24,25] The prosthesis functions by facilitating the passage of air from the lungs into the esophagus, which is later expelled through the oral cavity.[26,27] This air while traveling from esophagus to mouth creates vibration of tissues in the lower pharynx, which produces sound. This sound functions as the optional voice for patients who have undergone laryngectomy.[28–36]

Patients with tracheoesophageal puncture (TEP) can be prescribed with tracheoesophageal prosthesis for rehabilitation of speech.[37,38] As described by Singer and Blom, tracheoesophageal prosthesis is an excellent choice of treatment for voice reinstatement after total laryngectomy surgery.[39,40] During the surgical procedure, a small opening is made in the wall between the trachea and esophagus.[41,42] The tracheoesophageal prosthesis is inserted through this channel. This prosthesis has a tube-like channel in the center through which air will flow from tracheal end to esophageal end. During exhalation, air from lung can be directed through the pharynx with the assistance of this opening in the center of the prosthesis by closing off the stoma.[30,43–49] This redirection of air will aid to create vibrations during its passage through a conical segment of the esophagus. This makes speech possible for almost every patient. Tracheoesophageal puncture is classified as primary TEP and secondary TEP.[50,51]

Primary TEP is done at the time of laryngectomy, whereas secondary TEP is executed after a breach of time.[52–59] Secondary TEP has comparatively minor probabilities of fistula formation. Also wound infection is less, and it helps for 100% acquisition of fluent speech. The successful outcome of voice rehabilitation therapy subjects to employment of a suitable prosthesis which is precise. Precise measurement of dimensions across puncture site will help for expected voice rehabilitation due to meticulousness of fit of the prosthesis. It is necessary to master the procedure for precise measurement of the surgical site and fabrication of a custom-made tracheoesophageal prosthesis using medical-grade silicone for good clinical outcome and better prognosis.[60–67]

TECHNIQUE

Precise measurements of the deeply recessed stoma along with the tracheoesophageal puncture site need to be recorded (Fig.12.3). Fabricate two discs of identical diameters using modeling wax after a dialog with the surgeon as per his instructions regarding tracheoesophageal prosthesis. Fabricate a cylinder using the same wax with 4–5 mm lesser diameter.

Join the discs with cylinder in such a manner that the cylinder will remain exactly in the center of the two discs (Fig. 12.4). Get the dimensions of the wax pattern approved by the surgeon in context with tracheoesophageal prosthesis.

Investment of the wax pattern of the tracheoesophageal prosthesis in the lower part or drag of the conventional denture flasks is done using dental stone. Application of the separating medium should be done once dental stone in lower part of the flask will set.

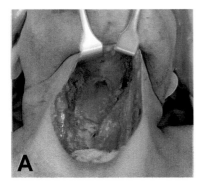
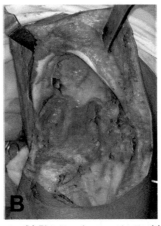
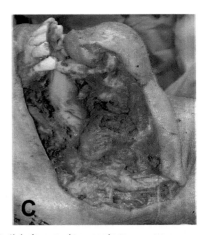

FIG. 12.1   (a) Total laryngectomy. (b) Pharyngolaryngectomy. (c) Partial pharyngolaryngectomy.

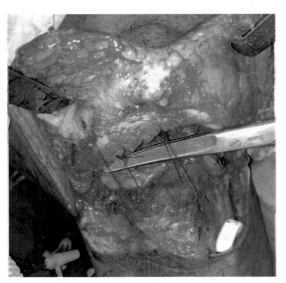
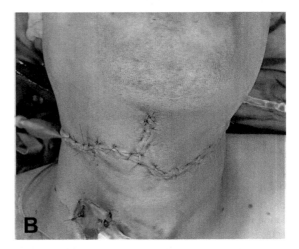

FIG. 12.2   (a) Reconstruction after total laryngectomy. (b) Surgical site closure after total laryngectomy.

Fit upper part of the flask, i.e., cope with the lower part of the flask. Pour dental stone in upper part of the flask followed by closure of the lid of the flask. Once dental stone is set completely, put the flasks in the dewaxing unit and carry out dewaxing in conventional manner (Fig. 12.5). Paint a thin layer of paraffin xylene solution after removal of the clay and allow it to dry. Solution of paraffin and xylene will work as a separating medium for silicone. Cut the suitable quantity of high-temperature vulcanizing (HTV) medical-grade silicone material MDX 4-4515, which is available in slab form (Fig. 12.6). Place small pieces of silicone in the hollowed out portion in the flask and close the flasks

under the force of few thousands pounds. The flasks should be tightened to close both parts in proper manner. Curing of the closed flask will be carried out in hot air over at a temperature of 235°C for 1.5 h and at a temperature of 150°C for 4.5 h. After completion of curing, cooling of the flasks under cold water should be done.

Open the flasks carefully and recover the prosthesis. Modify the diameter of hole in the prosthesis as per instructions of the surgeon so that the air directed to the pharynx will have minimum resistance (Fig. 12.7). Modification of the diameter in a tapering manner from one end to other end is done for safety purpose.

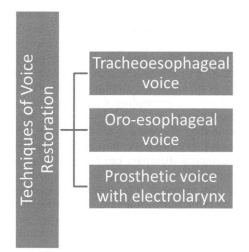

CHART 12.1 Techniques of voice restoration.

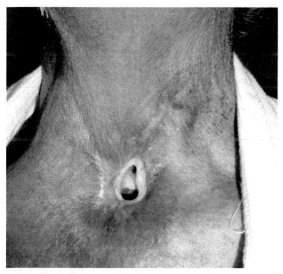

FIG. 12.3 Stoma showing the tracheoesophageal puncture.

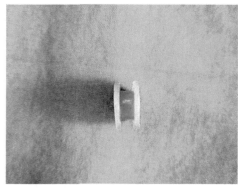

FIG. 12.4 Tracheoesophageal prosthesis in wax.

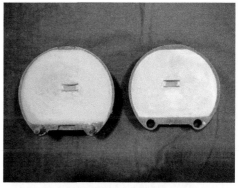

FIG. 12.5 Flask after dewaxing.

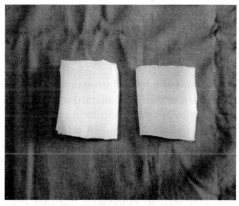

FIG. 12.6 HTV medical-grade silicone.

Finishing and polishing of the tracheoesophageal prosthesis is carried out. Polishing the cylindrical portion of the prosthesis effectively will help for smooth insertion through the tracheoesophageal puncture (Fig. 12.8). Sterilization of the prosthesis by autoclaving or with ethylene oxide is followed by adequate ventilation.

Suitable dimensions of the prosthesis are indispensable for successful speech outcome, and it is possible to achieve with the aid of custom made tracheoesophageal prosthesis.[68–71] The suitable size-related parameters for the prosthesis are still needed to be finalized precisely for better tracheoesophageal voice restoration. Because studies have shown that tracheoesophageal prosthesis length reduces over time for secondary punctures and it is necessary to make

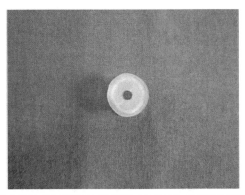

FIG. 12.7 Tracheoesophageal prosthesis showing channel for air passage.

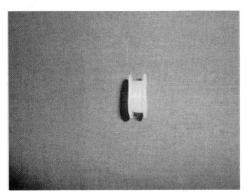

FIG. 12.8 Final polished prosthesis.

adjustments in coordination with a speech language pathologist.[72,73] There are a clinically significant circumstances, which have shown variations in prosthesis length.[74] Variation in the length is associated with an amplified risk toward necessity of repuncturing. Frequent removal of an implanted tracheoesophageal prosthesis followed by concurrent replacement of a new prosthesis can be achieved safely as well as competently with the help of retrograde technique. Retrograde technique helps to maintain the patency of the existing tracheoesophageal tract as well as restored voice.[41] Long-standing tracheoesophageal prosthesis may lead to esophageal mucosal bridge, which can be managed successfully using a scissor-type dissection knife. Apart from that, nowadays tracheoesophageal puncture is being performed as office-based procedure more frequently than operating room–based tracheoesophageal prosthesis. Apart from that, anterograde techniques have also been developed, which can be used in an effective manner

to achieve better speech outcome with the prosthesis. Studies have shown that the dimensions-related outcome for tracheoesophageal prosthesis is better in office-based procedure as compared with operating room–based procedure. The most probable reason for such type of outcome is the minor degree of inflammation of the tracheoesophageal partition wall in the office-based procedure.

The procedure of placement as well as retrieval of the prosthesis is performed under local pharyngealanesthesia.[75] Intravenous diazepam can be given to patients who are reluctant for the procedure due to nervousness. The pharyngoesophageal segment is visualized by using flexible esophagogastroscope in the upper segment of the esophagus. The site of placement of tracheoesophageal prosthesis is determined by transillumination. For precise visualization, endoscopic assessment is preferred. Also the precise site of puncture is confirmed by endoscopic examination. It is important to avoid injuries to posterior wall of the esophagus. Long-term use of tracheoesophageal prosthesis may lead to scar formation, which can affect the replacement of new prosthesis. Radiotherapy is not a contraindication for placement of tracheoesophageal prosthesis. But the timing of placement of tracheoesophageal prosthesis is important. The prosthesis should be place either during the primary surgery or few days before the commencement of radiation therapy. If it is placed after primary surgery, after commencement of radiation therapy or laryngectomy with flap reconstruction, prognosis of the treatment will be inferior.

The end of the prosthesis, which has smaller diameter, is placed toward esophagus from safety orientation.[76] Flanges of the prosthesis in the shape of discs generate effective seal and stop periprosthetic leakage. Flange of the prosthesis also avoids thorough intrusion of the prosthesis into the esophagus. Tracheoesophageal prosthesis is harmless and simple procedure of voice rehabilitation, and comparatively highly acceptable treatment option by patients. This treatment is more preferred by patients for rehabilitation of voice as compared with artificial larynx (electrolarynx) and esophageal speech.

Several clinical studies have been conducted regarding tracheoesophageal prosthesis.

Secondary tracheoesophageal prosthesis placement has the following advantages:

a. Clinical procedure can be performed without general anesthesia or target controlled infusion.
b. Traditional TEP set can be used.
c. This procedure is minimally traumatic.
d. This procedure doesn't require dilators.

e. Less probability of complications.

f. Voice prosthesis placement is possible after previous TEP closure.

g. Voice rehabilitation is comparatively faster.

It has been witnessed that secondary TEP is a safe as well as effective procedure to be executed in an office setting in a hospital, if that setup has easy availability of material if respiratory issues happen. Additionally, TEP technique may also be employed in patients with laryngectomy devoid of any contraindication to general anesthesia as well as rigid esophagoscopy to reduce the cost of tracheoesophageal puncture and voice prosthesis placement. Prosthetic voice restoration after total (pharyngo)-laryngectomy may be considered as a dependable option of relieving voice disability and improving the quality of life for the patients after laryngectomy. Failure of seal through or around the prosthesis is the most recurrent as well as simple complication. It has been observed that this procedure leads to minimal serious complications. It is necessary to deliberate specifically about every case so as to fulfill the characteristic outcome of the tracheoesophageal prosthesis in accordance with patient's expectations.[77]

Voice onset time is one of the fundamental parameters to perform acoustic analysis. It can be used as an important parameter to assess the differences in voice and articulation after total laryngectomy once patient's speech is restored by placement of tracheoesophageal prosthesis. Few studies have shown that there is absence of statistically significant difference in the articulation of voiceless plosives except "ka" sound when compared between control group and patients who have undergone total laryngectomy.[78] Additional research with precise planning is necessary to standardize the measured values and their applications in clinical practice by recruiting large sample size of patients and assessing several indicators related to characteristics such as quality and intelligibility of voice.

SUMMARY

Successful voice rehabilitation treatment depends on employment of a suitable tracheoesophageal prosthesis with accurate measurements. This technique is effective in precise fabrication of tracheoesophageal prosthesis in agreement with the surgeon and speech therapist toward natural phrasing of voice in addition to acoustically normal speech. Further studies with a larger sample size and a lengthier follow-up period are indispensable to approve the promising results of tracheoesophageal prosthesis.

REFERENCES

1. Singer MI, Blom ED. An endoscopic technique for the restoration of voice after laryngectomy. *Ann Otol Rhino Laryngol.* 1980;89:529–533.
2. Emerick KS, Tomycz L, Bradford CR, et al. Primary versus secondary tracheoesophageal puncture in salvage total laryngectomy following chemoradiation. *Otol -Head Neck Surg.* 2009;140(3):386–390. https://doi.org/10.1016/j.otohns.2008.10.018. PMID: 19248948.
3. Hotz MA. Success and predictability of provoxprosthesis voice rehabilitation. *Arch Otol Head Neck Surg.* 2002;128:687–691.
4. Light J, Silverman SI, Garfinkel L. The use of an intraoral training aid in the speech rehabilitation of laryngectomy patients. *J Prosthet Dent.* April 1976;35(4):430–440.
5. Murry T. Biophysical requirements for new and projected procedures and devices for voice rehabilitation after total laryngectomy. *Can J Otolaryngol.* 1975;4(4):571–578.
6. Bertl K, Zatorska B, Leonhard M, et al. Oral microbial colonization in laryngectomized patients as a possible cofactor of biofilm formation on their voice prostheses. *J Clin Periodontol.* September 2013;40(9):833–840.
7. Yang S, Bunn C, Kramer S, Thorpe E. The dynamic tracheoesophageal prosthesis length. *J Voice.* July 2023;37(4):633.e1–633.e6.
8. King AI, Stout BE, Ashby JK. The Stout prosthesis: an alternate means of restoring speech in selected laryngectomy patients. *Ear Nose Throat J.* February 2003;82(2):113–116, 118.
9. Etienne H, Fabre D, Gomez Caro A, et al. Tracheal replacement. *Eur Respir J.* February 14, 2018;51(2):1702211.
10. Madi MY, Peller M, Presti M, Bazarbashi AN. Endoscopic management of tracheoesophageal prosthesis-induced esophageal mucosal bridge. *Endoscopy.* December 2023;55(S 01):E625–E626.
11. Ghevariya V, Bansal R. Tracheoesophageal voice prosthesis: endoscopic appearance. *Gastrointest Endosc.* January 2015;81(1):236. discussion 236–7.
12. Burks CA, Feng AL, Deschler DG. Management of the embedded tracheoesophageal prosthesis: retrograde removal and replacement. *Ann Otol Rhinol Laryngol.* July 2021;130(7):840–842.
13. Kim HS, Khemasuwan D, Diaz-Mendoza J, Mehta AC. Management of tracheo-oesophageal fistula in adults. *Eur Respir Rev.* November 5, 2020;29(158):200094.
14. Apert V, Carsuzaa F, Tonnerre D, et al. Speech restoration with tracheoesophageal prosthesis after total laryngectomy: an observational study of vocal results, complications and quality of life. *Eur Ann Otorhinolaryngol Head Neck Dis.* March 2022;139(2):73–76.
15. Ricci E, Riva G, Dagna F, Seglie E, Cavalot AL. In-clinic secondary tracheoesophageal puncture and voice prosthesis placement in laryngectomees. *Eur Ann Otorhinolaryngol Head Neck Dis.* October 2018;135(5):349–352.

16. Babin E, Heutte N, Grandazzi G, Prévost V, Robard L. Quality of life and supportive care in head and neck cancers. *Bull Cancer*. 2014;101:505–510.

17. Coul BMRO, Hilgers FJM, Balm AJM, et al. A decade of postlaryngectomy vocal rehabilitation in 318 patients: a single institution's experience with consistent application of provox indwelling voice prostheses. *Arch Otolaryngol Neck Surg*. 2000;126:1320–1328.

18. Finizia C, Bergman B. Health-related quality of life in patients with laryngeal cancer: a post-treatment comparison of different modes of communication. *Laryngoscope*. 2001;111:918–923.

19. Jacobson BH, Johnson A, Grywalski C, et al. The voice handicap index (VHI): development and validation. *Am J Speech Lang Pathol*. 1997;66–70.

20. Woisard V, Bodin S, Puech M. The voice handicap index: impact of the translation in French on the validation. *Rev Laryngol Otol Rhinol*. 2004;125:307–312.

21. Ioannidis JPA. The proposal to lower p value thresholds to .005. *JAMA*. 2018;319:1429–1430.

22. Laccourreye O, Fakhry N, Franco-Vidal V, et al. Statistics in scientific articles published in the European annals of otorhinolaryngology head and neck diseases. *Eur Ann Otorhinolaryngol Head Neck Dis*. 2020;10:1016.

23. Terada T, Saeki N, Toh K, et al. Voice rehabilitation with provox2™ voice prosthesis following total laryngectomy for laryngeal and hypopharyngeal carcinoma. *Auris Nasus Larynx*. 2007;34:65–71.

24. Laccourreye O, Ménard M, Crevier-Buchman L, Couloigner V, Brasnu D. In situ lifetime, causes for replacement, and complications of the provox™ voice prosthesis. *Laryngoscope*. 1997;107:527–530.

25. Yenigun A, Eren SB, Ozkul MH, Tugrul S, Meric A. Factors influencing the longevity and replacement frequency of provox voice prostheses. *Singapore Med J*. 2018;56:632–636.

26. Guibert M, Lepage B, Woisard V, et al. Quality of life in patients treated for advanced hypopharyngeal or laryngeal cancer. *Eur Ann Otorhinolaryngol Head Neck Dis*. 2011;128:218–223.

27. Pereira da Silva A, Feliciano T, Vaz Freitas S, et al. Quality of life in patients submitted to total laryngectomy. *J Voice*. 2015;29:382–388.

28. Schindler A, Mozzanica F, Ginocchio D, et al. Voice-related quality of life in patients after total and partial laryngectomy. *Auris Nasus Larynx*. 2012;39:77–83.

29. Metreau A, Louvel G, Godey B, Le Clech G, Jegoux F. Long-term functional and quality of life evaluation after treatment for advanced pharyngolaryngeal carcinoma. *Head Neck*. 2014;36:1604–1610.

30. Hilgers FJM, Balm AJM. Long-term results of vocal rehabilitation after total laryngectomy with the low-resistance, indwelling provox™ voice prosthesis system. *Clin Otolaryngol*. 1993;18:517–523.

31. Choussy O, Hibon R, Mardion NB, Dehesdin D. Management of voice prosthesis leakage with blom-singer large esophage and tracheal flange voice prostheses. *Eur Ann Otorhinolaryngol Head Neck Dis*. 2013;130:49–53.

32. Rossi VC, Fernandes FL, Ferreira MAA, et al. Larynx cancer: quality of life and voice after treatment. *Braz J Otorhinolaryngol*. 2014;80:403–408.

33. Ackerstaff AH, Hilgers FJM, Meeuwis CA, et al. Multi-institutional assessment of the provox 2 voice prosthesis. *Arch Otolaryngol Neck Surg*. 1999;125:167–173.

34. Bozec A, Poissonnet G, Chamorey E, et al. Results of vocal rehabilitation using tracheoesophageal voice prosthesis after total laryngectomy and their predictive factors. *Eur Arch Oto-Rhino-Laryngol*. 2010;267:751–758.

35. Chone CT, Spina AL, Crespo AN, Gripp FM. Speech rehabilitation after total laryngectomy: long-term results with indwelling voice prosthesis Blom-Singer. *Rev Bras Otorrinolaringol*. 2005;71:504–509.

36. Schuster M, Lohscheller J, Hoppe U, et al. Voice handicap of laryngectomees with tracheoesophageal speech. *Folia Phoniatr Logop*. 2004;56:62–67.

37. Lundström E, Hammarberg B, Munck-Wikland E. Voice handicap and health-related quality of life in laryngectomees: assessments with the use of VHI and EORTC questionnaires. *Folia Phoniatr Logop*. 2009;61:83–92.

38. Kazi R, Cordova JD, Singh A, et al. Voice-related quality of life in laryngectomees: assessment using the VHI and V-RQOL symptom scales. *J Voice*. 2007;21:728–734.

39. Terrell JE, Ronis DL, Fowler KE, et al. Clinical predictors of quality of life in patients with head and neck cancer. *Arch Otolaryngol Head Neck Surg*. 2004;130:401–408.

40. Pruyn JFA, Jong PC, Bosman LJ, et al. Psychosocial aspects of head and neck cancer—a review of the literature. *Clin Otolaryngol*. 2009;11:469–474.

41. Robinson RA, Simms VA, Ward EC, et al. Total laryngectomy with primary tracheoesophageal puncture: intraoperative versus delayed voice prosthesis placement. *Head Neck*. 2017;39:1138–1144.

42. Bach KK, Postma GN, Koufman JA. In-office tracheoesophageal puncture using transnasal esophagoscopy. *Laryngoscope*. 2003;113:173–176.

43. Brown DH, Hilgers FJ, Irish JC, Balm AJ. Post-laryngectomy voice rehabilitation: state of the art at the millennium. *World J Surg*. 2003;27:824–831.

44. Zenga J, Goldsmith T, Bunting G, Deschler DG. State of the art: rehabilitation of speech and swallowing after total laryngectomy. *Oral Oncol*. 2018;86:38–47.

45. Neumann A, Schultz-Coulon HJ. Management of complications after prosthetic voice rehabilitation. *HNO*. 2000;48:508–516.

46. Gitomer SA, Hutcheson KA, Christianson BL, et al. Influence of timing, radiation, and reconstruction on complications and speech outcomes with tracheoesophageal puncture. *Head Neck*. 2016;38:1765–1771.

47. Andrews JC, Mickel RA, Hanson DG, Monahan GP, Ward PH. Major complications following tracheoesophageal puncture for voice rehabilitation. *Laryngoscope*. 1987;97:562–567.

48. Izdebski K, Reed CG, Ross JC, Hilsinger Jr RL. Problems with tracheoesophageal fistula voice restoration in totally laryngectomized patients. A review of 95 cases. *Arch Otolaryngol Head Neck Surg*. 1994;120:840–845.

49. Manni JJ, Van den Broek P. Surgical and prosthesis-related complications using the gronin- gen button voice prosthesis. *Clin Otolaryngol Allied Sci.* 1990;15:515–523.

50. Silver FM, Gluckmann JL, Donegan JO. Operative complications of tracheoesophageal puncture. *Laryngoscope.* 1985; 95:1360–1362.

51. Wang RC, Bui T, Sauris E, et al. Long- term problems in patients with tracheoesophageal puncture. *Arch Otolaryngol Head Neck Surg.* 1991;17:1273–1276.

52. Daniilidis I, Nikolaou A, Markou C, Kotsani A. Voice rehabilitation after total laryngectomy. Voice prostheses or esophageal replacement voice? *Laryngo-Rhino-Otol.* 1998; 77:89–92.

53. Maddalena H, Pfrang H, Schohe R, Zenner HP. Speech intelligibility and psychosocial adaptation in various voice rehabilitation methods following laryngectomy. *Laryngo-Rhino-Otol.* 1991;70:562–567.

54. Edge S, Byrd DR, Compton CC, Greene F, Trotti A. *AJCC Cancer Staging Manual.* 7th ed. New York, NY: Springer; 2010.

55. Greene F, Balch CM, Fleming ID, April F. *AJCC Cancer Staging Manual.* 6th ed. NewYork, NY: Springer; 2003.

56. Scherl C, Mantsopoulos K, Semrau S, et al. Management of advanced hypopharyngeal and laryngeal cancer with and without cartilage invasion. *Auris Nasus Larynx.* 2017;44: 333–339.

57. Hoebers F, Rios E, Troost E, et al. Definitive radiation therapy for treatment of laryngeal carcinoma: impact of local relapse on outcome and implications for treatment strategies. *Strahlenther Onkol.* 2013;189:834–841.

58. Mucha-Małecka A, Chrostowska A, Urbanek K, Małecki K. Prognostic factors in patients with T1 glottic cancer treated with radiotherapy. *Strahlenther Onkol.* 2019;195:792–804.

59. Dinapoli N, Parrilla C, Galli J, et al. Multidisciplinary approach in the treatment of T1 glottic cancer. The role of patient preference in a homogenous patient population. *Strahlenther Onkol.* 2010;186:607–613.

60. Uno T, Itami J, Kotaka K, Toriyama M. Radical radiotherapy for T3 laryngeal cancers. *Strahlenther Onkol.* 1996;172:422–426.

61. Herrmann IF. New aspects in the therapy of laryngeal tumors from the surgeon's viewpoint. *Strahlenther Onkol.* 1987;163:511–518.

62. Garth RJN, McRae A, Rhŷs Evans PH. Tracheo-esophageal puncture: a review of problems and complications. *J Laryngol Otol.* 1991;105:750–754.

63. Petersen JF, Lansaat L, Timmermans AJ, et al. Postlaryngectomy prosthetic voice rehabilitation outcomes in a consectutive cohort of 232 patients over a 13 year period. *Head Neck.* 2019;41:623–631.

64. Kress P, Schäfer P, Schwerdtfeger FP. The custom-fit voice prosthesis, for treatment of periprothetic leakage after tracheoesophageal voice restoration. *Laryngo-Rhino-Otol.* 2006;85:496–500.

65. Lewin JS, Hutcheson KA, Barringer DA, et al. Customization of the voice prosthesis to prevent leakage from the enlarged tracheoesophageal puncture: results of a prospective trial. *Laryngoscope.* 2012;122:1767–1772.

66. Al Kadah B, Papaspyrou G, Schneider M, Schick B. Novel modification of voice prosthesis. *Eur Arch Oto-Rhino-Laryngol.* 2016;273:697–702.

67. Remacle MJ, Declaye XJ. Gax-collagen injection to correct an enlarged tracheoesophageal fistula for a vocal prosthesis. *Laryngoscope.* 1988;98:1350–1352.

68. Lorenz KJ. The development and treatment of periprosthetic leakage after prosthetic voice restoration: a literature review and personal experience. Part II: conservative and surgical management. *Eur Arch Oto-Rhino-Laryngol.* 2015; 272:661–672.

69. Geyer M, Tan N, Ismail-Koch H, Puxeddu R. A simple closure technique for reversal of tracheoesophageal puncture. *Am J Otolaryngol.* 2011;32:627–630.

70. Hilgers FJM, Balm AJM, Gregor RT. Voice rehabilitation after laryngectomy with the provox voice prosthesis. Surgical and technical aspects II. *HNO.* 1995;43:261–267.

71. Lorenz KJ, Kraft K, Graf F, Pröpper C, Steinestel K. Importance of cellular tight junction complexes in the development of periprosthetic leakage after prosthetic voice rehabilitation. *HNO.* 2015;63:171–172, 174–178.

72. Pattani KM, Morgan M, Nathan CO. Reflux as a cause of tracheoesophageal puncture failure. *Laryngoscope.* 2009; 119:121–125.

73. Kummer P, Schuster CM, Rosanowski F. Prosthetic voice rehabilitation after laryngectomy. Failures and complications after previous radiation therap. *HNO.* 2006;54: 315–322.

74. Trudeau MD, Schuller DE, Hall DA. The effects of radiation on tracheoesophageal puncture. A retrospective study. *Arch Otol Head Neck Surg.* 1989;115:1116–1117.

75. Onbasi Y, Lettmaier S, Hecht M, et al. Is there a patient population with squamous cell carcinoma of the head and neck region who might benefit from de-intensification of postoperative radiotherapy? A monocentric retrospective analysis of a previously defined low-risk patient population treated with standard-of-care radiotherapy. *Strahlenther Onkol.* 2019;195:482–495.

76. Ursino S, Cocuzza P, Seccia V, et al. Pattern of dysphagia after swallowing-sparing intensity-modulated radiotherapy (IMRT) of head and neck cancers: results of a mono-institutional prospective study. *Strahlenther Onkol.* 2018;194:1114–1123.

77. Carpén T, Saarilahti K, Haglund C, et al. Tumor volume as a prognostic marker in p16-positive and p16-negative oropharyngeal cancer patients treated with definitive intensity-modulated radiotherapy. *Strahlenther Onkol.* 2018;194:759–770.

78. Azizli E, Alkan Z, Koçak I, Yiğit Ö. Voice onset time in patients using speech prosthesis after total laryngectomy. *J Voice.* November 2022;36(6):879.e1–879.e4.

FURTHER READING

1. Dumbrigue HB, Arcuri MR, LaVelle WE, Ceynar KJ. Polydimethyl siloxane materials in maxillofacial prosthetics: evaluation and comparison of physical properties. *J Prosthet Dent.* 1998;79:229–231.

CHAPTER 15

Regeneration of Hard and Soft Tissues

YASIR DILSHAD SIDDIQUI, BDS, MSC, PHD

Tissue regeneration and repair of oral and maxillofacial regions are the treatment of choice in various dental diseases. Traditionally, this treatment includes techniques of replacing missing or dead tissue with autologous grafts, which has been widely used in practice, but still has shortcomings such as chances to get infection and rejection after procedure that raise serious concerns for the operators and patients. Recent advancement that brought a unique concept of regenerative medicine utilizes self-healing ability of individuals along with tissue engineering, which aims to regenerate and repair compromised tissue and reverse condition from disease to health.[1]

Tissue engineering based on three components: (1) presence of stem/progenitor cells that has capability to differentiate into many cell types and synthesize new tissue matrix; (2) growth factors that promote and facilitate the tissue healing/regeneration; (3) the scaffold, required for the cellular differentiation, multiplications, and biosynthesis of extracellular matrix (ECM).[1]

Altogether, these components replace the damaged tissue and reverse function to original state.[2,3] It can be easily understood by conductive and inductive methods where polymeric barrier membrane seals off the intended area of tissue regeneration and facilitates growth of specific cells/tissues.[4] For instance, application of barrier membranes enhances the growth of periodontal supporting cells while preventing gingival epithelial cells and connective tissue cells from entering the area of regeneration,[5] whereas inductive method involves growth factors that send biological messages to cells near the site of damage to facilitate the formation of new tissue.[4] For instance, morphogenic proteins (BMPs) as growth factor trigger cells to form new bone at places that usually are unable to regenerate.[6] This is possible through polymeric carriers transporting inductive factors, to the desired site of regeneration.[4] Transplantation of cells is another approach where cells are cultivated in a laboratory and transplanted into the desired target. This method requires interaction and cooperation between a doctor, engineer, and a cell biologist.[4] Numerous research has been carried out using stem cells, bioactive agents, and distinctive scaffold materials such as natural and synthetic polymers[7–11] and ceramics,[12] attempted to regenerate dental tissues specifically guided tissue regeneration,[13] pulp–dentin complex regeneration,[7] bone and cartilage tissue regeneration,[4,14] and tooth regeneration.[15,16]

BONE REGENERATION

Bone defects of the maxilla and mandible result from injuries, infections, and birth defects, which pose challenging situation for maxillofacial surgeons attempting to gain comprehensive regeneration and functional restoration.[4] Conventional surgical methods such as autografts, allografts, and synthetic biomaterials are the treatment of choices but still have limitations such as tissue rejection and infection. Bone tissue engineering technique emerged as a prominent area of research to confront the inadequacies of conventional methods. In this, autologous bone grafts conditioned by adequate vascularization supplied with stem cells mainly MSCs originating from bone marrow or adipose/dental tissues provide a solution for reconstructing large size bone defects.[4,17] MSCs are considered primary component in bone regeneration due to their ability to induce bone regeneration by mimicking biological processes,[18] and to differentiate into bone forming cells such as osteoblasts that initiate the process of mineralization. Other methods of tissue engineering may be employed for successful bone regeneration such as conductive (i.e., barrier membrane), inductive (i.e., BMPs) and cell transplantation (i.e., MSCs).[4] Two schemes are used for cell transplantation: (1) MSCs are directly transplanted to the defect site and combine with scaffolds, (2) MSCs isolated from patients, cultured ex vivo and seeded onto suitable internal 3D scaffolds, which, in controlled culture conditions, proliferate and predifferentiate.[19] Other studies reported suitable results when DPSCs with collagen sponge scaffolds are fabricated in the human mandible.[20] Recently, the use of human gingival stem cells (GMSCs) complexed with 3D scaffolds was promising to provide a new therapeutic approach to improving bone tissue regeneration and healing of cranial bones.[21]

CARTILAGE REGENERATION

The temporomandibular joint (TMJ) is an articulation formed between the temporal bone and mandibular condyle, which is commonly affected by many diseases, such as osteoarthritis that can lead cartilage destruction.[4] Cartilage is devoid of blood vessels and has limited capacity for intrinsic healing and repair. Many surgical approaches are being used for TMJ disorders, but most are assertive and dangerous for the patient. From simple arthrocentesis to joint replacement, they cannot produce integral regeneration.[1] Recent advancement in tissue engineering making it possible to make integral regeneration using cells seeded with biocompatible scaffold, bioactive agents, and ability of host to accept the scaffolds considered promising to facilitate tissue regeneration.[22] Both natural and synthetic polymers can be used for the regeneration of soft cartilage tissue such as collagen, gelatin, hyaluronic acid, fibrin, silk, agarose, polylactic acid, or polyvinyl alcohol, which are suitable materials that can be used in cartilage tissue engineering,[21] whereas stem cells extracted from synovial capsules surrounding the joints have been proven favorable for generating neocartilage. In recent studies, it was demonstrated that human DPSCs in porous chitosan scaffolds are useful for regenerating chondrogenic cells.[23]

TOOTH REGENERATION

Regeneration of the whole tooth is a vastly improving area of research that represents the final objective of tooth tissue engineering.[1] Multiple studies have been performed with varying success in this area of study. The focus is to replace missing teeth with newly regenerated teeth using patients' own stem cells that could eliminate the risk of rejection as the new tooth would not be a foreign tissue.[24] Young et al. were the first to successfully regenerate tooth structure from third molar tooth buds.[25] Biodegradable scaffolds containing pig tooth bud cells were transplanted into rats, and 20–30 weeks later, defined tooth structure was present, although the size of the tooth was very small.[25] Recently, Wu et al., demonstrated that in pigs, tooth-like organs with dentin and enamel can be developed by seeding the reaggregated germ cells on biodegradable polymers and grafting cell aggregates to

subcutaneous tissue.[26] In another study, autologous transplantation of a bioengineered tooth germ in a postnatal canine model has reported functional tooth restoration.[1] This represented a relevant advancement in whole-organ replacement therapy as well as a practical model for future attempts.[27] There are many complex factors and challenges that still exist such as how to program the stem and progenitor cells to develop into tooth-specific cell types.[28,29] Research is currently progressing toward this desired outcome.

PERIODONTAL TISSUE REGENERATION

Periodontitis is an inflammatory disease that leads to destruction of soft and hard tissues around teeth.[30] Regeneration of tissues damaged by periodontitis has long been considered a key goal of periodontal treatment. Various products and techniques have been explored to achieve periodontal regeneration, and these have generally involved various membranes, and implantation of bone substitutes into periodontal defects. Yet, despite efforts to improve periodontal regeneration, each of these procedures remains technique sensitive and clinically unpredictable. Two major strategies for periodontal regeneration have been outlined: guided tissue regeneration (GTR) and tissue engineering.[31] GTR is a regenerative technique utilizing a barrier membrane, and their role is to prevent ingrowth of epithelial cells into the bone defect. These membranes are classified into nonabsorbable and absorbable membranes category.[32,33] In periodontal regeneration, the tissue engineering strategy may take one of two approaches: scaffold-free or scaffold-based.[34] The scaffold-free approach uses cells or cell aggregates transplanted onto the wound area with no carrier cell. Whereas cell sheet technique has been developed as a scaffold-free strategy for cell delivery and has been tried in various tissue regenerations, including for periodontal tissue.[35] Cell sheet engineering aims to prevent ECM degradation by isolating cells using enzymes and completely retaining them to ensure normal cell function.[35] In animal studies, periodontal regeneration was effective when SCs were implanted into periodontal defects.[34] Tissue engineering approaches may be improved by the use of bioactive molecules or growth factors. A study by Nevins et al. concluded that purified recombinant human platelet-derived growth factor BB (rhPDGF-BB) demonstrated effective periodontal regeneration.[36] Periodontal ligament stem cells (PDLSCs) considered as subpopulation of the mesenchymal stem cells. Successful periodontal regeneration was noted after transplantation of periodontal ligament stem cells in surgically created bone defect in rats.[37] Recently, specialized proresolving mediators (SPMs) such as resolvin, lipoxin, and maresins have been studied for periodontal regeneration. These SPMs promote resolution of inflammation by regulating polymorphonuclear leukocyte (PMN). Besides, SPMs facilitate stem cell activations presumably alveolar bone stem/progenitor cells and periodontal ligament stem/progenitor cells, and induce regeneration of periodontal tissues.[38]

DENTIN AND DENTAL PULP REGENERATION

For healthy and vital teeth, the hard dentin shell provides a strong physical framework for the soft pulp core inside. Dentin and pulp have to be understood as a physiological unity. Anatomically and functionally closely interlinked, the dentin—pulp complex counters external impacts and reacts sensitively to all kinds of stimuli, e.g., caries or trauma.[39] Many in vivo and in vitro studies have successfully engineered dentin and dental pulp tissue. Dental caries or trauma causes damage to the dentin followed by necrosis of dental pulp. There are many approaches to engineer lost dentin and pulp such as specific bone morphogenetic proteins can be utilized, allowing the newly synthesized odontoblasts to form new dentin. A study conducted by M. Nakashima concluded that reparative dentin can be developed in the cavity of amputated pulp capped with a bone morphogenic protein.[40] Thus, BMP plays a tremendous role and could be the primary inductive factor in odontoblast differentiation.

The earliest research on pulp tissue regeneration was performed by Nygaard-Ostby et al., who intentionally overinstrumented breaching apical foramina to induce bleeding from the periapical area into the root canal, followed by a short obturation to allow tissue growth into the canal space. The histological examination of the extracted teeth revealed that fibrous connective tissue and cellular cementum formed in the canal space.[41,42] Recently, Siddiqui et al. demonstrated successful vital pulp-like tissue regeneration and bacterial load reduction in contaminated root canals following topical resolvin D2 (RvD2) treatment. Vital pulp-like tissue was regenerated with significant increases in DMP1 expression and mineralization. The net outcome of RvD2-augmented root canal therapy was continued calcification around root apex, prevention, and reversal of periapical periodontitis.[43] Periapical tissues contain a higher concentration of stem cells compared with the blood from the systemic circulation.[43] Thus,

instrumentation beyond the apex induces bleeding inside canals and formation of blood clot creates a 3-D fibrin scaffold that may contain stem cells derived from peripheral blood, periodontal ligament, bone marrow, granulation tissue, or periapical lesions.[44]

CONCLUDING REMARKS AND FUTURE PERSPECTIVES

In recent decades, major progress has been achieved in regenerative medicine and in tissue engineering, contributing pivotal roles in various clinical applications. Tissue engineering based on stem or progenitor cells is the promising approach to restore and maintain the integrity of dental and maxillofacial tissues.[1] Clinical applications of dental SCs have proven their utility and benefits over conventional methods that possess risk of transplant rejection. Regeneration of the entire tooth using SCs is the principal objective for replacing dental implants and other prosthesis, attempting to regenerate natural teeth in the near future that impacts on the quality of dental health. Future studies are needed to develop suitable delivery devices that can successfully deliver cells to the sites of interest. Further, large-scale collaborative efforts between bioengineers, nanotechnologists, cell biologists, and molecular biologists are needed for the well-controlled, favorable, and cost-effective outcome of tissue engineering approach.

REFERENCES

1. Matichescu A, Ardelean LC, Rusu L-C, et al. Advanced biomaterials and techniques for oral tissue engineering and regeneration—a review. *Materials.* 2020;13(22):5303.
2. Upadhyay R. Role of biological scaffolds, hydro gels and stem cells in tissue regeneration therapy. *Adv Tissue Eng Regen Med Open Access.* 2017;2(1):00020.
3. Zhang K, Wang S, Zhou C, et al. Advanced smart biomaterials and constructs for hard tissue engineering and regeneration. *Bone Res.* 2018;6(1):1–15.
4. Kaigler D, Mooney D. Tissue engineering's impact on dentistry. *J Dent Educ.* 2001;65(5):456–462.
5. Nyman S, Lindhe J, Karring T, Rylander H. New attachment following surgical treatment of human periodontal disease. *J Clin Periodontol.* 1982;9(4):290–296.
6. Urist MR. Bone: formation by autoinduction. *Science.* 1965;150(3698):893–899.
7. Huang GT. Pulp and dentin tissue engineering and regeneration: current progress. *Regen Med.* 2009;4(5):697–707.
8. Raz M, Moztarzadeh F, Shokrgozar MA, Azami M, Tahriri M. Development of biomimetic gelatin—chitosan/hydroxyapatite nanocomposite via double diffusion method for biomedical applications. *Int J Mater Res.* 2014;105(5):493–501.

9. Naghavi Alhosseini S, Moztarzadeh F, Kargozar S, Dodel M, Tahriri M. Development of polyvinyl alcohol fibrous biodegradable scaffolds for nerve tissue engineering applications: in vitro study. *Int J Polym Mat Polym Biomater*. 2015;64(9):474−480.

10. Fahimipour F, Rasoulianboroujeni M, Dashtimoghadam E, et al. 3D printed TCP-based scaffold incorporating VEGF-loaded PLGA microspheres for craniofacial tissue engineering. *Dent Mater*. 2017;33(11):1205−1216.

11. Tahriri M, Moztarzadeh F, Hresko K, Khoshroo K, Tayebi L. Biodegradation properties of PLGA/nano-fluorhydroxyapatite composite microsphere-sintered scaffolds. *Dent Mater*. 2016;1(32):e49−e50.

12. Onomura A, Mizuno D, Hisada A, et al. Differential effect of scaffold shape on dentin regeneration. *Ann Biomed Eng*. 2010;38(4):1664−1671.

13. Goyal B, Tewari S, Duhan J, Sehgal P. Comparative evaluation of platelet-rich plasma and guided tissue regeneration membrane in the healing of apicomarginal defects: a clinical study. *J Endod*. 2011;37(6):773−780.

14. McGuire TP, Rittenberg BN, Baker GI. Restorative dentistry-TMD special report-conclusion-surgery for disorders of the temporomandibular joint. *Oral Health*. 2005; 95(7):51−66.

15. Ohara T, Itaya T, Usami K, et al. Evaluation of scaffold materials for tooth tissue engineering. *J Biomed Mater Res*. 2010;94(3):800−805.

16. Lim J-Y, Yi T, Choi J-S, et al. Intraglandular transplantation of bone marrow-derived clonal mesenchymal stem cells for amelioration of post-irradiation salivary gland damage. *Oral Oncol*. 2013;49(2):136−143.

17. Wu V, Helder MN, Bravenboer N, et al. Bone tissue regeneration in the oral and maxillofacial region: a review on the application of stem cells and new strategies to improve vascularization. *Stem Cell Int*. 2019;2019.

18. Trubiani O, Marconi GD, Pierdomenico SD, Piattelli A, Diomede F, Pizzicannella J. Human oral stem cells, biomaterials and extracellular vesicles: a promising tool in bone tissue repair. *Int J Mol Sci*. 2019;20(20):4987.

19. Iaquinta MR, Mazzoni E, Bononi I, et al. Adult stem cells for bone regeneration and repair. *Front Cell Dev Biol*. 2019;7.

20. Park Y-J, Cha S, Park Y-S. Regenerative applications using tooth derived stem cells in other than tooth regeneration: a literature review. *Stem Cell Int*. 2016;2016.

21. Diomede F, Gugliandolo A, Cardelli P, et al. Three-dimensional printed PLA scaffold and human gingival stem cell-derived extracellular vesicles: a new tool for bone defect repair. *Stem Cell Res Ther*. 2018;9(1):104.

22. Jazayeri HE, Tahriri M, Razavi M, et al. A current overview of materials and strategies for potential use in maxillofacial tissue regeneration. *Mater Sci Eng C*. 2017;70: 913−929.

23. Shetty L, Badhe R, Bhonde R, Waknis P, Londhe U. Chitosan and stemcells: a synchrony for regeneration. *J Dent Res Rev*. 2020;7(5):95.

24. Oshima M, Tsuji T. Whole tooth regeneration using a bioengineered tooth. In: *New Trends in Tissue Engineering and Regenerative Medicine Nagoya*. IntechOpen; 2014:109−119.

25. Young C, Terada S, Vacanti J, Honda M, Bartlett J, Yelick P. Tissue engineering of complex tooth structures on biodegradable polymer scaffolds. *J Dent Res*. 2002;81(10): 695−700.

26. Wu Z, Wang F, Fan Z, et al. Whole-tooth regeneration by allogeneic cell reassociation in pig jawbone. *Tissue Eng*. 2019;25(17−18):1202−1212.

27. Ono M, Oshima M, Ogawa M, et al. Practical whole-tooth restoration utilizing autologous bioengineered tooth germ transplantation in a postnatal canine model. *Sci Rep*. 2017; 7:44522.

28. Thesleff I. From understanding tooth development to bioengineering of teeth. *Eur J Oral Sci*. 2018;126:67−71.

29. Yelick P, Sharpe P. Tooth bioengineering and regenerative dentistry. *J Dent Res*. 2019;98(11):1173−1182.

30. Page RC, Schroeder HE. Pathogenesis of inflammatory periodontal disease. A summary of current work. *Labor Investig J Tech Method Pathol*. 1976;34(3):235.

31. Liang Y, Luan X, Liu X. Recent advances in periodontal regeneration: a biomaterial perspective. *Bioact Mater*. 2020;5(2):297−308.

32. Murphy KG, Gunsolley JC. Guided tissue regeneration for the treatment of periodontal intrabony and furcation defects. A systematic review. *Ann Periodontol*. 2003;8(1): 266−302.

33. Needleman I, Worthington HV, Giedrys-Leeper E, Tucker R. Guided tissue regeneration for periodontal infra-bony defects. *Cochrane Database Syst Rev*. 2006;2.

34. Zhou LN, Bi CS, Gao LN, An Y, Chen F, Chen FM. Macrophage polarization in human gingival tissue in response to periodontal disease. *Oral Dis*. 2019;25(1):265−273.

35. Seciu A-M, Craciunescu O, Zarnescu O. Advanced regenerative techniques based on dental pulp stem cells for the treatment of periodontal disease. In: *Periodontology and Dental Implantology*. IntechOpen; 2018.

36. Nevins M, Camelo M, Nevins ML, Schenk RK, Lynch SE. Periodontal regeneration in humans using recombinant human platelet-derived growth factor-BB (rhPDGF-BB) and allogenic bone. *J Periodontol*. 2003;74(9):1282−1292.

37. Iwasaki K, Akazawa K, Nagata M, et al. The fate of transplanted periodontal ligament stem cells in surgically created periodontal defects in rats. *Int J Mol Sci*. 2019; 20(1):192.

38. Cianci E, Recchiuti A, Trubiani O, et al. Human periodontal stem cells release specialized proresolving mediators and carry immunomodulatory and prohealing properties regulated by lipoxins. *Stem Cells Translat Med*. 2016;5(1):20−32.

39. Widbiller M, Schmalz G. Endodontic regeneration: hard shell, soft core. *Odontology*. 2020:1−10.

40. Nakashima M. The induction of reparative dentine in the amputated dental pulp of the dog by bone morphogenetic protein. *Arch Oral Biol*. 1990;35(7):493−497.

41. Ostby BN. The role of the blood clot in endodontic therapy an experimental histologic study. *Acta Odontol Scand.* 1961;19(3–4):323–353.

42. Nygaard-Ostby B, Hjortdal O. Tissue formation in the root canal following pulp removal. *Eur J Oral Sci.* 1971;79(3):333–349.

43. Siddiqui YD, Omori K, Ito T, et al. Resolvin D2 induces resolution of periapical inflammation and promotes healing of periapical lesions in rat periapical periodontitis. *Front Immunol.* 2019;10:307.

44. Lovelace TW, Henry MA, Hargreaves KM, Diogenes A. Evaluation of the delivery of mesenchymal stem cells into the root canal space of necrotic immature teeth after clinical regenerative endodontic procedure. *J Endod.* 2011;37(2):133–138.

CHAPTER 16

Application of Various Tissue Grafts

CYNTHIA BERNARDO D'LIMA, B.SC., DIP. TISSUE BANKING •
PANKAJ KHARADE, MDS, FJPS

INTRODUCTION

Tissue grafts have been used for decades in surgical reconstruction and regeneration of tissue defects. Autografts, allografts, xenografts, and synthetic biomaterials are the numerous alternatives used for reconstructive surgeries.

Bone grafts can be classified based on material groups[1]:

Allograft-based bone graft comprises allograft bone, used alone or in amalgamation with other materials (e.g., Grafton, OrthoBlast).

Factor-based bone graft can be natural or with recombinant growth factors, used alone or in mixture with other materials such as transforming growth factor-beta (TGF-beta), platelet-derived growth factor (PDGF), fibroblast growth factors (FGF), and bone morphogenic protein (BMP).

Cell-based bone grafts use cells to produce new tissue alone or are added onto a support matrix, for example, mesenchymal stem cells.

Ceramic-based bone graft substitutes include calcium phosphate, calcium sulfate, and bioglass used alone or in combination, for example, OsteoGraf, ProOsteon, OsteoSet.

Polymer-based bone graft uses degradable and nondegradable polymers alone or in combination with other materials, for example, open porosity polylactic acid polymer.

There are definite biologic mechanisms that offer a validation for bone grafting. They are osteoconduction, osteoinduction, and osteogenesis.[2]

AUTOGRAFTS

Autografts remain the gold standard as there is no risk of disease transmission, cause rapid healing, and do not induce immune rejection. Bone autografts promote osteoconduction, osteoinduction, osteogenesis, and rapid healing. However, autografts have disadvantages such as donor site morbidity, increased surgical and hospitalization cost, and limited availability specially in children and where there are massive defects. Bone autografts from the iliac crest, mandibular symphysis (chin area), anterior mandibular ramus (coronoid process), rib, or the fibula are normally used.[3] Autografts of tooth and dentin,[4–6] skin,[7] bone,[8] and nerves have been reported in literature.

Autogenous bone grafts are preferred for the reconstruction of small vertical defects as shown in Fig. 16.1. Instruments such as bone scraper can be used to harvest autogenous bone in a conservative manner.

Allografts and xenografts have the risk of transmitting various diseases, the potential to develop incompatibility reactions, chronic granulomatous inflammations, and religious restrictions.[9] Allografts are advantageous for their biocompatibility and host acceptance, but they may have limited availability as compared with xenografts. Xenografts are available in larger quantities and various sizes. However, some researchers have discussed the theoretical risk of zoonotic infectious microorganisms being transferred from the graft to the recipient, especially bovine spongiform encephalopathy or porcine endogenous retroviruses and *Clostridium difficile*.[10] There is no way to adequately screen xenografts for the presence of these viruses.[11] Some examples of xenografts are bovine bone and pericardium, porcine skin, bone and heart valves, and fish collagen membranes.

ALLOGRAFTS

Allografts could be procured from living as well as deceased donors. Preserved tissue allografts such as bone, cartilage, tendons, tooth and dentin, dura mater, heart valves, skin, and amnion that are processed and distributed by tissue banks have been widely used for reconstructive surgeries. Prions and some viruses are

Prosthetic Rehabilitation of Head and Neck Cancer Patients. https://doi.org/10.1016/B978-0-323-82394-4.00006-9

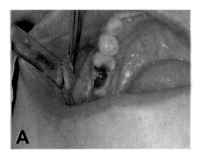
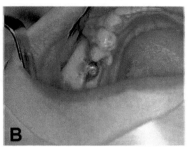
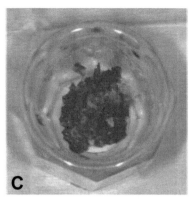

FIG. 16.1 (a) Small vertical bone defect in the buccal cortical plate. (b) Placement of dental implant. (c) Autogenous bone harvested for grafting using bone scraper.

highly resistant to many sterilizing methods; hence, careful donor screening and selection is important to avoid the risk of disease transmission. A review of the social and medical history, physical examination, serology tests, and autopsy results are mandatory in the case of deceased donors. In case tissues are obtained from living donors, the social/medical history and serology tests are mandatory. The minimum serology tests required as per the Standards of the Asia Pacific Association of Surgical Tissue Banking (APASTB) are the HIV1 and 2, hepatitis B, hepatitis C, and syphilis.[12] There are various methods of tissue processing, which aim at reducing the microbial bioburden, eliminating the serodiagnostic window for viral infections, and reducing the host immune response in allograft transplantation. The primary cause of host immune response in allograft transplantation are the cells of the blood and bone marrow, primarily the leukocytes. Reduction or removal of these cells by subjecting the tissues to various processing methods such as washing off the blood and bone marrow, processing using chemicals, freezing, freeze drying (lyophilization), and radiation sterilization reduces the leukocytes and hence reduces the immune reactions.

Processing of the tissues using the principles of good manufacturing practices and a robust quality management system, including terminal sterilization of the tissue allografts, will help reduce the risk of transmissible infections and ensure quality grafts (Fig. 16.2).

Donor evaluation, donor consent, serology tests, quality control tests of the produced grafts, and quality assurance at every step of the processing procedure including documentation to ensure complete traceability from the donor tissue to the graft utilization are the basic requirements for graft production.

Country- or region-specific tissue banking standards and regulations must be followed.

Allografts can be classified based on the anatomy, the processing methods, the sterilization methods used, and the type of graft produced. Classification of tissue allografts on the basis of the following:

- **Anatomy:** Includes bone grafts (cortical/cancellous/ corticocancellous/osteochondral), tooth and dentin grafts, tendons, ligaments, cartilage, placental membrane grafts, skin, and heart valves.
- **Processing methods:** Fresh frozen tissues, processed frozen tissue, lyophilized/dehydrated sterilized tissues, cryopreserved tissues, aseptic processing of grafts, mineralized bone/demineralized bone.
- **Type of grafts produced:** Bone strips, bone blocks, bone chips, mineralized and demineralized bone granules and blocks, mineralized and demineralized tooth and dentin granules and blocks, biological dressings (amnion, chorion, amnion chorion membrane and skin), putty and pastes.
- **Sterilization methods:** Various types of sterilization methods such as gamma irradiation, ETO sterilization, autoclaving, and peracetic acid have been used. However, the sterilization method of choice is gamma irradiation because of its many advantages. There is no rise in temperature during the radiation process; hence, it does not induce any chemical or physical changes in the grafts. There is no residual toxicity; hence, no quarantine period is required. Gamma radiation is able to penetrate into the grafts through the final package. The exposure time is the only variable parameter; hence the process can be controlled precisely. Gamma radiation reduces the antigenicity of the processed grafts. According to the International Atomic Energy Agency, a dose of

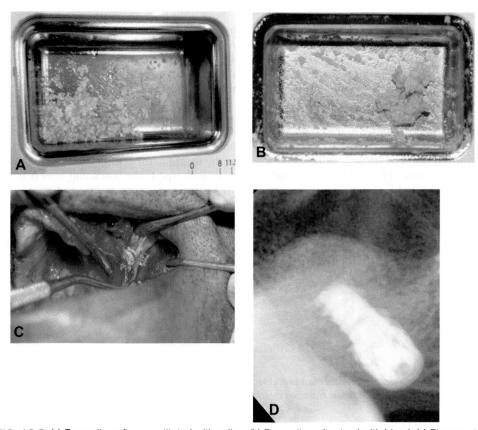

FIG. 16.2 (a) Bone allograft reconstituted with saline. (b) Bone allograft mixed with blood. (c) Placement of bone allograft followed by amniotic membrane in maxillary sinus. (d) Radiograph showing bone formation in maxillary sinus after placement of allograft.

25 kGy is a reference dose to ensure sterilization of tissue grafts. However, tissue banks use different validated irradiation doses for sterilization to preserve the tissue properties and ensure sterilization.

Advantages of allografts include avoidance of donor site morbidity, decreased operating time, reduced cost of surgery, and hospitalization. Allografts can be made available in different sizes as per the need of the patients, thus allowing the clinician to use a size-appropriate graft and therefore minimize waste. Allografts can be preserved and stored for a long duration. Freeze-dried allografts can be stored and transported at ambient temperatures. Banked allografts are readily available in large quantities.

ALLOPLASTS

Alloplastic grafts may be prepared from synthetic hydroxyapatite crystals, which may be made from bioactive glass. Hydroxyapatite is a naturally available mineral, which is the main mineral constituent of bone. Hydroxyapatite is a synthetic bone graft, which is frequently used nowadays because of its osteoconductive properties, hardness, and acceptability by the host bone. Some synthetic bone grafts are made of calcium carbonate but it is not frequently used because it is completely resorbed in a short time and may result in bone fracture. The use of tricalcium phosphate in amalgamation with hydroxyapatite gives the benefits of osteoconduction and resorbability.

Flexible hydrogel–hydroxyapatite (HA) composite has a mineral to organic matrix ratio similar to that of human bone.

Artificial bone can be fashioned from ceramics such as calcium phosphates (e.g., HA and tricalcium phosphate), bioglass, and calcium sulfate and is biologically active depending on its solubility in the physiological environment. These materials are combined with growth factors, ions such as strontium, or mixed with bone marrow aspirate to upsurge biological activity. The presence of elements such as strontium can result in advanced bone mineral density (BMD) and improved osteoblast proliferation (Figs. 16.3—16.7).

MUSCULOSKELETAL TISSUES

The musculoskeletal system consists of the bones, muscles, tendons, ligaments, joints, cartilage, and other connective tissue, which could be banked. Donated bone includes the femur, tibia, fibula, humerus, radius, ulna, rib, femoral head, and iliac crest.

Bone is the chief supporting tissue of the body and is composed of mineralized extracellular matrix and three types of cells: osteocytes, osteoblasts, and osteoclasts. All bones are lined by layers of connective tissues containing osteogenic cells: periosteum on the external surface and endosteum of the internal surface.

60%—70% of the dry weight of bone is made up of inorganic matter mainly calcium phosphate in the form of hydroxyapatite crystals with a mixture of carbonate, citrate, magnesium, potassium, and sodium. 90% of the dry weight of the organic bone matrix is composed of collagen type I. The remaining 10% is made up of proteoglycans, glycoproteins, and noncollagenous

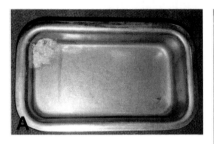 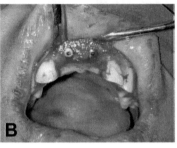 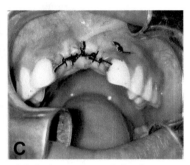

FIG. 16.3 (a) Hydroxyapatite crystals mixed with blood. (b) Hydroxyapatite crystals for bone augmentation in anterior maxilla. (c) Altered soft tissue morphology after placement of hydroxyapatite crystals.

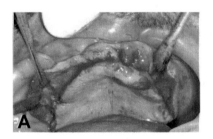 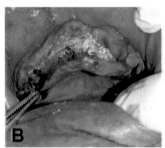 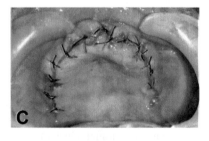

FIG. 16.4 (a) Edentulous ridge with deficient bone. (b) Combination of alloplast and biologic membrane for bone augmentation of edentulous ridge. (c) Altered morphology of edentulous ridge after placement of hydroxyapatite crystals.

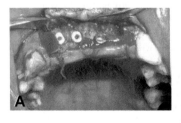 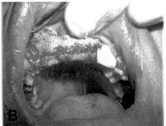 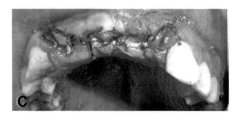

FIG. 16.5 (a) Anterior maxilla with deficient bone for implant placement. (b) Anterior maxilla augmented with alloplast. (c) Anterior maxilla after placement of hydroxyapatite crystals.

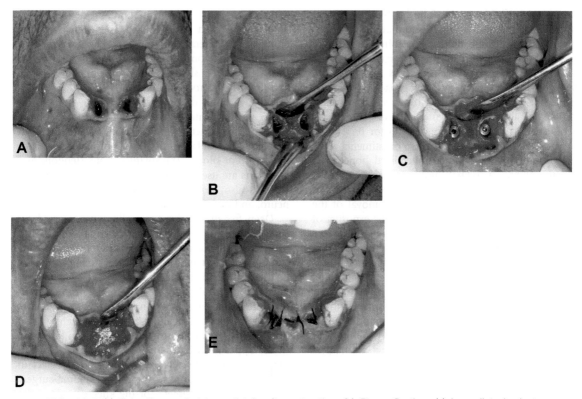

FIG. 16.6 (a) Extraction socket immediately after extraction. (b) Flap reflection. (c) Immediate implant placement after extraction. (d) Extraction socket grafted with alloplast after implant placement. (e) Extraction socket closed with sutures.

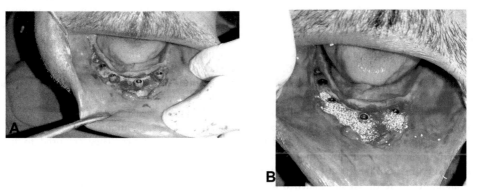

FIG. 16.7 (a) Resorption of bone and exposure of implants due to cystic lesion. (b) Placement of alloplast for regeneration of resorbed bone after enucleation of the cyst.

proteins. Glycoproteins and noncollagenous proteins play an important role in calcification. Along with hormones and vitamins, they are responsible in bone homeostasis, remodeling, fracture healing, and rebuilding bone grafts.[13]

Healing at the graft host junction takes place due to the processes of osteoconduction and osteoinduction. Osteoconduction is the ingrowth of capillaries, perivascular tissue, and osteoprogenitor cells from the host bed to the graft structure, which penetrate into nonviable osteones by a revascularization process followed by resorption of the grafted bone and new bone formation, a process known as creeping substitution. Osteoinduction is the process of new bone formation by the transformation of primitive mesenchymal precursor cells into chondroblasts and osteoblasts. This inductive capacity is primarily due to the presence of bone morphogenetic proteins (BMPs), and also other molecules, proteins, and growth factors such as transforming growth factor β.[8] Hence, care must be taken to preserve these constituents while bone is processed. Processed mineralized bone grafts are osteoconductive and basically act as a scaffold. Demineralized bone matrix has both osteoinductive and osteoconductive properties due to the removal of the inorganic component, which results in the exposure of the growth factors, thereby hastening the healing process. The healing process of bone graft involves inflammation, revascularization, osteogenesis, remodeling, and incorporation into the host skeleton, which results in a mechanically efficient structure.[14]

Subjecting bone to various processing methods helps reduce the bioburden, closes the serodiagnostic window, and reduces the immunogenicity of the grafts. Freeze drying is known to reduce the mechanical strength of the bone, and hence, massive bone and load bearing allografts should be processed and used as frozen grafts. Freeze-dried bone allograft can be stored at ambient temperature and is easy to transport.

Tissue banks follow different procedures for processing bones. Gajiwala et al. described the processing of lyophilized bone: bones are washed and pasteurized at 60°C for 3 h, cleaned of all soft tissue and cut into the required shapes and sizes, washed free of blood and bone marrow, treated with 70% ethanol to extract lipids that may inhibit osteogenesis and serve as a virucidal agent. The bones are then washed free of ethanol, lyophilized, packed, and sterilized by gamma irradiation at a dose of 25 kGy.[15]

The processing of frozen bone follows a similar procedure, skipping the lyophilization process. The processed bones are triple packed and then sterilized in the frozen state in dry ice. After sterilization, the allografts are preserved in the deep freezer until use. Radiographs of the allografts are recorded and matched with that of the recipient's resected bone before use.

For preparing bone granules, the processed bone is lyophilized, granulated, and sieved to obtain desired particulate sizes as required for the clinical use. For demineralization of bone granules, the processed granulated bone is demineralized using 0.5/0.6N hydrochloric acid and washed with phosphate buffer saline until the pH is neutral. The demineralized granules

are then lyophilized, sieved to obtain the desired particulate sizes, packed, and sterilized. The residual calcium content of demineralized bone should not exceed 8%.[16] For the preparation of bone blocks, the bones are cut into the desired shapes and sizes while processing, and the similar process is followed.

Bone is often destroyed by infection, trauma, tumors, and implanted materials and has to be replaced to restore the structure and function. Bone is the most commonly transplanted tissue than any other tissue or organ except blood. Transplanted bone, tendon, and ligaments are used extensively in orthopedic surgeries. Bone is also used in oral and maxillofacial, dental, neuro, and plastic surgeries.

Deep frozen massive bone allografts are used for limb salvage surgeries in cancer patients and are also used for reconstructing large bony defects. They provide structural support and biomechanical strength and may be used with a prosthesis, an osteosynthesis, or a vascularized fibular graft. They are used for reconstruction after tumor resection, revision arthroplasty, and after trauma. Osteochondral allograft may be used for partial joint reconstruction at the knee or ankle in children and in the upper limb in adults.[17] Osteoarticular allograft may be used in the reconstruction of joint defect in limb salvage procedure in tumor and trauma surgery and revision joint surgery for the knee or ankle joint and used less frequently for elbow or shoulder joint. Frozen bone is also used in anterior spine surgery after complete or partial vertebrectomy. Frozen femoral heads are used in the reconstruction of less severe bone loss, in primary or revision joint surgery, e.g., acetabular reconstruction and in trauma surgery. Frozen bones can also be morselised and used for packing of cavities caused by trauma or disease.

Lyophilized bone allografts being weaker than deep frozen bone allografts can only be used for packing of cavities in various clinical conditions. Demineralized bone being the weakest of all bone allografts is mainly used in the form of granules, chips, or blocks in oral and maxillofacial surgeries. They are used to fill cavities from pathology, like cyst and tumor, bony defects around dental or maxillofacial implant fixtures, sinus lift surgeries, augmentation of the atrophic mandible or maxilla, grafting in nonunion or malunion of fracture site of mandible or maxilla, grafting in cleft alveolus, cleft palate defects, and periodontal defects. For larger defects, or for structural support, they are used in combination with autografts, frozen allografts, or freeze-dried allografts.[18]

The advantages of bone allografts include the benefits of allografts in general and also include the following: the bone allograft achieves the quality of the host bone after incorporation. Immunologic response is very minimal after processing and storage of bone allografts; hence, immunosuppressive drugs are not required. Soft tissue and ligament attachment are possible with allografts used in tumor resection and revision arthroplasty.[19]

TOOTH AND DENTIN GRAFTS

The quest of finding the ideal graft has driven research in the direction of inventing a number of bone graft substitutes. Autogenous tooth used as a bone substitute (AutoBT) was developed from extracted tooth and has been in clinical use since 2008 in Korea.[5] The rationale for the use of teeth as a bone graft substitute is that dentin and bone have similarities in terms of structural and biochemical properties. Moreover, demineralized dentin matrix (DDM) has shown to possess exogenous bone morphogenetic proteins (BMPs) and other growth factors that promote bone remodeling. Several noncollagenous proteins such as osteocalcin (OCN) and osteopontin (OPN) are mutual in bone and dentin; however, dentin phosphoprotein is a noncollagenous protein found specifically in dentin.[20] It has been observed that autogenous mineralized dentin particles can be grafted instantaneously after extraction of tooth and should be considered an excellent option to preserve the extraction socket.[21] Dentin graft can also be used to augment bone in maxillary sinus as well as restoration of bone defects.

Autogenous DDM has demonstrated promising results, but it comes with its own practical challenges. Especially in routine dental practice, its chair-side preparation can be tedious and time-consuming. The amount of autografts obtained is unpredictable as it depends on several clinical conditions, such as dental caries, restorations, and prostheses in the harvested teeth. Hence, whole tooth and dentin allografts prepared from extracted human teeth overcome the shortcomings of autografts and are a better alternative as allografts are a ready source of grafts.[22,23]

There are very few studies reported in literature on the clinical use of tooth and dentin allografts. In 2017, the first randomized, controlled, prospective, clinical pilot study comparing freeze-dried tooth and dentin allografts with freeze-dried bone allografts (FDBA) in alveolar ridge preservation was reported. Joshi et al. described the processing of grafts as follows: donated whole teeth were cleaned using an ultrasonic scaler. In case of dentin grafts, the dentin was separated using carbide straight fissure bur by trimming superficial enamel and cemental portion. Processing of all

teeth was done immediately postextraction. The teeth and dentin were washed and processed, freeze-dried, and granulated to a particle size of 300–500 μm, packed and sterilized by gamma irradiation at a dose of 25 kGy.

The study found that the mineralized whole tooth and dentin allografts consistently showed superior results both clinically and radiographically, as compared with FDBA in achieving minimum volumetric alveolar bone loss in alveolar ridge preservation procedure. Histological analysis also confirmed better results for new bone formation by teeth allografts. However, between whole tooth allografts and dentin allograft treated sites, there was no statistically significant difference.[22]

A comparative clinical evaluation was performed by Um et al. between demineralized dentin matrix autografts and demineralized dentin matrix allografts to analyze buccal marginal bone resorption, around dental implants for guided bone regeneration. The allografts and autografts in guided bone regeneration showed comparable clinical results in terms of buccal marginal bone resorption during the first year of functional loading.[23]

A case report that evaluated the efficacy of whole tooth allograft in combination with autologous fibrin glue to treat alveolar ridge defect in maxillary right canine region confirmed substantial gain in alveolar bone width and height. Comparison of baseline and 4-month postoperative scans revealed a gain of 5.31 and 4.27 mm in ridge width and height, respectively. The results strengthened the benefits of using tooth allograft mixed with autologous platelet concentrates in improving alveolar bone profile. Optimal integration of graft particle compounded with uneventful clinical healing demonstrated the potential of whole tooth allografts to be used as an alternative to conventional bone grafts.[24]

The use of tooth autografts is widespread. The study by Um et al. showed comparable results between the autografts and allografts. Hence, banking tooth allografts will ensure a ready supply of material when required without probably compromising on the clinical results. Teeth can be collected from healthy donors to be processed into allografts in a tissue bank. It is observed that tooth has much lower fat content and no marrow compared with bone, which makes processing of the allografts easier. Extracted teeth is a biomedical waste and is easily available. Tooth allografts are economical, natural, biocompatible, versatile, and predictable grafting material and can serve as a better alternative to most of the conventional allografts. This opens up a whole new avenue of deciduous as well as permanent exfoliated and extracted teeth banking.[22]

However, the quantity of extracted teeth for allograft preparation is limited as compared with bone (Fig. 16.8).

PLACENTAL MEMBRANE ALLOGRAFTS

Amniotic membrane obtained from the human placenta has been used as a biomaterial for surgical reconstruction for almost a 100 years. The amniotic membrane is composed of two layers, the amnion and the nonplacental chorion. The amnion is the innermost of the two fetal membranes and is in contact with the contents of the amniotic sac, namely the amniotic fluid, the fetus, and the umbilical cord. The chorion is the outermost of the two fetal membranes and is in contact with the amnion on its inner aspect and the maternal decidua on its outer aspect. The amnion consists of five layers. These are, from within outward: epithelium, basement membrane, compact layer, fibroblast layer, and spongy layer. The amniotic epithelium is a single layer of cells and lies nearest to the fetus. The basement layer is one of the thickest membranes found in all human tissue and contributes to the structural integrity. The compact layer forms the main fibrous skeleton of the amniotic membrane. Collagen types I and III are situated in the fibroblast layer and maintain the mechanical integrity of membrane. Collagen types V and VI form filamentous connections between interstitial collagens and the epithelial basement membrane. The spongy layer has abundant content of proteoglycans and glycoproteins and a nonfibrillar meshwork of mostly type III collagen. There is no presence of nerves and blood vessels in the amniotic membrane, and its nutrition is obtained directly by diffusion out of the amniotic fluid.

The chorion consists of four layers. These are, from within outward: cellular layer, reticular layer, pseudo-basement membrane, and trophoblast. The cellular layer of the chorion is frequently imperfect or completely absent from the chorion when examined at term. The reticular network is composed of collagens I, III IV, V, VI and proteoglycans. The basement membrane contains collagen IV, fibronectin, and laminin. The trophoblast layer consists of 2–10 layers of trophoblasts, which contact with the decidua. The spongy layer of the amnion is loosely connected to the chorion; hence, the amnion is easily separated from the chorion by means of blunt dissection.[25,26] Chorion is estimated to be 200 μm thick as compared with amnion, which is 50 μm thick.[27]

Placental membranes have an advantage of being an immune-privileged tissue and are mechanically strong and elastic owing to the collagens.[27] The proteoglycans probably perform a barrier function, account for the biochemical properties of the membrane,[28] and are involved in all cellular processes with molecular interactions at the cell surface.[29] The fibronectin is involved in cellular processes including tissue repair, blood clotting, cell migration, and adhesion and in the maintenance of normal tissue order.[30,31] The laminin functions as structural components and initiates intracellular signaling events that regulate cellular organization and differentiation.[32]

Amnion and chorion membranes have antimicrobial properties, inhibiting the growth of a number of bacteria including pathogens. The antibacterial effects of the chorion are superior to amnion. The antimicrobial effect of amnion and chorion is significantly different on various bacteria.[33,34]

Both amnion and chorion contain numerous and similar growth factors and cytokine composition, which

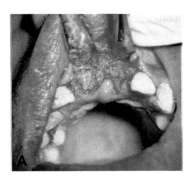
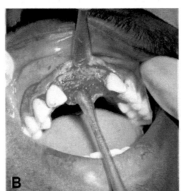
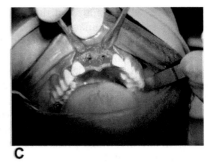

FIG. 16.8 (a) Placement of dentin graft in extraction socket of right central incisor. (b) One month after placement of dentin graft in the same extraction socket. (c) Implant placement in the bone formed after dentin graft.

results in their ability to repair tissues.[35] However, chorion contains more growth factors and more cytokines per square centimeter as compared with amnion likely due to the overall increased thickness of chorion.[36] The presence of higher concentration of cytokines and growth factors in chorion, its superior antimicrobial effects, and thickness as compared with amnion could be an added advantage when chorion allografts are produced for use in oral surgeries.[37]

Placental membranes allografts have the ability to adhere well to the surface of wounds and seal the wound and the exposed nerve endings, thereby offering protection against bacterial infections, preventing heat and fluid loss, and reducing pain at the site by preventing nerve stimuli and inflammation. They also promote epithelialization, enhance soft tissue healing,[26,38] lack antigenicity, and are nontoxic. The wound dressing can be easily changed, is cost effective, and has a long shelf life and simple storage requirements. These characteristics meet the requirements of an ideal wound dressing as described by Ghomi et al.[39] The amnion is a translucent membrane, and the progress of the wound healing can be viewed unlike conventional dressings. However, processed chorion is thicker and more opaque. The bilayered amnion chorion membrane (ACM) is more opaque and thicker than chorion and has the properties of both the amnion and the chorion membranes, which could be used to an advantage. Like in the case of all biological material, the choice between these three grafts too should be decided carefully depending on the desired clinical outcome.

There are reports in the literature about various methods of preservation and storage of amniotic membrane, including dehydration by freeze drying and air drying, sterilization by gamma irradiation, cryopreservation using 10% dimethyl sulfoxide (DMSO),[40] preservation in Dulbecco Modified Eagles Medium/glycerol (1:1) and 50%−85% glycerol.[41]

AMNION

Amnion allografts were used as biological dressings in the treatment of burns as early as 1913, varicose ulcers, decubitus ulcers, and open infected wounds. Mijewski et al. used amnion grafts as a biological dressing to minimize or prevent air leakage post lung surgery in cancer patients. Preserved amnion grafts have been widely used in ophthalmology for the treatment of deep ulcerations of the cornea and sclera and conjunctive melanoma. It has been used in otolaryngology for replacing the nasal mucosa in Rendu−Osler−Weber disease, as tympanic membrane grafts, for treatment of severe epistaxis and for covering head and neck sites

after flap necrosis. Amnion allografts are also used in the modulation of peripheral nerve regeneration and in reconstructive surgery of the vagina following resection for diffuse carcinoma in situ (CIS) as well as for severe, erosive vulvovaginal burns.[42] It has been used in the reconstruction and management of wounds of the oral cavity and as a barrier membrane for guided tissue regeneration in oral surgeries.[37] The use of amnion has also been reported in the reconstruction of the bladder, and omphalocele and preventing tissue adhesion in surgery of the head, abdomen, pelvis, and larynx.[35] Amnion has also been used in the treatment of leukoplakia[43] and moist desquamation following radiation therapy in cancer patients (Figs. 16.9 and 16.10).[44]

CHORION

Though the use of amnion has been reported in a number of clinical conditions, the human chorionic membrane was until recently routinely discarded worldwide. D'Lima et al. were the first to describe the processing of chorion. The chorion layer was separated from the placenta, washed free of blood and blood clots, pasteurized with normal saline at 60°C for 1 h. The tissues were then treated with 70% ethyl alcohol for 0.5 h, and washed with normal saline until free of ethyl alcohol. The processed tissues were then lyophilized and sterilized by gamma irradiation at a dose of 25 kGy. The chorionic membrane has been extensively used in India as a barrier membrane for sinus lift procedures, implant, and periodontal surgeries (for guided tissue regeneration in periodontal pocket therapy, gingival biotype enhancement, root coverage, gingival recession, and alveolar ridge preservation). As chorion is thicker, stiffer, and easier to handle as compared with amnion, it has been an added advantage in oral surgeries. However, more research needs to be done on the use of chorion in areas other than oral surgeries (Figs. 16.11−16.13).[37]

FIG. 16.9 Amnion.

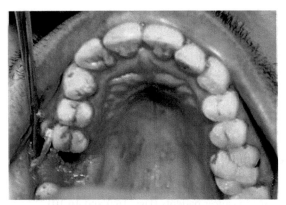

FIG. 16.10 Amnion used for guided bone regeneration.

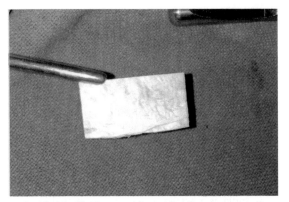

FIG. 16.11 Chorion used for guided tissue regeneration.

AMNION CHORION MEMBRANE

In 1940, De Rotth described the transplantation of amnion chorion membrane (ACM) for the first time in the repair of conjunctival defects.[45] The first commercially available human placental allografts composed of dehydrated ACM for the use in dentistry was released in 2008. It has been used as a barrier membrane for guided tissue regeneration in periodontal intrabony defects.[46] Processed dehydrated ACM grafts have been utilized clinically to promote healing in a variety of applications including skin and corneal wounds, periodontal surgery, and soft tissue repair, with no known adverse events. ACM has shown improved healing of diabetic foot ulcers and venous leg ulcers as compared with the clinical standard compression therapy in randomized controlled clinical trials. ACM allografts have more recently been used in the treatment of orthopedic tissue injuries such as plantar fasciitis, tendinopathy, and vertebral fusion procedures.[47] It has successfully been used in vaginoplasties in cases of vaginal agenesis and vaginectomy following malignancy.[48] Ahuja et al. used ACM in the treatment of burns in pediatric population and found that it had an excellent rate of healing comparable to split thickness skin grafts with less rate of hypertrophic scar and contracture.[49]

Lyophilized ACM grafts have also been used in patients with laryngeal squamous cell carcinoma for closing postlaryngectomy pharyngocutaneous fistula (PCF), which is a severe complication after laryngectomy. These grafts had advantages over other existing treatment methods as they are noninvasive, prevent donor morbidity, and were effective in closing PCF without further surgical intervention.[50] In a study where dehydrated ACM allograft was used as nerve wrap around the prostatic neurovascular bundle, its use appeared to hasten the early return of continence and potency in patients following robot-assisted radical prostatectomy.[51]

Subach and Copay studied the use of dehydrated ACM on the formation of soft tissue scarring in the epidural space on patients who subsequently underwent reexploration after posterior lumbar instrumentation. The ACM barrier was clearly useful in limiting

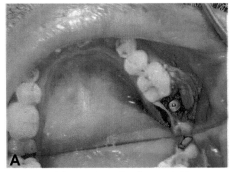
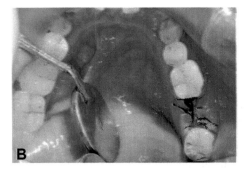

FIG. 16.12 (a) Use of chorion for guided bone regeneration after graft placement. (b) Closure of the grafted defect.

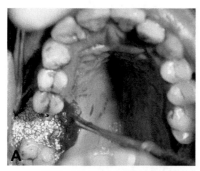 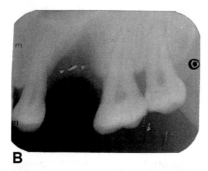 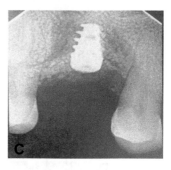

FIG. 16.13 (a) Grafting with alloplast after maxillary sinus lift. (b) Radiograph showing deficient bone for implant placement. (c) Radiograph after sinus lift and implant placement.

epidural fibrosis and promoting dissection in revision spinal surgery in patients and did not lead to any adverse events such as infection or spinal fluid leak. Compared with other barriers, ACM performed better in revision surgery.[52]

In a case study where processed lyophilized ACM was evaluated against processed lyophilized chorion for root coverage and gingival biotype enhancement, it was found that on both the ACM and chorion operated sides, 100% root coverage was seen even 3 months after surgery. Preoperative gingival thickness on either treated side was 1.04 mm. Three months later, gingival thickness at the site where ACM was used was 1.46 mm whereas the chorion side had gingival thickness of 1.28 mm. Gingival tissues at both the sites appeared healthy, with no visible signs of inflammation. It was observed that the ACM being bilayered and thicker than the chorion gave a pronounced gingival biotype improvement (Fig. 16.14).[53]

ADVANTAGES OF PLACENTAL MEMBRANES

- Placental grafts are nontoxic, nonantigenic, antiin-flammatory, antimicrobial, and bioresorbable.
- They have analgesic effect due to coverage of exposed nerve endings.
- They promote epithelialization, establishing angio-genesis by vessel proliferation, and have pluripotent properties.
- They can easily stick to the wound bed and closely adapts to the contours of the underlying surface, whether the irregular contours of the body or when placed over bone graft and proximal bony walls and do not compromise blood flow. They are very pliable membranes.

- During surgery, it does not easily displace from underneath the overlying flap.
- They have good mechanical strength and elasticity.
- Being bioresorbable, the technique does not require a second surgical procedure, thereby improving clinical results and cost-effectiveness, and decreasing patient morbidity.
- The amnion is a translucent membrane and has an advantage in wound dressing as the healing can be observed. If the dressing is intact, it needs not be changed unlike conventional dressings.
- A biomaterial that can be easily obtained, processed, and transported and the dehydrated membranes can be stored at ambient temperature.
- It is economical, easy to apply, and readily available.

Placental grafts are currently being used mainly for bone regeneration in the oral and maxillofacial surgeries and as a biological wound dressing. They offer the surgeon a wider choice based on their thickness and properties to achieve the desired clinical outcome. The use of placental membranes is expanding rapidly in fields of tissue repair and regeneration, surgical reconstruction, tissue engineering, and stem cell research.

SKIN GRAFTS

Skin is the largest organ of the human body. The functions of the skin include barrier function, thermoregulation of the human body, sensory, excretion, immune function, production of melanin, and vitamin D.[54]

Skin is composed of two major layers: the epidermis and the dermis. The epidermis, the outermost layer, is primarily composed of stratified squamous epithelium of keratinocytes and comprises over

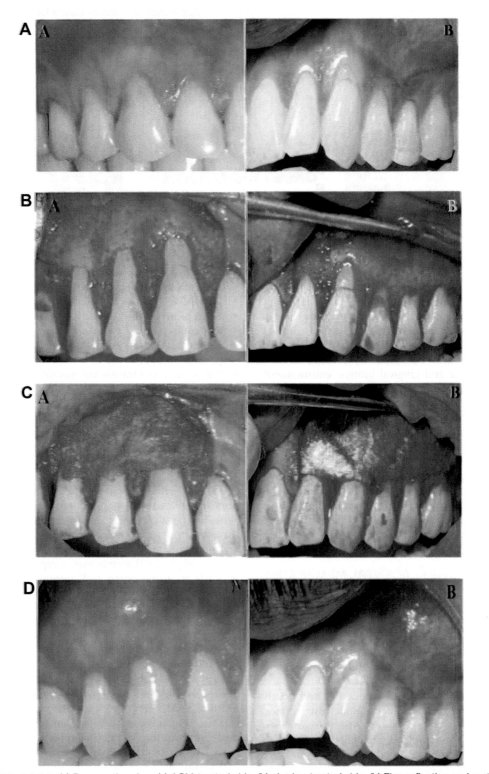

FIG. 16.14 (a) Preoperative view: (a) ACM-treated side, (b) chorion-treated side. (b) Flap reflection and root planning. (c) (a) Placement of ACM over 13,14,15 (b) Placement of chorion on 22,23. (d) 3-month postoperative view. (a) ACM-treated side, (b) Chorion-treated side.

90% of epidermal cells. Keratinocytes bind the epidermal structure together and are responsible for the barrier function. Pigment-containing melanocytes, antigen-processing Langerhans cells, and pressure-sensing Merkel cells are present within the epidermis. The epidermis is avascular. The dermis consists of papillary dermis, and the deeper layers of the dermis are called the reticular dermis. The mechanical properties of the skin are contributed by the dermis. It is composed of fibroblasts, which lie within an extracellular specialized matrix and collagens, elastin, proteoglycans, fibronectin, and other components. The basement membrane connects the epidermis and

dermis. It is composed of various integrins, laminins, collagens, and other proteins that play important roles in regulating epithelial–mesenchymal interaction. The dermis contains microvascular and neural networks. Sebaceous glands, eccrine glands, apocrine glands, and hair follicles develop as downgrowths of the epidermis into the dermis. In addition, the dermis also contains blood vessels, lymphatic vessels, and sensory nerve endings. The tissue lying underneath the dermis is the hypodermis (subcutis). It is composed primarily of adipose tissue and separates the dermis from the underlying muscular fascia (Figs. 16.15–16.21).[55]

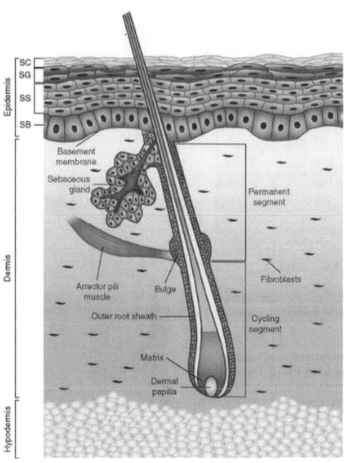

FIG. 16.15 Anatomy of the skin. Skin is composed of three layers, starting with the outermost layer: the epidermis, dermis, and hypodermis. Epidermis is a stratified squamous epithelium that is divided into four layers, starting with the outermost layer: stratum corneum (SC), stratum granulosum (SG), stratum spinosum (SS), and stratum basale (SB). Outer root sheath of the hair follicle is contiguous with the basal epidermal layer. Stem cell niches include the basal epidermal layer, base of sebaceous gland, hair follicle bulge, dermal papillae, and dermis.[55]

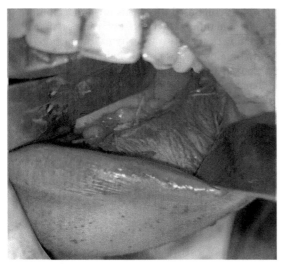

FIG. 16.16 Reconstruction of resected mandible with radial forearm flap.

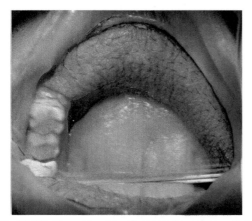

FIG. 16.17 Reconstruction of resected mandible with free fibula flap.

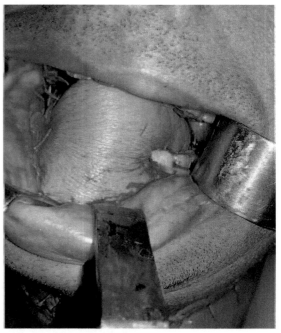

FIG. 16.18 Reconstruction of resected tongue with radial forearm flap.

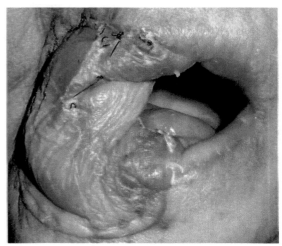

FIG. 16.19 Reconstruction of composite defect with forehead flap.

The skin is capable of regeneration and restoration of its functions if the damage is superficial. Damage and/or loss to large areas of the skin such as extensive burns can cause severe systemic complications, and even death. Hence, lost skin should be replaced temporarily or permanently by skin substitutes and/or skin grafts. Cultured autologous keratinocytes sheet grafts usually take about 3 weeks after harvesting of the skin and initiation of the cultures.[54] Autografts are the gold standard for skin grafting, but this is only possible in a few cases. In most cases, allografts are the best alternative.

The common methods of skin allograft preservation are in glycerol, by cryopreservation and lyophilization. Glycerolized and lyophilized skin grafts are not viable but retain structural and mechanical properties, whereas cryopreserved skin allografts are viable grafts. Frozen grafts stored between −15 to −80°C are viable but have reduced cell viability. Glycerol preserved allografts are used as temporary dressings, are easier to process as compared with cryopreservation, have a certain

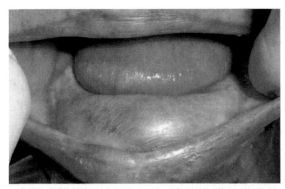

FIG. 16.20 Reconstruction of resected mandible with free fibula flap.

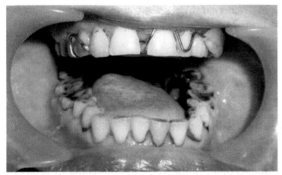

FIG. 16.21 Reconstruction of resected tongue with radial forearm flap.

degree of antibacterial and antiviral activities, and have reduced immunogenicity. They can easily be distributed by maintaining the cold chain. Hence, they are used alone or in combination with cryopreserved skin for treating difficult, posttraumatic and surgical wounds, and deep loss of substance (e.g., tendon coverage).

A split-thickness skin graft includes the epidermis and part of the dermis. The thickness of the graft depends on the donor site and the clinical use. Split thickness grafts are usually used to cover large areas. The rate of autorejection is low. The area of the graft can be expanded greatly by using a skin mesher. Reepithelialization from the dermis and surrounding skin contributes to the healing of the donor site. If appropriate dressings are used, it hastens the healing process and the same site can be harvested again after 6 weeks, if required.

A full-thickness skin graft is composed of the epidermis and the entire dermis. A composite graft includes the skin and underlying cartilage or other tissue.[56]

Viable allograft is often regarded as the gold standard in temporary skin coverage,[57] possessing many of the qualities of the ideal wound dressing as described by Ghomi et al.[39]

Skin allografts if used early prevents mortality and morbidity caused by disseminated burn wound sepsis, by creating a protective barrier against microorganisms. Allograft skin also reduces the pain of an exposed wound, decreases evaporative loss of water, electrolytes, and protein, improves re-epithelialization, prepares the wound bed for definitive closure, and leads to improved cosmesis.[58] Using dermal allografts is of main importance in the management of wound healing, as the less immunogenic dermal component takes to the wound bed. Viable skin allografts remain a major therapeutic choice for extensive deep burns and hard-to-heal wounds and have significantly improved clinical outcomes with respect to unviable allografts and synthetic medications.[56]

Allograft skin is used temporarily until the donor sites have healed. It is used between sessions of harvesting and pending definitive surgical coverage of deep full-thickness burns or spontaneous healing of partial-thickness skin loss.[58] In addition to burns, it has been used in cases of skin loss caused by orthopedic trauma with bone–tendon exposure, surgery (after the debridement of extensive, necrotizing soft tissue infections), dental surgery, maxillofacial reconstruction, reconstruction of critical areas of the face, nasal septum or tympanic reconstruction, as temporary coverage (after laser-resurfacing and dermabrasion), and in the cases of disease (such as toxic epidermal necrolysis, congenital bullous epidermolysis, diabetic ulcers, venous ulcers, pressure, and trophic ulcers). Dermal allografts have been used for soft tissue augmentation, dural repair, hernia repair and eyelid reconstruction, autoimmune and infectious skin loss, pyoderma gangrenosum, and Mohs surgery.[56,57,59]

Applying skin grafts early during burn recovery has several patient benefits including reduced length and cost of hospitalization, pain reduction in the patients, and speedy recovery. thereby decreasing the amount of complications and reducing scar formation. Skin grafts are considered lifesaving tissue transplants.

NERVE GRAFTS

The brain and the spinal cord make up the central nervous system. Nerve roots exit from the spinal cord to both sides of the body. The spinal cord carries signals back and forth between the brain and the peripheral nerves. Peripheral nerves transfer signals across a vast network and deliver data from tissues and organs to and from the brain to every part of the body.

A peripheral nerve injury can result from trauma injury, disease, removal of neuroma to reduce pain or surgical repair of nerves that are cut in surgical procedures. Peripheral nerve injuries can involve sensory, motor, or mixed nerves and can be debilitating for patients, lead to pain and loss of motor function and/or sensation. Regeneration following peripheral nerve injuries depends on several factors, including the local environment for neurons to reach their synaptic targets. Therefore, the goal of treatment is to help facilitate the swift migration of these cells to provide axonal regrowth past the site of injury for reinnervation. Current options for bridging nerve gaps include autograft, nonprocessed allograft with immunosuppression, decellular nerve allografts and autogenous (i.e., vein) or bioabsorbable conduits (e.g., collagen, polyglycolic acid, caprolactone).[60]

Damaged peripheral nerves can be surgically repaired using allografts, helping to restore nerve function and improve patient quality of life. Only peripheral nerves from extremities are currently donated and transplanted.

The use of nerve allografts is reserved for devastating or segmental nerve injuries.[61] Nerve allograft is one of the most promising substitutes for nerve autografts. Cadaveric nerve allografts are abundantly available in various sizes; length and motor/sensory-specific nerves may be obtained. They contain both viable donor Schwann cells (SCs) and endoneurial microstructure and are similar to nerve autografts in terms of providing regenerative support. However, the use of fresh nerve allografts requires systemic immunosuppression, which predisposes the graft recipients to opportunistic infections, neoplasia, and toxicity-induced side effects. Processing nerve allografts to remove cellular components reduces graft immunogenicity. However, with the lack of viable SCs, the acellular allografts are limited to short gap distances of 3 cm. Though acellular, the allografts are able to revascularize and repopulate with host cells, thus providing an environment that is conducive for regeneration. Despite inherent differences, all processing techniques simultaneously aim to reduce graft immunogenicity by eliminating cellular constituents and enhance regenerative capacity through preservation of native extracellular matrix (ECM).[62] Processed acellular frozen nerve allografts are now commercially available.

Peripheral nerve surgery involves the direct repair of peripheral nerves after trauma, reconstruction of nerve gaps, and the management of painful nerve conditions such as end neuroma. There are a variety of situations where direct microsurgical repair is not possible or not the preferred option. Processed nerve allograft can be used in the management of nerve gaps without the disadvantages of using autografts. In a study, Nirjan et al. used nerve allografts for the reconstruction of painful neuromata in patients with neuropathic pain and sensitization, reconstruction of gaps following tumor resection to prevent neuropathic pain, in cases of insufficient donor nerve availability, previous failed autologous grafting, late-presenting cases with large gaps where surgery was for pain management or prevention rather than functional recovery, replantation where the amputated part may not survive, gap management in a mixed nerve when distal motor nerve transfer was employed for critical functions and acute detensioning repairs in noncritical sensory nerves.[63]

Thus, processed nerve allografts can be used to repair the damaged nerve or reconstruct peripheral nerve pathways, which can lead to restoration of sensory and motor function at the area of the injury. Moreover, it is readily available in unlimited quantity and is thus an attractive choice for neural repair. However, nerve graft banking is not widely practiced.

Tissue allografts results in faster healing and improve the quality of life of the recipients. Allografts are used in almost all fields of medicine with the orthopedic surgeries having the highest demand. The percentage-wise use of allografts in the various fields of medicine is shown in Graph 16.1.[19]

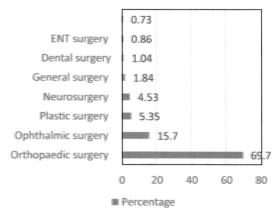

GRAPH 16.1 Use of allografts in the various fields of medicine.

SUMMARY

Transplanted tissues are used in almost all fields of surgery for reconstruction and regeneration of tissue defects. Autografts, allografts, and xenografts are the types of tissue grafts used for surgical reconstruction. Autografts are the gold standard as there is no risk of disease transmission, causes rapid healing, and does not induce immune rejection. However, it results in donor site morbidity, increased surgical and hospitalization cost, and has limited availability. Preserved tissue allografts such as bone, cartilage, tendons, tooth and dentin, dura mater, heart valves, skin, and amnion are processed and distributed by tissue banks for use in reconstructive surgeries. Bone is the most commonly transplanted tissue in the human body.

Tissue banks must follow the principles of good manufacturing practices and have a quality management system to ensure the production of sterile quality grafts. Allografts could be procured from living as well as deceased donors. Careful donor screening and selection is important to avoid the risk of disease transmission. The minimum serology tests required are HIV1 and 2, hepatitis B, hepatitis C, and syphilis. Different methods of tissue processing are followed by tissue banks, which aim at reducing the microbial bioburden, eliminating the serodiagnostic window for viral infection, and reducing the host immune response in allograft transplantation. Donor evaluation, donor consent, serology tests, quality control tests of the produced grafts, and quality assurance at every step of the processing procedure including documentation to ensure complete traceability from donor tissue to graft utilization is the basic requirement for graft production.

In the case of bone allografts, healing at the graft host junction takes place due to the processes of osteoconduction and osteoinduction. Processed mineralized bone grafts are osteoconductive. Demineralized bone matrix has both osteoinductive and osteoconductive properties. Freeze drying is known to reduce the mechanical strength of the bone, and hence, massive bone and load bearing allografts should be processed as frozen grafts. Freeze-dried bone allograft can be stored at ambient temperature and easy to transport. Demineralized bone being the weakest of all bone allografts is mainly used in the form of granules, chips, or blocks in oral and maxillofacial surgeries.

Autogenous tooth, a bone graft substitute, has been in clinical use since 2008. The rationale for the use of whole teeth and dentin as bone graft substitute is that dentin and bone are similar in terms of structural and biochemical properties. Very few clinical studies have been performed on tooth and dentin allografts. The studies showed no difference between tooth and dentin allografts, and tooth allografts showed better results as compared with mineralized bone allografts. Studies also showed comparative results between demineralized dentin allografts and autografts.

Amnion, chorion, and the bilayered amnion chorion membranes are the placental membrane grafts used in surgical reconstruction. Placental membranes are mechanically strong, elastic, and antimicrobial and have numerous growth factors and cytokines. They adhere well to the surface of wounds, sealing the wound, and the exposed nerve endings, thereby offering protection against bacterial infections, preventing heat and fluid loss, and reducing pain and inflammation. They also promote epithelialization, enhance soft tissue healing, and lack antigenicity. They are bioresorbable, nontoxic, easily processed, and available. The chorionic membrane has a higher concentration of cytokines and growth factors, superior antimicrobial effects, and is thicker as compared with amnion, which could be an added advantage when chorion allografts are used in oral surgeries.

Amnion and amnion chorion membranes have been used in various clinical applications over the years, whereas the use of chorion is more recent. The chorion has been extensively used in India as a barrier membrane in oral surgeries.

Damage and/or loss to large areas of the skin such as extensive burns can cause severe systemic complications, and even death. Hence, lost skin should be replaced temporarily or permanently by skin substitutes and/or skin grafts. The gold standard to obtain permanent wound closure is autologous grafting. However, autografting is not always possible, and allografting is often the best alternative. Allograft skin is used as a temporary dressing while awaiting the healing of autograft donor sites between sessions of harvesting. Skin grafts are considered lifesaving tissue transplants.

Peripheral nerves from extremities are currently donated, recovered, and used for transplantation. Allogenic nerve allograft is one of the most promising substitutes for nerve autograft. Cadaveric nerve allografts are available in great abundance and offer the potential for size/length and motor/sensory specificity. Processing nerve allografts remove cellular components and reduce graft immunogenicity. Processed acellular frozen nerve allografts are commercially available.

QUESTIONS

1. What is a bone graft?
2. What happens if graft is not placed after extraction?

3. Mention indications for use of amnion.
4. What are contraindications of graft placement?
5. Classify bone graft material based on source of origin.
6. What are the requirements for bone graft to be successful?
7. Explain the terms osteogenic, osteoinductive, and osteoconductive.
8. What is the difference between repair and regeneration?
9. What are advantages of placental membranes?
10. Explain in detail the gold standard graft material.
11. What are bone substitute materials?
12. What are complications of graft placement?
13. Describe management of complications in graft placement.
14. Describe bone regeneration issues related to bone grafting biomaterials.
15. Describe guided bone regeneration.

REFERENCES

1. Laurencin C, Khan Y, El-Amin SF. Bone graft substitutes. *Expert Rev Med Devices.* 2006;3:49−57.
2. Giannoudis PV, Dinopoulos H, Tsiridis E. Bone substitutes: an update. *Injury.* 2005;36(Suppl 3):S20−S27.
3. Kumar P, Vinitha B, Fathima G. Bone grafts in dentistry. *J Pharm BioAllied Sci.* 2013;5(1):125−127. https://doi.org/10.4103/0975-7406.113312.
4. Indurkar MS, Awad MS, Gajiwala AL, Samant U, D'Lima C. AutoBT: a new paradigm in periodontal regeneration. *J Int Med Den.* 2018;5(2):51−55. https://doi.org/10.18320/JIMD/201805.0251.
5. Kim YK, Lee J, Um IW, et al. Tooth-derived bone graft material. *J Korean Assoc Oral Maxillofac Surg.* 2013;39:103−111. https://doi.org/10.5125/jkaoms.2013.39.3.103.
6. Murata M, Akazawa T, Mitsugi M, et al. Autograft of dentin materials for bone regeneration. In: Pignatello R, ed. *Advances in Biomaterials Science and Biomedical Applications.* Rijeka: IntechOpen; 2013:391−403.
7. Jaller JA, Herskovitz I, Borda LJ, et al. Evaluation of donor site pain after fractional autologous full-thickness skin grafting. *Adv Wound Care.* 2018;7(9):309−314. https://doi.org/10.1089/wound.2018.0800.
8. Marino JT, Ziran BH. Use of solid and cancellous autologous bone graft for fractures and nonunions. *Orthop Clin N Am.* 2010;41:15−26. https://doi.org/10.1016/j.ocl.2009.08.003.
9. Kakabadze A, Mardaleishvili K, Loladze G, et al. Reconstruction of mandibular defects with autogenous bone and decellularized bovine bone grafts with freeze dried bone marrow stem cell paracrine factors. *Oncol Lett.* 2016;13:1811−1818.
10. Yamamoto T, Iwase H, King TW, Hara H, Cooper DKC. Skin xenotransplantation: historical review and clinical potential. *Burns.* 2018;44(7):1738−1749. https://doi.org/10.1016/j.burns.2018.02.029.
11. Jacobsen G, Easter D, eds. *Allograft vs. Xenograft Practical Considerations for Biologic Scaffolds.* San Diego: The University of California; 2008. School of Medicine.
12. *APASTB Standards of Tissue Banking.* 2nd ed. Asia Pacific Association of Surgical Tissue Banking; 2016.
13. Dziedzic-Goclawska A. Application of ionising radiation to sterilise connective tissue allografts. In: Phillips GO, ed. *Radiation and Tissue Banking.* Singapore: World Scientific Publishing Co. Private Limited; 2000:57−99.
14. Cypher TJ, Grossman JP. Biological principles of bone graft healing. *J Foot Ankle Surg.* 1996;35(5):413−417. https://doi.org/10.1016/S1067-2516(96)80061-5.
15. Gajiwala AL, Agarwal M, Puri A, D'Lima C, Duggal A. Reconstruction tumour defects: lyophilised, irradiated bone allografts. *Cell Tissue Bank.* 2003;4:109−118.
16. *AATB Standards for Tissue Banking.* 14th ed. American Association of Tissue Banks; 2016.
17. Delloye C, Cornu O, Druez V, Barbier O. Bone allografts: what they can offer and what they cannot. *J Bone Joint Surg Br.* 2007;89(5):574−579. https://doi.org/10.1302/0301-620X.89B5.19039.
18. Phillips GO ed. Multi-Media Distance Learning Package on Tissue Banking, Module 6- Distribution and Utilisation, National University of Singapore.
19. Natarajan MV. Introduction to bone banking and allografts. https://www.tnmgrmu.ac.in/images/7th-vice-chancellor/bonebanking.pdf.
20. Murata M. Collagen biology for bone regenerative surgery. *J Korean Assoc Oral Maxillofac Surg.* 2012;38:321−325.
21. Um I-W, Kim Y-K, Mitsugi M. Demineralized dentin matrix scaffolds for alveolar bone engineering. *J Indian Prosthodont Soc.* 2017 Apr-Jun;17(2):120−127. https://doi.org/10.4103/jips.jips_62_17.
22. Joshi CP, D'Lima CB, Samat UC, et al. Comparative alveolar ridge preservation using allogenous tooth graft versus freeze-dried bone allograft: a randomized, controlled, prospective, clinical pilot study. *Contemp Clin Dent.* 2017;8:211−217.
23. Um IW, Ku JK, Kim YM, et al. Allogeneic demineralized dentin matrix graft for guided bone regeneration in dental implants. *Appl Sci.* 2020;10(13):4661.
24. Joshi CP, D'Lima CB, Karde PA, Mamajiwala AS. Ridge augmentation using sticky bone: a combination of human tooth allograft and autologous fibrin glue. *J Indian Soc Periodontol.* 2019;23(5):493−496. https://doi.org/10.4103/jisp.jisp_246_19.
25. Bourne G. The foetal membranes a review of the anatomy of normal amnion and chorion and some aspects of their function. *Postgrad Med J.* 1962;38:193−201.
26. Niknejad H, Peirovi H, Jorjani M, et al. Properties of the amniotic membrane for potential use in tissue engineering. *Europ Cells Mat.* 2008;15:88−99.

27. Chua WK, Oyen ML. Do we know the strength of the chorioamnion? A critical review and analysis. *Europ J Obst Gynaec Reprod Biol.* 2009;144:128−133.

28. Dua HS, Gomes JAP, King AJ, Maharajan VS. The amniotic membrane in ophthalmology. *Surv Ophthalmol.* 2004;49(1):51−77.

29. Perrimon N, Bernfield M. Cellular functions of proteoglycans-an overview. *Semin Cell Dev Biol.* 2001;12:65−67.

30. Rouslahti E. Fibronectin. *J Oral Pathol.* 1981;10:3−13.

31. Baum BJ, Wright WE. Demonstration of fibronectin as a major extracellular protein of human gingival fibroblasts. *J Dent Res.* 1980;59(3):631−637.

32. Tunggal P, Smyth N, Paulsson M, et al. Laminins: structure and genetic regulation. *Microsc Res Tech.* 2000;51:214−227.

33. Kjaergaard N, Hein M, Hyttel L, et al. Antibacterial properties of human amnion and chorion in vitro. *Eur J Obstet Gynecol Reprod Biol.* 2001;94:224−229.

34. Zare-Bidaki M, Sadrinia S, Erfani S, Afkar E, Ghanbarzade N. Antimicrobial properties of amniotic and chorionic membranes: a comparative study of two human fetal sacs. *J Reprod Infertil.* 2017;18(2):218−224.

35. Francisco JC, Cunha RC, Simeoni RB, et al. Amniotic membrane as a potent source of stem cells and a matrix for engineering heart tissue. *J Biomed Sci Eng.* 2013;6:1178−1185.

36. McQuilling JP, Vines JB, Kimmerling KA, Mowry KC. Proteomic comparison of amnion and chorion and evaluation of the effects of processing on placental membranes. *Wounds.* 2017;29(6):38−42.

37. D'Lima C, Samant U, Gajiwala AL, Puri A. Human chorionic membrane: a novel and efficient alternative to conventional collagen membrane. *Trends Biomater Artif Organs.* 2020;34(1):33−37.

38. Ravishanker R, Bath AS, Roy R. "Amnion Bank"-the use of long term glycerol preserved amniotic membranes in the management of superficial and superficial partial thickness burns. *Burns.* 2003;29(4):369−374. https://doi.org/10.1016/S0305-4179(02)00304-2.

39. Ghomi ER, Khalili S, Khorasani SN, Neisiany RE, Ramakrishna S. Wound dressings: current advances and future directions. *J Appl Polym Sci.* 2019;136:17. https://doi.org/10.1002/APP.47738.

40. Perepelkin NMJ, Hayward K, Mokoena T, et al. Cryopreserved amniotic membrane as transplant allograft: viability and post-transplant outcome. *Cell Tissue Bank.* 2016;17(1):39−50. https://doi.org/10.1007/s10561-015-9530-9.

41. Sangwan VS, Burman S, Tejwani S, Mahesh SP, Murthy R. Amniotic membrane transplantation: a review of current indications in the management of ophthalmic disorders. *Indian J Ophthalmol.* 2007;55:251−260.

42. Mijewski M, Pietraszek A. The application of deep-frozen and radiation-sterilized human amnion as a biological dressing to prevent prolonged air leakage in thoracic surgery. *Ann Transplant.* 2005;10(3):17−20.

43. Sham ME, Sultana N. Biological wound dressing—role of amniotic membrane. *Int J Dent Clin.* 2011;3(3):71−72.

44. Gajiwala AL, Sharma V. Use of irradiated amnion as a biological dressing in the treatment of radiation induced ulcers. *Cell Tissue Bank.* 2003;4:147−150.

45. De Rotth A. Plastic repair of conjunctival defects with fetal membrane. *Arch Ophthalmol.* 1940;23(3):522−525.

46. Holtzclaw DJ, Toscano NJ. Amnion-chorion allograft barrier used for guided tissue regeneration treatment of periodontal intrabony defects: a retrospective observational report. *Clin Adv Per.* 2013;3(3):131−137.

47. Lei J, Priddy LB, Lim JJ, Koob TJ. Dehydrated human amnion/chorion membrane (dHACM) allografts as a therapy for orthopedic tissue repair. *Tech Orthop.* 2017;32(3):149−157.

48. Nisolle M, Donnez J. Vaginoplasty using amniotic membranes in cases of vaginal agenesis or after vaginectomy. *J Gynecol Surg.* 1992;8(1):25−30.

49. Ahuja N, Jin R, Powers C, Billi A, Bass K. Dehydrated human amnion chorion membrane as treatment for pediatric burns. *Adv Wound Care.* 2020;9(11):602−611. https://doi.org/10.1089/wound.2019.0983.

50. Kakabadze Z, Mardaleishvili K, Loladze G, et al. Clinical application of decellularized and lyophilized human amnion/chorion membrane grafts for closing postlaryngectomy pharyngocutaneous fistulas. *J Surg Oncol.* 2016;113:538−543.

51. Patel VR, Samavedi S, Bates AS, et al. Dehydrated human amnion/chorion membrane allograft nerve wrap around the prostatic neurovascular bundle accelerates early return to continence and potency following robot-assisted radical prostatectomy: propensity score—matched analysis. *Eur Urol.* 2015;67:977−980.

52. Subach BR, Copay AG. The use of a dehydrated amnion/chorion membrane allograft in patients who subsequently undergo reexploration after posterior lumbar instrumentation. *Adv Orthoped.* 2015:6. https://doi.org/10.1155/2015/501202. Article ID 501202.

53. Joshi CP, Panjwani AA, D'Lima CB, Dani NH. Comparative evaluation of amnion-chorion membrane and chorion membrane for root coverage and gingival biotype enhancement: a case report. *EC Den Sci.* 2017;14(6):255−259.

54. Koller J. Basic anatomy and physiology of human skin. In: Phillips GO, ed. *Advances in Tissue Banking Vol 5. The Scientific Basis of Tissue Transplantation.* Singapore: World Scientific Publishing Co. Pte. Ltd.; 2001:123−138.

55. Wong DJ, Chang HY. Skin tissue engineering. In: *StemBook.* Cambridge (MA): Harvard Stem Cell Institute; 2009. https://doi.org/10.3824/stembook.1.44.1, 2008.

56. Tognetti L, Pianigiani E, Ierardi F, et al. Current insights into skin banking: storage, preservation and clinical importance of skin allografts. *J Biorepository Sci Appl Med.* 2017;5:41−56. https://doi.org/10.2147/BSAM.S115187.

57. Imahara SD, Klein MB. Skin grafts. In: Orgill D, Blanco C, eds. *Biomaterials for Treating Skin Loss.* Cambridge, UK: Woodhead Publishing and CRC Press LLC; 2009:58−79.

58. Seah CS. Skin graft and skin equivalent in burns. *Ann Acad Med Singap.* 1992;21(5):685–688.

59. Leon-Villapalos J, Eldardiri M, Dziewulski P. The use of human deceased donor skin allograft in burn care. *Cell Tissue Bank.* 2010;11:99–104. https://doi.org/10.1007/s10561-009-9152-1.nerves.

60. Tang P, Chauhan A. Decellular nerve allografts. *J Am Acad Orthop Surg.* 2015;23(11):641–647. https://doi.org/10.5435/jaaos-d-14-00373.

61. Ray WZ, Mackinnon SE. Management of nerve gaps: autografts, allografts, nerve transfers, and end-to-side neurorrhaphy. *Exp Neurol.* 2010;223(1):77–85. https://doi.org/10.1016/j.expneurol.2009.03.031.

62. Moore AM, MacEwan M, Santosa KB, et al. Acellular nerve allografts in peripheral nerve regeneration: a comparative study. *Muscle Nerve.* 2011;44(2):221–234. https://doi.org/10.1002/mus.22033.

63. Nijran A, Challoner TJ, Jordaan P, Power D. The role of processed nerve allograft in peripheral nerve surgery. *J Musc Surg Res.* 2019;3(1):110–115. https://doi.org/10.4103/jmsr.jmsr_86_18.

Index

Note: Page numbers followed by f indicate figures, t indicates tables.